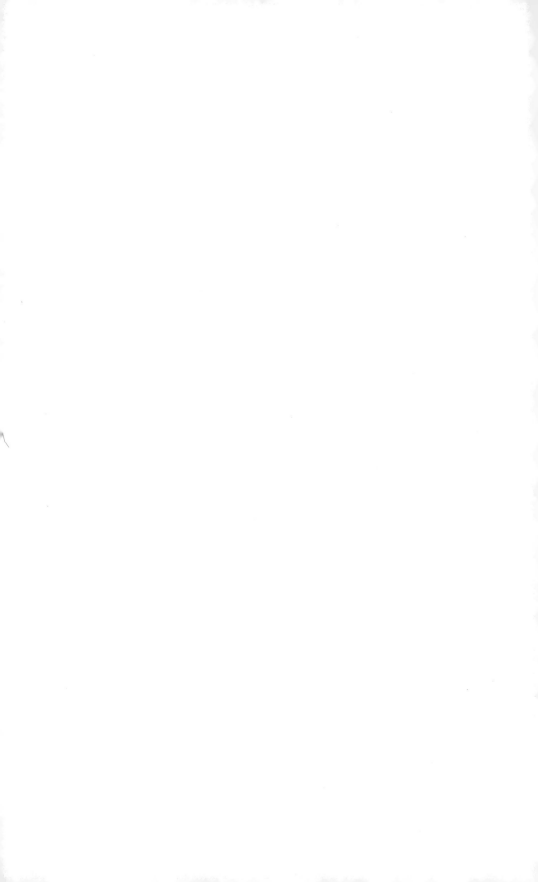

SAFE DIVING

Allan Kayle graduated from the Medical School of the University of the Witwatersrand, Johannesburg, in 1965. He joined the full-time staff of the Department of Physiological Chemistry and was awarded the PhD degree in 1972.

In 1981 he completed his advanced sport diving training under the auspices of the National Association of Underwater Instructors and attended a South African Navy course in submarine medicine in Simon's Town. In 1983 he was granted a permit by the National Monuments Council to salvage the historical wreck of HMS *Birkenhead* which sank off the Cape coast in 1852. His book *Salvage of the Birkenhead* was published in 1990. He writes regular feature articles on the technical and medical aspects of diving for *Divestyle* magazine and was a contributor to the *South African Second Underwater Handbook* published in 1989.

Dr Kayle is a member of the International Affairs Committee of the Undersea Hyperbaric Medical Society and the Scientific Board of DAN Europe and is diving medical officer to South African Underwater Engineering for the Mossgas saturation diving offshore oil project. He is President-elect of the newly formed Southern African Hyperbaric and Undersea Medical Association and is currently working on new methods of atmospheric purification in submarines. In 1993 he was nominated by Scuba Schools International for their highest award − their Platinum Pro 5000.

Safe Diving

A Medical Handbook for Scuba Divers

Allan Kayle

VIKING

VIKING

Published by the Penguin Group
27 Wrights Lane, London W8 5TZ
Viking Penguin, a division of Penguin Books USA Inc, 375 Hudson Street, New
York, New York 10014, USA
Penguin Books Australia Ltd, Ringwood, Victoria, Australia
Penguin Books Canada Ltd, 10 Alcorn Avenue, Toronto, Ontario, Canada M4V 3B2
Penguin Books (NZ) Ltd, 182-190 Wairau Road, Auckland 10, New Zealand
Penguin Books, Amethyst Street, Theta Ext 1, Johannesburg, South Africa

Penguin Books Ltd, Registered Offices: Harmondsworth, Middlesex, England

First published in 1994

ISBN 0 670 85386 0

Typeset by Iskova Image Setting
Colour reproduction by Dando & Van Wyk, Johannesburg
Cover design by Hadaway Illustration & Design

Printed and bound by National Book Printers, Goodwood, Cape

This book is dedicated to my daughter Alexandra who, like me, is a dreamer; to my wife Jean Anne who manages to keep my feet on the ground even when my head is under water; to all those divers whose ingenuity and courage from the time of Alexander the Great have made the sport possible; and to all modern scuba divers who delight in the underwater world.

Contents

Foreword

Some books for divers seem to be written for instructors, others for research specialists or book reviewers, and a few for all three. This one is really written for committed and serious divers from Openwater I to Instructor level, diving medical technicians, and even diving physicians who have just recently entered the field of diving medicine. The text presents all areas of diving medicine from early history to recent scientific developments.

Approximately one-third of the text is devoted to the important issue of fitness to dive. Today's divers are considerably more knowledgeable than those of thirty years ago about the physiology and medicine of diving, as evidenced by their regular attendance at diving symposia and their ever-increasing demand for educational materials. Those medical conditions that militate against pursuing diving as a recreational or professional activity are very clearly discussed and, for some conditions, excellent examples are used, often with pleasant humour to stress the issue.

The classification of decompression disorders has been the subject of considerable discussion and review by diving physicians recently, and a descriptive approach was proposed by Francis and Smith (Describing Decompression Illness) which does not need formal acceptance of a mechanism or site. It utilises a description of symptoms, their rate of progression and their response to treatment, rather than the older classification of Type I or Type II decompression sickness. The author uses this classification of decompression disorders in his sections on treatment. The system is simple and it works.

The understanding of safe and efficient diving is greatly aided by this exceptionally complete and well-written book. *Safe Diving* is thoroughly recommended to all divers from student level to instructor — and to those physicians or diving medical technicians who may be required to provide medical treatment to those who venture under the sea.

Leon J. Greenbaum, Jr., PhD
Executive Director
Undersea and Hyperbaric Medical Society
Bethesda, Maryland
United States of America

Introduction

Over the past ten years I have seen and chatted to thousands of divers. We've spoken about bends and arterial gas embolism, bone necrosis and oxygen toxicity, nitrogen narcosis and middle ear problems. Over a sea of beer we've sailed through the hazards of squeezes and squalls, swum through kelp, and coughed through lung injuries and carbon monoxide.

Gradually it occurred to me that there is still a lot of mystery about diving. Most divers know of the dangers, but not so many really know what to do when they occur. This book is for the diver who has enough knowledge to feel insecure when faced by a diving emergency. It is a look at diving from a victim's point of view. It explains basic medical fitness to dive and explores the advisability of diving with an underlying illness. Attention is devoted to diseases peculiar to divers, plus a no-nonsense approach to diving accidents and ailments — how to help and get help when a potential disaster threatens. For the sake of completeness, diving laws, tables, and therapeutic recompression tables are included at the end of the book.

One major change has been the elimination of Type I and Type II decompression sickness from diving medicine jargon. This was mooted by D.J. Smith and T.J.R. Francis and approved at the Undersea and Hyperbaric Medical Society in 1990 and at the European Undersea Biomedical Society in 1991.

Henceforth all new gas injuries during or after ascent will be called acute decompression illness which now includes arterial gas embolism.

Many medicines and drugs are mentioned in this book. Their generic names have been used instead of their more popular trade names. There were three reasons for doing this. The first was the fact that many pharmaceutical companies often make the same generic compound but market it under a different name. Secondly, for some unknown reason, many companies change the trade name of their product in different countries. The third and most important reason was to force the diver to obtain professional medical advice in identifying and obtaining a particular generic drug, and to seek help about the wisdom of using that drug in his or her particular case.

None of the drugs or medications named in this book should be used without consulting your doctor in advance for a prescription and proper consideration of any allergic or untoward side-effect in your individual case. The same applies to all members of any diving group. It is essential that qualified confirmation about the safety of any medicine or drug incorporated in a medical kit be obtained individually by each and every diver.

AIDS has been given special attention because of the escalating spread of the epidemic and the potential danger of assisting a bleeding victim who may be HIV-positive. The awful consequences of contracting the disease while saving a life have made safety precautions necessary in handling wounds and administering CPR.

This book belongs in the cubby hole of your 4X4 or in the waterproof compartment of your dive boat. Keep it handy should you have a medical question or problem, or to guide you if things get rough. I hope you never really need it.

History of Diving

Man has always dived. From simple plunges for fish and food, breathhold diving became a pearl, shell and food industry in about 4500 BC. Diving for sponges began during ancient Greek times and has continued to this day. The wisdom of the ancient Greeks even incorporated the legal rights of divers — the deeper the dive, the greater their share of profits.

Breathhold diving

The Greek and Roman navies dominated early recorded diving history. Breathhold divers were used in the Trojan wars around 1190 BC, sabotaging wooden enemy ships by drilling holes, cutting anchor lines, and constructing submerged wooden port defences against assailing ships. Alexander the Great's engineer and architect, Philo of Byzantium, recommended replacing anchor ropes with chains to foil enemy divers.

Using divers, Pompey's son Gnaeus refloated ships sunk by the Romans to obstruct entrance to the harbour of Oricus in Greece, and then captured the port. Mark Antony attempted to impress Cleopatra during a fishing competition by having his divers secretly load his hook with a steady supply of fish. Cleopatra reacted by ordering one of her divers to attach a salted fish to his hook!

During the sixteenth to eighteenth centuries, the native divers of Margarita Island were reported to be able to dive to 30 metres of sea water (msw) for 15 minutes, all day and every day. They claimed their stamina was due to the use of tobacco!

The pearl diving industry still uses the basic technique of breath-holding; for example, the Ama or diving women of Japan where the technique has been employed for over two thousand years, and the pearl divers of the Tuamoto archipelago.

Snorkels

The first major technical advance was the use of a bamboo or reed as a snorkel when hunting in water. This allowed the diver to replenish his air requirements while stealthily approaching his prey, but restricted depth to just below the surface. The method was reported by Aristotle in ancient

Greece, by Columbus as used by the North American Indians to hunt for wild fowl, and was also used by Australian aborigines to trap wild duck.

Leonardo da Vinci made drawings of breathing tubes. The breathing device amounted to a snorkel but as the dead space was large, carbon dioxide would have accumulated. He also designed a diver's fin and suggested that divers could breathe from 'a wine skin to contain the breath' − the first scuba design? In 1680 Borelli in Italy examined da Vinci's designs and disagreed with them. He felt that exhaled air would have to be cleansed before rebreathing and proposed that cooling it through a copper tube would be effective. He was not too far off the mark. Modern rebreathing sets use breathing gases stored in ultra-cold liquid form, exhaled carbon dioxide and water vapour being frozen out.

Diving bells

After snorkels, the next advance in boosting underwater endurance was the development of open diving bells. Alexander the Great is rumoured by Ethicus to have built one in 3 BC, but the stories relating to it are surely the antecedents of modern fishing tales. Alexander apparently entered a 'glass barrel' and was 'swallowed by the sea'. On his return he proclaimed, 'Sir Barons, I have just seen that this whole world is lost and the great fish mercilessly devour the lesser.' One fish seen was so big that it took three days to swim past the appalled Alexander in his submerged bell!

During the 1500s weighted wooden chambers, air-filled but with a bottom opening, were built. In 1620 Sir Francis Bacon described one. 'It is a sort of metal barrel lowered into the water, open end downward. The diver can put his head in and so recover his breath.' The air could not be purified or replaced, however, and it was not until 1691 that Edmund Halley, the astronomer of comet fame, extended the scope of these open bells and managed to damage an ear drum in the doing. He patented an open diving bell that could be replenished with air. As efficient pumps had yet to be invented, his bell was supplied by weighted barrels of air which the divers hauled down from the surface. Keeping the barrels well below the bell allowed the barrel air to escape through hoses and up into the bell. He also freed divers of the need to breathhold from the bell by designing hose systems to supply the diver with air from the bell. Primitive, but they managed dives to 20 msw for one and a half hours. Using his bells, fifty bronze cannons, each weighing half a tonne, were recovered from the *Wasa*, a Swedish warship sunk in 30 msw.

Surface air supply

When dependable hand-operated air pumps became available during the late 1700s, it became possible to supply a submerged diver with air from the surface. Helmets were first used. The early ones were really only miniature open bells − an inverted bucket over the head. Excess air pumped into these helmets escaped through the open bottom and created a flushing system. The diver could breathe as long as he stood. If he stooped or stumbled, the helmet simply flooded.

Next came the idea of tailoring the diving bell to the shape of a man — providing him with a watertight cover and an air supply. The first diving suit appeared — a copper helmet with glass viewports, firmly attached to a full rubber suit. It was designed by Augustus Siebe who called it a 'closed dress'. Now more commonly known as the *standard diving dress* or *standard rig*, it enabled a diver to move freely without water entering his helmet. Incoming air was pumped down a hose into the helmet and surplus air escaped through an outlet valve. Siebe's design has evolved into the modern surface-supplied dry suit and hard hat.

But with the closed dress suit and resultant longer dives came the bends, previously described in caisson workers — men who worked in fixed underwater pressurised chambers and tunnels. At first the cause was unknown, then the great French physicist Paul Bert suggested that nitrogen bubbles were the cause and showed that a gradual ascent from depth would avoid the onset of the condition, and that recompression relieved the pain. A British scientist, John Haldane, was appointed to investigate the problem and continue Bert's work. Haldane noted that a diver could be lifted from 10 msw to the surface without bending, and postulated staged decompression stops, allowing enough time at progressively shallower stages for excess gas to be exhaled. The idea was tested on goats, then on men in pressurised chambers, and finally, in 1906, on sea dives to 64 msw. Haldane published his tables and in 1915 US Navy divers, breathing air, located and raised to the surface a sunken submarine at a depth of 93 msw. It is extremely doubtful whether a modern diver would even dream of diving, let alone working, to 93 msw with air as a breathing source. But it was done despite extreme narcosis, an oxygen partial pressure of over two atmospheres which should have caused underwater convulsions, and an enormous risk of acute decompression illness.

Scuba

The next step was the liberation of the diver from a surface air hose and a heavily weighted suit. During the nineteenth century compressors could only achieve a maximum pressure of 40 atmospheres, which meant a very limited time under water. Modern scuba divers now return to the surface when their cylinder pressure is 50 atmospheres because they are running out of air! But at the time 40 atmospheres was all they had and they worked with it. In the early 1800s, an American engineer, Charles Condert, carried his air compressed in a copper tube coiled around his body. The air was released into a hood covering the upper part of his body. A small hole was supposed to allow the escape of exhaled carbon dioxide. Condert died using his system in 1831.

In 1865 two French technicians, Benoit Rouquayrol and Auguste Denayrouze, invented an aerophore, a full face mask supplied from the surface, but fitted with an air receiver carried on the back so that the diver could uncouple himself from his hosing for a few minutes. It was the first

Self-Contained Underwater Breathing Apparatus or SCUBA.

At the same time, work was proceeding to develop oxygen rebreathing sets and the first practical one was built by an Englishman, Fleuss, in 1878. It was a closed circuit set that supplied pure oxygen to the diver and removed exhaled carbon dioxide by using a rope soaked in potassium hydroxide. The system was dangerous as the effects of oxygen toxicity were largely unknown. It was the forerunner of military oxygen sets, submarine escape sets, fire-fighting sets, and mine rescue equipment.

In 1918 Ogushi in Japan patented a scuba system using a cylinder carried on the back. The diver controlled his air supply by triggering air flow into his mask with his teeth. Then in 1933 a Frenchman, Yves Le Prieur, designed a system where the diver carried the cylinder on his chest and released air into his mask by manually opening a tap. Le Prieur's system was adopted by the French Navy.

In 1943 scuba as it is now known was developed. An engineer, Gagnan, had devised a reducing valve for use in gas-powered cars. Together with Jacques Cousteau, he modified this valve to construct the first underwater demand valve, triggered by the diver's breathing and automatically compensating for changes in depth and pressure. It was simple and reliable and heralded the beginning of sport scuba diving.

During the 1950s complex self-monitoring closed circuit sets were developed and over the years have been upgraded into ultra-sophisticated electronically controlled systems, accurately regulating the required gas flow from oxygen and diluent helium cylinders.

Chariots

Since the times of the ancient Greeks wars have stimulated diving developments and the First World War was no exception. Human torpedoes or chariots — small open submarines manned by divers with mines — were developed by the Italians, and were successful in sinking an Austrian battleship in Pola Harbour. The fact that the battleship was already in friendly hands was unfortunate. Not to be deterred, and despite the fact that Winston Churchill had refused the Royal Navy permission to develop their own chariots, the Italian Navy again used their chariots in World War Two and successfully damaged two British battleships and tankers harboured in Alexandria. Conditions for these divers were dangerous and, as depths beyond the maximum 10 msw using pure oxygen were often necessary, a method of reducing decompression time after air-breathing during a mine-laying or mine-clearing operation became vital.

Mixed gases

Nitrogen-oxygen (nitrox) mixtures using semi-closed rebreathing sets were developed by the Admiralty Experimental Diving Unit together with Siebe, Gorman and Co., Ltd. Increasing the oxygen ratio in the mix reduced nitrogen uptake and removed or shortened decompression commitments. The main difficulty in using air or nitrox was nitrogen narcosis if depths beyond 60 msw were needed. As early as 1919, Professor Elihu Thompson had suggested that nitrogen narcosis could be eliminated by using helium as a breathing gas. The cost at that time was prohibitive ($US 2000 per cubic foot), but when natural helium wells were located the price dropped to 3 cents per cubic foot and, by 1940, dives to 128 msw had been done in Lake Michigan.

At the same time Arne Zetterstrom, a Swedish engineer, was working with highly explosive hydrogen as a potential breathing gas. He showed that hypoxia and the risk of explosion could be avoided by diving on air to 30 msw, changing the breathing mix to four per cent oxygen in nitrogen and then switching to four per cent, or less, oxygen in hydrogen (hydrox). Zetterstrom dived on his mix in the sea in 1945. He reached 160 msw safely but on his ascent his tenders mistook his instructions and accidentally hauled him up too fast. He died of hypoxia and acute decompression illness. Work on hydrogen continued, however, and has led to animals being safely pressurised to over 1 000 msw on hydrox.

Saturation diving

Great depths require very long decompression times and saturation diving was conceived by Albert Behnke after World War Two. Behnke was one of the great pioneers in diving medicine. He was the man who first postulated the *oxygen window* to explain Haldane's empirical concept of tissue nitrogen-supersaturation. He suggested that nitrogen, a metabolically inert gas, was responsible for 'compressed air intoxication' at depths. This clouding of consciousness with nitrogen narcosis was previously attributed to oxygen, claustrophobia, and even unidentified impurities in the air from the compressors. Behnke also first presented the now outmoded Type I and Type II classification system for decompression sickness, was the first to use hyperbaric oxygen in its treatment, and pioneered work on cerebral oxygen toxicity.

Behnke proposed that caisson workers should be kept at depths and live under pressure for the duration of their work and be slowly decompressed only once, at the end of their task.

After the reports of chamber tests on mice and men at the US Naval Submarine Research Laboratory, openwater saturation was tried by the French in September 1962. Robert Stenuit spent 24 hours at 60 msw in the Sea-Link project off the French Riviera. During the same month Captain Jacques Cousteau initiated the Conshelf I habitat experiments, and two men spent seven days at 10 msw. The next year Cousteau's Conshelf II supported five men for one month at 10 msw; then two men for one week at 26 msw. The subsea race was on and, in 1964, the Americans launched Sealab I, the first of a series. Sealab II followed in 1965, with the former astronaut Scott Carpenter spending one month at 60 msw in a heliox atmosphere. By 1968 surface chamber dives to 250 msw for 48 hours were being done in America, with deeper excursions to 310 msw − in preparation for Sealab III. It was proposed to set up the Sealab III habitat at 180 msw. A fatal error in sodalime canisters caused diver death before the habitat was ever used. The ill-fated Sealab III, costing millions of dollars, was abandoned brand-new at the bottom of the sea and the project was shelved.

Habitats and Bells

At this stage saturation diving had split into two paths. One was habitat work and research, but the huge disadvantage was lack of mobility. Habitats do not lend themselves to uprooting and moving to a new job at a distant destination. The other path used a pressurised personnel transfer capsule or PTC (popularly called a diving bell), which transported divers from their living quarters in the surface deck decompression chamber (DDC) on the support ship to the work site at the bottom of the ocean. There the divers could open a hatch at the bottom of the bell and enter the sea to perform their duties. Initially the research was navy-funded, but a huge amount of private money became available when it was realised that a method had been found to reach and tap hitherto impossible riches − the subsea oil and natural gas fields. Saturation diving has now grown to the point where dive companies are prepared to tender for contracts requiring divers to work at 600 msw. When one considers that this is twice the maximum diving depth of a Daphne-class submarine, one can appreciate the vast expansion in diving technology that has occurred in the past forty years.

Armoured suits

The prolonged decompression time needed for deep saturation diving led to a further development. For work where a short but very deep dive is needed, armoured suits were developed. These are a hybrid between a diver and a one-man submarine, allowing the diver to work in an armoured suit which can take the full pressure of the water. The inside of the suit is maintained at one atmosphere. No decompression is needed. The JIM and WASP suits which permit work at 450 msw are examples.

Fluid breathing

The ultimate concept is fluid breathing, analogous to fish gills, with a diver breathing oxygen-enriched liquid into and out of the lungs, so avoiding the need for diluent nitrogen or helium gas, and eliminating the risk of bending. The depth range would be almost unlimited, and oxygen could even be extracted from the surrounding water. The physical and technical problems are obvious, but man is very ingenious and perhaps will one day return to the sea, breathing a liquid, with unlimited bottom times, and free to surface from any depth.

Diving Medicals and Scuba Diving

All qualified scuba divers receive their training at clubs affiliated to the relevant national union, such as SAUU in South Africa and BSAC in Britain; or at private schools under the auspices of institutions such as the American-based NAUI, SSI or PADI. Training courses cover the whole gamut — from basic to instructor certification. In most cases the divers emerge from their courses with adequate understanding and only needing additional diving time and experience to complete their metamorphosis into *Homo scubiens*.

But, are they safe under water? Divers trained by most national unions are compelled to undergo a medical examination before training to ensure that their state of health meets the particular, and often peculiar, demands of diving. The reputable private schools do the same, and these medicals should be repeated every two years if under forty, or annually if older. But there is always the law of the buck. It costs money to have a medical and a chest X-ray — these raise the price of the diving course and most divers are poor. They are on a tight budget to pay for their course, buy a wet suit, an ABLJ, a scuba cylinder, demand valve and so on. They investigate the diving school market.

'Hey,' they say, 'here's a school that doesn't need a medical unless you're over forty. We're only nineteen, and we run marathons — hell, we're fit enough! Why waste money on a medical? We'd rather use the bucks to buy a mask!'

Here's why. Here are some stories and they are all true.

• Joe had just returned from Israel where he had done a one-day 'resort course' and had fallen in love with the sport. He approached a diving school and was told to have a medical. He said he had recently had one in Israel and had been passed A1. The school believed him. During their openwater diver training, Joe completed his bottom time and ascended normally with his instructor. At the surface, he suddenly started choking and gasping and lost consciousness. All attempts at resuscitation were futile. Post-mortem revealed air bubbles in the arteries of his brain and heart. Joe had suffered an arterial gas embolus from a ruptured lung on a controlled ascent. Discussion with his family revealed that he had had a previous spontaneous pneumothorax. Joe had lied and died for his ambition to dive.

• Mike was an athlete. He was a long-distance runner and a league squash player. He was 23 years old. At his medical he appeared a perfect physical specimen — muscular, lean and powerful. He was asked to pass a specimen of urine.

'I can't,' he replied. 'I went just before I came here. I'll bring one later.'

'No,' he was told. 'Have some water and read a magazine.'

Mike passed his specimen after further argument. It was loaded with sugar plus ketones.

'I didn't want to tell because I knew I would fail,' he said ruefully. 'I am a diabetic on insulin.'

• Tim had completed his openwater one course and was keen to advance his training. He had changed diving schools and was told to have a medical. He had 'not needed an examination' with his first school — he was only nineteen. At his medical he was tense and reticent, revealing his history only with persuasion. Eventually the dam broke. He had been diagnosed as having multiple sclerosis and had been admitted to hospital twice in the previous year. On both occasions he had attempted suicide by alcohol overdose. He could not face the horror of his illness. His breathing muscles and his limbs had been paralysed and he had needed an artificial ventilator. He had been on huge doses of cortisone. He was on antidepressants and was seeing a psychiatrist. He had completed his openwater one course between his admissions to hospital.

Unbelievable? Here is another.

• Pete arrived for his medical with his form filled out and his X-rays in his hand. Like all would-be divers, he was excited and impatient to have his medical behind him. The X-rays showed a tumour at the root of his left lung. The 26-year-old Pete was referred to his doctor as an emergency.

All diving schools require their students to sign an indemnity form, releasing the school from any financial or legal obligation should a diving accident occur. But there is an unwritten inescapable moral obligation — ensuring that their students are medically fit to dive. Their students have families, fiancées, wives, husbands and children who need them and care for them. It is a woeful and terrible task to inform these people that their loved one is dead. Does a diving instructor actually have to see the uncomprehending anguish on the face of a four-year-old and the weeping mother before accepting and implementing this moral responsibility?

The number of sport divers is increasing daily. Accidents and deaths are going to happen. All newcomers to the sport are dying to dive. They have no idea of the hazards. They are thinking of beaches and palm trees and beautiful coral in crystal-clear water. They admiringly look to qualified divers for informed advice. Tell them to have a medical. Don't let them dive to die.

Age, Sex and Body Build Implications in Scuba Diving

The basic health demands of diving are simple. A diver's psyche and body must safely be able to handle the physical loads of pressurised gases in and out of solution, and the inherent dangers of the sea.

Age Limits

Except for the very young and the very old, age *per se* is not an absolute limiting factor in sport diving.

Children under twelve years of age should probably not dive, and certainly no deeper than 9 msw or without adult supervision. There are two main reasons. Bone growth and lengthening occurs at the epiphyseal cartilage near the ends of each limb bone. Any bubble formation in these very sensitive growth plates could led to stunting or deformation of further growth. Final bony fusion of limb epiphyseal cartilage usually occurs between the ages of 13 and 16 years in girls, and between 15 and 18 years in boys. Children are also adventurous and liable to dive, without mature consideration of risks, beyond safe time, depth, and sea condition limits. Buoyancy can be a real problem in children, and even in small adults. At the beginning of the dive the scuba cylinder is full of compressed air and negatively buoyant − the child sinks easily. At the end of the dive the nearly empty and now-buoyant cylinder can initiate an uncontrollable ascent.

Adults over the age of forty should also exercise additional caution. They are invariably less fit and fatter than younger divers, and have less efficient cardiovascular and pulmonary systems with resultant decreased effectiveness of tissue nitrogen degassing after a dive. Very conservative depth/dive durations should be followed, with a mandatory 5-minute stop at 5 msw after any dive. Decompression-stop dives should otherwise be avoided in older divers.

Sex

There are specific differences peculiar to women divers, not because of any lack of ability or understanding, but simply because women are women.

These differences are due to both physical and psychological factors. Some are advantageous, some disadvantageous, and others are myths.

Physical factors

Fat distribution. In general, women have a greater natural distribution of fatty tissue underlying the skin as compared to men. Their relative lean body mass (their mass minus that of fat) is less than that of males. As a result women generally tolerate cold conditions better than men do and hypothermia often takes longer to develop in women. Their relatively increased amount of fatty tissue also provides a potentially greater store for nitrogen retention, and the risk of bends is theoretically higher in women than in men. In practical terms, however, this difference is rarely encountered, provided standard diving tables are followed.

Menstruation. Let's explode a myth. Many female divers refrain from diving during their periods − the reason being that sharks will detect bleeding and eat them up. This is untrue. The use of internal tampons provides a convenient method of controlling flow and the incidence of shark attacks on women who are menstruating is actually lower than that on non-menstruating women.

But what happens to tampons when women dive? Will pressure force a tampon beyond ready recovery by the user? Will the little string disappear, making an embarrassing visit to a doctor necessary? No. Tampons are porous and unaffected by water depth. Tampons are safe for diving.

Heavy periods can cause other problems, however. Regular blood loss with inadequate dietary replacement of iron may cause iron deficiency and anaemia. This can place the female diver at risk at times when strength and stamina are demanded, for example swimming against powerful currents. Women with heavy flows should seek medical advice to confirm that their iron stores and haemoglobin are adequate.

Some women experience severe abdominal pain, irritability, nausea and vomiting with or just before their periods. These are a potential source of danger under water − inability to swim properly due to cramps, hasty and unwise responses, and inhalation of vomit may occur. The decision to dive must allow for these. If drugs are required to control these symptoms, the answer is easy: do not dive at period time.

Breast implants. Here is another myth. It is commonly believed that breast implants will implode or explode or burst as a result of the pressure changes incurred while diving (or even flying in aeroplanes!). They won't. Only gas spaces obey Boyle's Law and undergo substantial pressure-volume changes, and implants are filled with saline or silica gel. They are not inflatable pneumatic bladders. They will absorb some inert gas during a dive, however, and inconsequential small bubble formation inside an implant can occur.

Oral contraception. The majority of oral contraceptives contain combined derivatives of the female hormones oestrogen and progesterone. The basic idea of the pill is to stop cyclical ovulation and the release of a viable egg or ovum from an ovary each month. Without ovulation, no fertilisation can occur.

Considering the number of females actively enjoying sport diving, it is obvious that many hundreds of thousands or even millions of them must be taking oral contraceptives. For safety, however, it should be remembered that one of the side-effects of the pill is an increased tendency for platelets to clump, leading to abnormal blood clotting, especially inside calf veins where blood flow is slower and more sluggish than anywhere else in the body. Venous nitrogen bubbles after a dive also stimulate platelet aggregation around them so the risk of venous thrombosis in female divers does increase with the pill. A few precautions will help avoid the problem: safe diving techniques with care to avoid excessive bubble loading; ensuring that the calf muscles are not compressed; and sitting or lying with the knees extended after diving to allow easy venous return from the calves.

Pregnancy. The vast majority of female divers are of child-bearing age and so, not unexpectedly, the vast majority of them fall pregnant from time to time. They then want to know whether they should dive with descendants under their wet suits. A negative reply causes indignation: 'But my friend Zelda Saitowitz dived right through her pregnancy and even while she was breast feeding her twins!'

So, aside from being unaffected by the nitrogen equivalent of carbonated milk, who is this initially-smaller-than-a-kiwi-fruit-pip-sized result of parental genetic fusion to dictate maternal exposure to the hyperbaric environment? Why should foetal needs be any different from the mother's? Why shouldn't a pregnant woman dive until her bulk threatens to rend asunder her double-lined two-tone lycra suit? And what if she promises to do shallow dives and no decompression-stop dives?

It's to do with lungs. Unborn babies float in amniotic fluid, the protective liquid suspending them within the muscular wall of their mother's uterus. Their lungs are non-functional in a liquid environment and all of their oxygen, carbon dioxide and nitrogen needs are handled via the umbilical cord and placenta. The placenta is not just a lump of inconvenient flesh to be discarded after a delivery. It is an amazing union of mother and child, a unique organ composed half of mother's tissue and half of child's, with maternal capillaries looping to touch, but never joining, the baby's matching capillary loops. It is an intimate network of totally separate blood supplies, providing sustenance and oxygen to the baby, and removing metabolic end-products and carbon dioxide for excretion via maternal kidneys and lungs. The two circulations do not mix. They are the blood supplies of two different people – the mother's capillaries providing and nurturing, and the child's taking and excreting.

This giving and taking includes the gases of diving. The mother gives her child hyperbaric oxygen plus a hefty nitrogen load during the dive. The child offloads carbon dioxide and then tries to degas nitrogen after the dive. But junior hasn't got functional lungs and depends on the placenta to return nitrogen to the mother's blood. This is the first snag. Nitrogen decompression requires a gradient. It's fine for mom — she's got a gradient to 0.79 atmospheres at the beach. Junior has a gradient from himself (assuming a baby boy) to mom's nitrogen-loaded venous system and for the first few minutes of decompression mom may even continue to supply nitrogen to junior. In other words, there is a delay. Junior has to join the queue to degas. This means he has a higher residual nitrogen time than his mother, who is already putting on her wet suit for a repetitive dive because her tables or computer say it's fine. Baby bubbles loom! But things are even more dangerous. Junior also has normal shunts between the right and left sides of his heart (foramen ovale), and between the pulmonary artery and aorta (ductus arteriosus). Any foetal venous bubbles can easily embolise into the child's arterial system.

The next snag is biliousness. During the first three months of pregnancy, many women develop nausea and vomiting. If on land or on a boat, fluid loss results in relative or absolute dehydration. A decrease in total body water means a faster rate of tissue nitrogen loading during diving. This naturally includes junior. Then when mom decides to retch under water, inhalation of vomit and sea water may follow, progressing to hypoxia, near-drowning, or worse.

Saturation divers breathing oxygen at a partial pressure of higher than 0.5 ATA for prolonged periods are prone to develop acute pulmonary oxygen toxicity, with coughing, burning chest pain, breathlessness and eventually respiratory failure. Unborn babies live under conditions of relatively low oxygen partial pressure. Nature has supplied them with a special oxygen carrier, foetal haemoglobin, which has a very high affinity for oxygen. After birth, foetal haemoglobin is rapidly replaced with adult haemoglobin, which is maintained for life. Foetuses and newborn babies don't do well with high oxygen partial pressures. Cataracts in the lens of the eye can occur as well as acute respiratory distress, very similar to the acute pulmonary oxygen toxicity found in saturation diving. When a pregnant woman dives to 20 metres she receives oxygen at a partial pressure of 0.63 ATA. Her baby gets a little less, but the threat of oxygen toxicity is there. Congenital abnormalities in the newborn occur nearly six times more frequently in females who continue to dive regularly as compared to non-divers. The risk increases should the pregnant (and invariably fatter) mother suffer a bend or arterial gas embolism and require pure oxygen therapy under pressurised conditions in a chamber.

Later in pregnancy other problems arise. The expectant mother becomes clumsy and is liable to trip over her fins, lose her balance while hefting a heavy cylinder, or injure herself in a rocking ski-boat. The presence of a large belly makes breathing more difficult, and an agile physical response to underwater stress a doubtful prospect.

A normal baby and healthy mother warrant a nine-month lay-off from diving.

Lactation. The question sometimes arises, 'Is it safe to dive while breast feeding?' The answer is yes. Diving will not affect breast milk production nor predispose to milk retention and mastitis. Although diving will cause a temporarily increased nitrogen partial pressure in unreleased breast milk, feeding is done at ambient surface pressure and any excess gas load to the baby will be minimal, or relieved with a good burp.

Menopause. With the onset of menopause at around the age of fifty, female divers are exposed to an increased risk of osteoporosis, the decalcification of bone that renders them more liable to bony injury after relatively minor trauma. The skin and other tissues also become more fragile, with easy bruising and skin bleeding. It has become very common for women to take calcium, vitamins and female hormone replacement therapy near the onset of menopause. Care to avoid venous thrombosis, as with oral contraceptives, should be remembered.

Physical mismatching. A large part of sport diver training is devoted to diver rescue and resuscitation. The novice diver learns how to share an air supply, assist an unconscious diver to the surface and get him aboard a boat. But what happens if she weighs 47 kilograms and he weighs 126 kilograms? Such buddy pairs do occur and it then becomes necessary to ensure that they always dive with another pair. Three could easily do what a slightly built partner would struggle or fail to accomplish.

Psychological factors

Women divers usually fall into one of two groups. Most are extremely safe divers, lacking the male macho need to demonstrate strength and ability, and dive efficiently, intelligently and well. They take few risks and are very considerate buddy partners.

The others fall into the fragile league. Staunch in their belief in male chivalry, they encourage or request their male partners to prepare their equipment, fill their air cylinder from the compressor, carry their gear to the boat, and plan the dive schedule from the tables. With time, they forget how to fill a cylinder, calculate air depth-time durations, or even how to plan a dive. Should problems arise they are then incapable of providing an intelligent solution. These ladies become a liability to their buddies and incompetent in an emergency. There is no place for sloppiness in diving – a member of a buddy pair may have to rely on the other for his or her life one day.

Body Build

There are three basic body builds – the skinny ectomorphs, the muscular mesomorphs, and the tubby endomorphs – with varying combinations of each. Ectomorphs have very little body fat for insulation and their diving Achilles' heel is hypothermia. Skinny divers should always wear a wet suit. The tubby endomorphs are amply insulated and have the further advantage of buoyancy — their shape approximates that of a sphere and, in accordance with Archimedes' Principle, they displace the maximum volume of water per given mass. This means that compression of their wet suits at depth will have less effect in creating negative buoyancy.

But the disadvantages of fatty insulation unfortunately outweigh inherent warmth and floating power. A large fat reserve means a large potential nitrogen storage capacity as nitrogen is about five times more soluble in fat than in blood or muscle tissue. So fat divers are more prone to the bends. They are also more prone to high blood pressure, heart disease and diabetes, which could disqualify them from diving altogether. In addition, being less agile they are more liable to injury in a boating or diving emergency requiring a rapid physical response. The mesomorphs are intermediate, with reasonable insulation, easy buoyancy, and good physical power and agility when needed.

It is extremely difficult and requires great dedication to change one's body build. Few have this determination and even fewer are blessed with a naturally pure mesomorphic body. But like any sport, efficient diving does place demands on habits. Good eating habits with minimal intake of animal fats, regular exercise, minimal alcohol and no smoking will help keep an average sport diving enthusiast in good condition for safe diving, even if the belt buckle is a notch or two too wide.

Cardiovascular Requirements in Scuba Diving

The cardiovascular system is the distribution network for diving gases dissolved in blood. The heart, arteries, arterioles, capillaries, venules, veins and blood comprise a highly sophisticated hydraulic system whose efficiency is an inflexible essential for safe diving.

The Heart

The heart is the most efficient pump known. Aside from having to work without maintenance or respite for seventy-plus years, it can automatically adjust both its rate and the volume of blood delivered per beat to suit circulatory demands. It has a resting capacity of 60 to 100 ml per ventricle and beats at an average of between 60 and 80 times per minute. This means a blood output of 3.6 to 8.0 litres per minute at rest. The ventricles can dilate and increase the volume per stroke, and at maximal exercise an accelerated heart can pump about 40 litres of blood per minute. It is a double pump, the right side supplying only the lungs, and the more heavily muscled and thicker left side providing blood to the systemic circulation — that is, to every other organ and tissue in the body.

As the blood flow per minute is the same through the left and right sides of the heart, it follows that the lungs receive a blood flow per minute equal to that of the rest of the entire body put together. This prodigious blood flow through the lungs is distributed into an enormous pulmonary capillary bed. It must be appreciated that capillaries are not just thin-walled blood vessels. They form a gigantic network between the arterial and venous systems and their one-cell-thick walls allow extremely rapid transfer of oxygen and nitrogen to tissues, and carbon dioxide and nitrogen release from tissues. It has been estimated that the total surface area of all the capillaries in a human adult is around 6 300 m^2 or 68 000 ft^2. Or, if all the capillaries were laid out flat, they would cover an area 19 kilometres long and 0.3 metres wide! Such is the scope of the gas exchange surface in the average human body.

The left side of the heart consists of the powerful left ventricle and the left atrium. The right side of the heart comprises the right atrium and right ventricle, which contract synchronously with the left. Filling of the ventricles between beats is mainly passive, the atria contracting just before the ventricles are ready to beat. Atrial contraction completes ventricular filling, 'topping up' the ventricles in preparation for the next rush of blood into the arteries of the body and lungs.

Arteries

The body's arterial system is a branching network, dividing into smaller and smaller arteries, and then subdividing into even smaller arterioles and finally capillaries. Arteries and arterioles carry freshly oxygenated and − when diving − freshly nitrogen-loaded blood from the lungs to the tissues of the body. The arterial system is pressurised, the power of pressurisation coming from the ventricles. This pressurisation is known as blood pressure.

Blood Pressure

Measured in millimetres of mercury, the normal upper arm blood pressure ranges between 100/60 and 140/90. The blood pressure in the pulmonary artery to the lungs is much lower, being only about 20/10. The top figure represents arterial pressure during ventricular contraction or systole. The bottom figure represents arterial pressure during ventricular relaxation or diastole. Arteries are elastic and stretch during ventricular contraction. It is their elastic recoil during ventricular relaxation that maintains the lower diastolic pressure. If arteries were rigid pipes, blood pressure would drop to zero between beats.

Capillaries

Systemic arterial pressure cannot be transmitted directly into the thin-walled capillaries. They would burst. A progressive drop-off in pressure occurs due to the resistance of arteriolar branching. At the capillaries, the pressure is very low. These thin-walled capillaries surround every cell system in the body in a net-like fashion. Through the capillary walls:
− oxygen passes to the tissue cells,
− carbon dioxide passes from the cells to the blood,
− nourishment, for example glucose, passes from the blood to the cells,
− waste products from the cells pass into the blood,
− nitrogen passes into and from cells in divers.

Veins

The venous system follows capillaries, and tiny venules join to form progressively larger veins carrying carbon dioxide and nitrogen from the tissues to the right side of the heart and then to the lungs for exhalation. Venous blood is the only route to the lungs for nitrogen degassing during decompression after a dive.

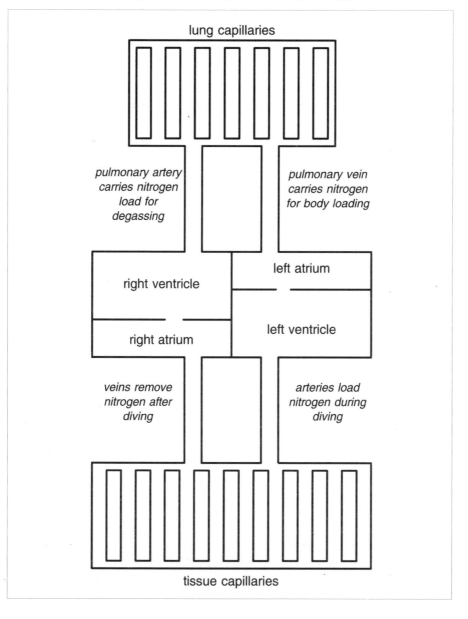

Nitrogen transport in divers

Diving Implications of Cardiovascular Disease

A significant percentage of the population suffer or will suffer from cardiovascular disorders. It is essential that would-be divers, or qualified divers who later develop vascular disease, know whether they may safely scuba dive. Some cardiovascular conditions are relatively innocuous, or with suitable medication may have little effect on surface lifestyle, exercise capability and fitness. Indeed, in many cases people first have to have a heart attack before quitting smoking and deciding to eat, drink and exercise properly. Diving, however, places special, and even unique, demands on the cardiovascular system.

Cold Water Stress

If a diver is subjected to cold by swimming in water between 5°C and 25°C, a variety of changes occur — some moderate, others dramatic, and a few potentially lethal.

Diving reflex

Immersion of the face in cold water stimulates the so-called diving reflex, with slowing of the heart and breathholding. This is one of the reasons generally given for hypothermic survival after cold water near-drowning. While operative in diving mammals such as seals and whales, and to some degree in infants and young children, in most adults immersion in water at 5°C causes a dramatic increase in heart rate, a rise in the volume of blood pumped per heart beat, intense spasm of the arterioles in the periphery of the body, and a substantial and rapid rise in blood pressure.

Gasping reflex and hypocapnia

Sudden immersion in cold water may lead to profound gasping and even hyperventilation. Aside from the risk of inhaling water and commencing the drowning process, hyperventilation causes the blood carbon dioxide level to fall, a condition called *hypocapnia*; and should the diver have coronary artery disease, a potentially fatal sequence of events begins.

Carbon dioxide in solution is acidic, and together with alkaline sodium bicarbonate forms the main buffering system of blood, keeping the pH of blood slightly alkaline at 7.4. With a drop in the carbon dioxide level with hyperventilation, blood becomes even more alkaline. This then affects calcium salts in solution. They come out of solution and bind to blood proteins. A fall in dissolved calcium salts results in intensely painful cramps in the limbs, especially hand, foot and calf muscles. Swimming ability falls and predisposes to panic with further acceleration of heart rate. Drowning impends. In addition, the heart itself is sensitive to changes in blood calcium, becoming much more irritable and prone to abnormal rhythms including ventricular fibrillation.

Add a combination of cold, gasping, hyperventilation, water inhalation, limb cramps, panic, accelerated heart rate, an elevated blood pressure, an increase in oxygen requirements and an irritable heart muscle to coronary artery disease or high blood pressure, and you have a recipe for death. To complicate matters, the adrenal glands respond to cold water stress, even at 10°C, with as much as a tripling of the release of circulating noradrenaline. Aside from contributing to the accelerated heart rate and increased blood pressure, this also can trigger runs of sudden irregular ventricular beats and even cardiac arrest, leading to sudden death. It is probable that a large proportion of middle-aged male deaths attributed to drowning in cold water are really due to ventricular fibrillation or cardiac arrest.

Hypertension (High Blood Pressure)

For sport divers, the absolute maximum blood pressure permissible without any treatment is 145/95 mm Hg (many diving physicians would balk at 140/90 mm Hg). Beyond this figure the diver is medically unfit to dive. Exposure to cold water and the exercise needs of diving may cause an extreme rise in blood pressure, with severe heart loading, rapid exhaustion and even heart failure. Even if treated and controlled, hypertension is not simply high blood pressure. It can seriously affect the functioning of the kidneys, heart, brain and eye, and the diver must consult his or her physician to ensure that these organs are unaffected.

Treatment of high blood pressure poses problems too. Many drugs used to control hypertension have unpredictable effects on blood pressure, heart rate, exercise tolerance and sensitivity to hypothermia when combined with the profound cardiovascular reactions of cold water stress. The drugs commonly used are diuretics, beta-blockers, calcium channel antagonists and ACE inhibitors. While these terms will have little or no meaning to the average sport diver, current thinking allows the use of ACE inhibitors, and if possible these should be used by hypertensive sport divers after discussing the situation with their physicians. Diuretics, often used with mild hypertension, control blood pressure by increasing urine output. As cold water immersion also increases urine output, the diver may be faced with an excessive depletion of body fluids and undue nitrogen loading during the dive. Acute decompression illness may result. Beta-blockers are generally unacceptable for diving but small doses may be permitted if blood pressure control is good and a treadmill exercise tolerance test is absolutely normal. Calcium channel antagonists are probably safe with diving.

Heart Disease

The heart is the pump of life. Like any organ, it is subject to disease. Some abnormalities are congenital, being present at birth. Others are inherited − such as a predisposition to coronary artery disease and a familial tendency to an elevated blood cholesterol; and others are acquired following illnesses such as rheumatic heart disease. But a large percentage of heart disease sufferers have coronary artery disease mainly as a result of prolonged self-abuse − uncontrolled eating, drinking and smoking.

Congenital heart disease

There are a number of possible defects present at birth that affect the heart. Some are lethal, for example, absence of ventricles; or require complex surgery to correct valvular, chamber or vessel abnormalities. The majority are diagnosed soon after birth because the baby is blue or breathless or has a characteristic murmur. Congenital heart abnormalities almost invariably bar the person from diving, especially if a shunt is present between the left and right sides of the heart.

Patent foramen ovale (PFO). From time to time bends occur even though a diver has been meticulous in planning and executing the dive. None of the obvious predisposing causes of bends, such as exercise, dehydration, hot showers, rapid ascents, missed decompression stops, etc., can be blamed for the episode of acute decompression illness. Recent work has shown that a patent foramen ovale could be the underlying reason for many of these unexplained bends.

Before birth, a baby is surrounded by fluid within the mother's womb. The child has no air to breathe and the lungs are non-functional from the point of view of oxygen uptake. Oxygen is received through blood vessels in the umbilical cord. Until the child is born and takes its first breath, blood returning from the lungs to the left atrium of the heart has not been replenished with oxygen. The large pulmonary blood flow (equal in volume to the rest of the body's circulation) that exists after birth to reoxygenate venous blood is not required in the unborn child. Nature has solved the problem by introducing an opening or short-circuit in the muscle wall or septum between the right and left atria of the heart. Blood returning from the unborn child's body via the superior and inferior venae cavae enters the right atrium. Some blood is then pumped into the right ventricle and from there to the lungs. The rest passes through the opening between the two atria to enter the left atrium, then via the left ventricle to the aorta. This opening between the two atria is called the foramen ovale (oval window) and is found in all normal newborn babies. It acts as a flap valve, permitting blood flow from the right to the left atrium. Shortly after birth, the foramen ovale closes for ever and all venous blood from the body is obliged to pass through the right ventricle to the lungs for replenishment of oxygen and removal of carbon dioxide. In about 25-37 per cent of people, the foramen ovale does not close and a potential shunt remains between the right and left sides of the heart. This has little relevance in the average population, but can cause grave problems to divers.

The venous blood returning to the right atrium of the heart after an air dive always contains nitrogen bubbles. These are normally carried via the pulmonary arteries to the lungs where direct transfer of bubble nitrogen to the alveoli occurs (provided bubble loading is not excessive). The pressure within the right atrium is lower than that within the left atrium. If a PFO is present, the higher pressure in the left atrium keeps the flap-like foramen closed. Any increase in pressure within the chest cavity may cause blood in the right atrium to shunt through to the left atrium. This increase in pressure could occur by overinflating a buoyancy jacket, sneezing, coughing, vomiting or performing a Valsalva manoeuvre. Nitrogen bubbles are then shunted into the left atrium to be pumped into the general arterial circulation. The results of these nitrogen bubbles in the arterial system are identical to those of arterial gas embolism (AGE) following pulmonary barotrauma, with the brain and upper spinal cord being most commonly affected.

It would be time-consuming, expensive and impractical to subject every would-be diver to the tests required to determine a PFO, but theoretically one in every three or four divers has a PFO. Should a bend occur when a diver has complied with all recommended diving procedures, the possibility of a PFO and its investigation must be remembered. If a PFO is found, the diver must stop diving.

Atrial septal defect (ASD). An atrial septal defect is the commonest abnormal congenital heart defect. It is an abnormality of development of the septum of the heart between the right and left atria and absolutely excludes diving. Unlike the valve-like action of a PFO, which permits blood flow only from right to left atrium, an ASD is simply a hole or a series of holes in the wall dividing the two atria. Blood can flow in either direction through the defect and a right to left flow after diving will result in AGE. With modern medical facilities an ASD is usually diagnosed soon after birth and the affected child may be subjected to cardiac surgery to repair the defect. Sometimes an ASD spontaneously closes but if a history of ASD is present, an aspiring diver must first get confirmation from a cardiologist that no small shunt remains.

Ventricular septal defect (VSD). A VSD is the ventricular equivalent of an ASD. It is the second most common congenital cardiac abnormality. It is a defect or a series of defects in the septum dividing the two ventricles. With a VSD, blood flows from the high-pressure (120 mm Hg) left ventricle to the low-pressure (20 mm Hg) right ventricle. Any resistance to pulmonary blood flow (due to a tight suit, overinflated BC, or inadequate exhalation during ascent) can reverse flow to a right-to-left shunt, and AGE after diving is a major hazard, precluding diving. Spontaneous or surgical closure requires cardiological confirmation before any diving may be considered.

Patent ductus arteriosus (PDA). During foetal development a connection, the ductus arteriosus (arterial duct), normally exists between the aorta and pulmonary artery. It serves, like the foramen ovale between the atria, to reduce blood flow through non-functional lungs by shunting venous pulmonary artery blood to the aorta and systemic circulation. The ductus arteriosus normally closes during the first two years of life, totally separating the pulmonary artery from the aorta. If it persists, or is not surgically closed, a nitrogen-bubble shunt and AGE can occur after diving. A PDA excludes diving.

Coronary artery disease

Concern about the coronary arteries — two small arteries branching from the root of the aorta immediately above the heart — has generated numerous multimillion-dollar industries. Pharmaceutical products, health foods, sports equipment and clothing industries, diet programmes, high-powered fitness gymnasiums, masses of books and literature — all are a result of awareness and fear of sudden death due to coronary artery disease.

Cholesterol. Cholesterol is not all bad. Although universally maligned by health authorities, cholesterol is one of the normal animal fats. It is an integral part of the fatty or lipid layers of normal cell membranes in all animals, and is essential for normal membrane electrical and chemical function. Its chemical ring structure is also an essential building block in the synthesis of both male and female sex hormones; the production of the hormones cortisone and aldosterone in the adrenal glands; and the formation of bile salts, indispensable for normal digestion, in the liver. So, if cholesterol is so essential, why then is it so vilified and dangerous?

The problem with cholesterol is that, in excess, it is deposited as a shaggy coat on the inside of arterial walls. It slowly obstructs the free passage of blood through the arteries and creates a rough surface predisposing to blood clot and bubble formation. Within the narrow confines of the coronary arteries, cholesterol deposits predispose to a heart attack or a coronary artery bend.

What causes a high blood cholesterol? An uneducated guess would suggest that eating foods high in cholesterol results in a high blood cholesterol level. This is only fractionally true. It is a fact that organs with very active cell membranes, such as brain, kidney, liver and lung, are particularly rich in cholesterol. It is also true that on a weight-for-weight basis full cream cow's milk has less than a quarter of the cholesterol content of herring, haddock, cod and mackerel, and one-tenth of the cholesterol content of lobster. Medium-fat bacon has less total cholesterol than crab meat. But most animal foods are constantly condemned for their cholesterol-elevating effect, whereas fish is universally recommended. Why? The point is that, apart from offal, the cholesterol content of any animal or fish food (excluding egg yolks which contain 1.48 per cent cholesterol) is invariably much less than one-tenth of one per cent of the total food mass. It is the associated non-cholesterol fats in animal products such as beef, chicken skin, egg yolk, cream, bacon and butter that are responsible for elevating blood cholesterol. These fats are saturated fats and when eaten they stimulate excess cholesterol production in the liver. Saturation, in fat terms, refers to the amount of hydrogen bound to fatty acids. Saturated fats contain the maximum amount of chemically bound hydrogen — they are fully hydrogenated. Unsaturated fats possess less bound hydrogen. Fish flesh, although high in contained membrane cholesterol, has less total fat and this fat is low in hydrogen and highly unsaturated. Unsaturated fish fat reduces cholesterol production in man. Saturated animal fat stimulates cholesterol formation.

Vegetarians have the right end of the dietary stick. Cholesterol is not found in plants. The lipid-containing cell membrane of animals is replaced by fibre-rich, indigestible cellulose cell walls. But even this is an over-simplification because ingested cholesterol is generally not as important as consuming associated saturated fats. Avocado pears, coconut oil and olive oil contain mostly saturated fats and these therefore may stimulate liver cholesterol production. An Avocado Ritz, containing succulent crab and lobster in a delicate olive-oiled bed of lemon-tanged avocado is an exotic and expensive source of abundant cholesterol!

But eating saturated fats is not the whole story. There are many people who gorge on animal fats to the point of gross obesity and yet have normal or low cholesterol levels. There are strict vegetarians, bone-lean and athletic, who have enormously high cholesterol levels and die of heart disease at a young age. The difference is preset in the genes. A genetically inherited propensity to a high cholesterol cannot be prevented or even controlled by diet alone. Cholesterol-reducing drugs are required in addition to meticulous dietary control.

How is cholesterol transported in blood? Cholesterol, being a fat, is insoluble in water and blood. Before entering the bloodstream it is bound by the liver to a carrier. This carrier acts as a bridge between fat and water. It is called a lipoprotein and has a fat-soluble lipid portion which dissolves and carries cholesterol, and a water-soluble protein section which then dissolves the whole complex in blood. In the liver, cholesterol absorbed from the diet or manufactured in liver cells following a saturated fat load is bound to a low-density lipoprotein or LDL. An LDL-cholesterol complex is formed. The term LDL refers to the large lipid portion of the molecule which reduces the overall density of the complex (fat is less dense than water and floats just as cream does on milk). Up to 75 per cent of cholesterol is transported bound to LDL in blood. The problem with an elevated LDL-cholesterol level is that it has a precarious solubility in blood and tends to deposit out of solution and on to arterial walls. Thick, hardened, gruel-like plaques of LDL-cholesterol form. This is called atherosclerosis (from the Greek *athere* meaning groats or gruel, and *sklerosis* meaning hardening). For this reason, LDL-cholesterol is commonly referred to as 'bad cholesterol'.

On the good side, a high-density lipoprotein or HDL also exists. HDL has a much smaller lipid fraction in its molecule and is correspondingly denser with a higher blood-soluble protein portion. Cholesterol bound to HDL is tightly held in solution as HDL-cholesterol. HDL is even capable of removing cholesterol already deposited on arterial walls and conveying it to the liver for breakdown and excretion in bile. No deposition of HDL-cholesterol occurs and it is popularly referred to as 'good cholesterol'.

It is the ratio between LDL and HDL levels that is important, rather than the total cholesterol level. A high LDL:HDL ratio implies a high risk of developing coronary artery disease. If the protective HDL level increases, the ratio and the risk of a heart attack decrease.

What can one do to increase HDL? Being blessed with good genes and a naturally high HDL is the surest way of avoiding a heart attack. For the rest of humanity, prevention is the only cure.
- Avoid foods high in saturated fats and eat lots of fibre.
- Exercise regularly. Exercises (especially endurance activities) do help to reduce total cholesterol and increase HDL levels.
- Lose excess weight. Human fat is saturated fat and is a ready reserve for liver cholesterol synthesis.
- Stop smoking. Aside from directly causing lung and heart disease, smoking lowers HDL levels.
- Never use anabolic steroids to increase muscle bulk and power. These steroids are male hormones and drastically reduce HDL levels. Men have a naturally greater risk than premenopausal women of developing coronary artery disease. The female hormone oestrogen is protective until women reach menopause when the risk equalises between the sexes.

Is an elevated LDL-cholesterol level relevant in diving? Yes! Efficient circulation of blood is vital to diving and having arteries clogged with LDL-cholesterol cannot assist efficient gas transfer. Bubble formation commonly begins on uneven rough surfaces and craggy plaques of cholesterol form an ideal base for bubble development. When these deposits are in a coronary artery, disaster looms. High blood fats may also affect nitrogen transport and surface tension physics in blood and predispose to bubble formation and acute decompression illness on an otherwise totally safe dive profile.

Myocardial infarction (heart attack). Branches of the left and right coronary arteries supply the heart muscle itself with blood. As blood cannot adequately flow into powerfully contracting ventricular muscles, the coronary arteries are the only arteries in the body that supply their end-organ (heart muscle) with blood during ventricular relaxation. The elastic recoil of the aorta is the driving force for blood flow into the coronary arteries. Gradual obstruction of these arteries by shaggy fatty deposits on their walls, followed by sudden blockage due to the formation of a blood clot on the roughened surface, leads to a heart attack.

Deprived of essential oxygen, the portion of heart muscle beyond the block dies. If a major branch is involved, the person dies. Death is usually due to the sudden onset of abnormal heart rhythms, especially ventricular fibrillation, resulting in ineffectual pumping and cessation of the blood supply to the brain. Resuscitation must commence within four minutes of the onset of ventricular fibrillation or brain death will begin. (See management of cardiac arrest.)

Sport diving after a heart attack may be considered after one year, provided chest pain or irregular rhythms do not occur at maximal treadmill exercise testing; the stress ECG shows no strain pattern; and the diver is examined by a cardiologist twice a year and by a diving physician once a year. In addition, the diver must always wear a full wet suit and hood to avoid cold exposure. Swimming against a current or surf entries into powerful waves must be avoided, and staged decompression stops should be shunned (except for a mandatory 5-minute stop at 5 msw with all dives). Maximum permitted diving depth is 18 msw.

Coronary angioplasty. Advances in technology have revolutionised the management of coronary artery disease. Up to the early 1970s, sufferers from coronary artery disease were given oral palliative treatment only, and diving was an impossibility. Nowadays surgery has become the treatment of choice. A diagnosis of angina pectoris, the chest pain felt when coronary artery blood supply is inadequate, is followed by coronary angiography. Radio-opaque dye is injected into the coronary arteries. If a significant block is found and the arteries are amenable to surgery, there are two possible treatments — coronary angioplasty and coronary bypass surgery. If surgery is technically impractical because of very extensive coronary artery disease, palliative oral therapy is again the treatment of choice.

Coronary angioplasty dilates and opens narrowed coronary arteries by means of a small inflatable balloon at the tip of a long catheter introduced through a femoral artery in a groin and pushed via the aorta into the coronary arteries. In the early stages of a heart attack it is also often possible to inject streptokinase, an enzyme that dissolves blood clots, into the affected coronary artery and so abort the attack. High-energy laser techniques are being developed to vaporise obstructing fatty plaques and clots and restore coronary artery patency.

Diving after an angioplasty *may* be permitted by a diving physician, provided the restrictions described above for diving after a heart attack are adhered to.

Coronary bypass surgery. Recircuiting coronary artery blood flow is being performed routinely in many centres around the world. The operation involves the initial removal of lengths of superficial veins from the legs. These vein segments are then grafted to the coronary arteries, one end above and the other below the site of arterial obstruction. The area of disease is left alone and simply bypassed through the transplanted veins. In most cases the operation is virtually curative, in that the need for oral medication stops and the patient can resume a fully active lifestyle with minimal restrictions.

In the case of sport divers, return to diving may be considered provided the conditions outlined above for diving after a heart attack are met. The question of pleural scarring after open chest surgery leading to pulmonary barotrauma with diving must be discussed by the diver and his physician in each case.

Disorders of rhythm and rate

There are many disorders of heart rhythm and rate, the commonest being a too-fast or too-slow heart rate. The majority are not indicative of underlying disease, and merely reflect excesses in lifestyle. Immoderation in the use of alcohol, nicotine and caffeine, and anxiety and stress all cause a rapid resting heart rate, often with occasional extra abnormal beats. These extra beats disappear with effort. A very slow heart rate often occurs in super-fit athletes, but increases normally during exercise.

Any other unusualness in heart rhythm or rate requires investigation to exclude underlying disease such as an overactive thyroid gland, high blood pressure or coronary artery disease. The nature and severity of the cause will determine further fitness to dive. Uncontrolled abnormalities of rhythm and rate, or those due to or requiring drug therapy, must exclude diving.

Valvular disease

Any abnormalities of the valves of the heart are invariably first detected because of characteristic murmurs heard on clinical examination.

Very common in young people is a pulmonary flow murmur, of no clinical significance, merely reflecting vigorous blood flow through the pulmonary valve of the heart. It is not a contraindication to diving. Another common murmur, and usually posing no threat to divers, is that of the billowing mitral leaflet syndrome (click-murmur syndrome; Barlow's syndrome). The murmur is due to a rather floppy leaflet of the mitral valve between the left atrium and ventricle. It is detected by hearing a classic murmur and click when listening to the heart through a stethoscope. In some cases palpitations occur, with runs of rapid heart beats, and if beta-blockers are needed the person may be unfit to dive. Some congenital valve abnormalities need not necessarily exclude diving. A bicuspid aortic valve, where the aortic valve guarding against reflux of blood back into the left ventricle has two cusps instead of three, is an example. If not incompetent on assessment by a cardiologist, the person may dive.

In young people, the commonest pathological murmurs are due to valvular scarring and distortion by rheumatic heart disease; and in older divers, to the hardening and calcification of the aortic and mitral valves. If narrowing or leaking of the affected valves is considered significant by a physician, diving is prohibited. Bubble initiation is a real risk on actively moving valves that have lost their smooth surfaces.

Cardiac surgery, with the implantation of artificial heart valves, also bars diving in most cases. People who have had such surgery commonly use anticoagulants to prevent clotting on the valves, and the risk of massive haemorrhage with any barotrauma plus the effects of cold water stress, exercise, and the demands of nitrogen loading and degassing, make diving unacceptable.

Pacemakers

Electronic pacemakers, inserted under the skin and taking over the control of heart rate, are used when cardiac or coronary artery disease presents with possibly life-threatening abnormal rhythms. The problems of diving with a pacemaker are the original reasons for inserting it, the effects of pressure on a possibly non-pressure-resistant electronic instrument, and the need for the pacemaker to accelerate heart rate during diving exercise. Variable rate pacemakers are available but before any decision to dive with a pacemaker is possible, detailed discussion between the manufacturer, the cardiologist, the diving physician and the patient is essential.

Bleeding disorders

Any disorder that predisposes to a bleeding tendency usually means immediate and total disqualification from diving. Whether due to the use of anticoagulant drugs, liver disease, bone marrow problems, or inherited disorders such as haemophilia, a tendency to haemorrhage could be fatal with diving. Any pressure-volume changes with depth could result in uncontrolled bleeding in the lungs, middle ears, sinuses and gut. The regular infusion of fresh-frozen plasma into the blood of haemophiliacs and allied bleeders can only offer some protection under normal surface circumstances. It can never handle the potential catastrophe of pulmonary barotrauma or trauma due to boat propellers or marine animal bites. But there are divers who dive while on anticoagulant treatment. Their rationale is that they always dive carefully and safely. The risk is entirely in their own hands. It cannot be medically condoned. No one can guarantee that an emergency under water will not occur.

Blood donors

After donating blood, donors should wait a period of 48 to 72 hours before diving. The reason is not related simply to blood loss and a lower total oxygen-carrying capacity by haemoglobin. Under diving conditions the available oxygen is at a higher partial pressure than at the surface and a significant amount can dissolve in plasma. The reason is related to the loss of about one-sixth of the total *fluid* volume of blood, the *only* route for inert gas carriage from tissues to alveoli. After two to three days it is safe for divers to recommence diving as blood fluid volume balance will have been restored, even though the cellular and protein elements still have to be replaced.

Peripheral vascular disease

A number of diseases, such as arteriosclerosis and diabetes, affect the small peripheral vessels of the body. This effect reduces the blood supply to the tissues of arms and legs, especially the lower legs, feet and hands, which become permanently cold with decreased hair and nail growth. Under exercise conditions the oxygen supply becomes very inadequate and muscle cramping occurs, classically in the calf muscles with walking. The affected person has to stand and wait until the acidic products of metabolism, such as lactic acid, can be removed from the area and the oxygen debt repaid. Diving aggravates this because cold water causes spasm of already inadequate blood vessels, worsening of blood supply, and easy cramping. Tissue degassing is also affected and diving is dangerous.

Chillblains are a minor and temporary form of peripheral vascular disease. Spasm of the blood supply to the fingers and toes occurs in cold weather. These digits become cold, pale and numb. The skin becomes painful and itchy and then rebound flushing occurs. In severe cases blistering or even sores can develop. Diving in cold water intensifies this and the fingers can become very pallid, totally numb and difficult to move. Restoration of the blood supply after the dive is accompanied by intense burning and itching plus red flaring of the skin as spastic vessels dilate. Wearing gloves and bootees while diving often helps. Taking vitamin B6 also assists in improving peripheral blood supply.

Varicose veins

Varicose veins generally cause no problem with diving. The surrounding water pressure provides even support to dilated and tortuous veins. Severe cases should be treated surgically as the veins may bleed profusely with accidental trauma, and coral cuts on the legs and bumping and scraping on boats are very common injuries among divers.

Pulmonary Requirements of Scuba Diving

In contrast to the hydraulically operated cardiovascular system, the respiratory system is a pneumatic system. It is a simple double bellows. There are two lungs, each surrounded by a tough but flexible double sheath, the pleura. The lungs are encased by the rib cage and the diaphragm, a powerful flat sheet of muscle dividing the chest or thorax from the abdomen below.

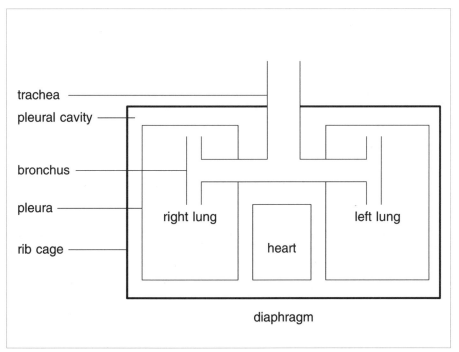

Diagrammatic representation of the pulmonary system

Although the lungs and heart actually fill the thorax, the pleural cavity is a potential space between the lungs and the ribs.

Breathing Mechanics

The lung bellows work as follows:

The intercostal muscles between the ribs contract and pull the ribs outwards. At the same time, the diaphragm contracts downwards. This means that the volume of the chest increases. A vacuum forms in the potential space between the lungs and the rib cage. The lungs expand to fill this space and air is sucked into the lungs – this is *inspiration*. The muscles of the chest wall and diaphragm then relax and the rib cage springs back to its resting position. Air is squeezed out of the lungs – this is *expiration*. Inspiration is active, and expiration passive, under resting conditions. During exercise, additional chest muscles assist with the need for rapid inhalation, and exhalation becomes active too.

Respiratory Tree

Like the arterial network, the respiratory system is a branching system. Inhaled air passes into the trachea, the ridged pipe in the front of the throat below the larynx. In the chest, the trachea divides into two bronchi. Each bronchus passes to a lung. Within the lung, bronchi subdivide until the terminal bronchioles. Each of the millions of terminal bronchioles ends in a grape-like cluster of alveoli.

Alveoli

It is important to understand the physical scope of the lungs. Alveoli are not just air-filled sacs dangling from bronchioles. The total number of alveoli has been estimated at 750 000 000, with a total surface area for gas exchange equal to that of the playing surface of eight full-size snooker tables, or 25 times that of the total surface area of the skin. Around the alveoli is a capillary network processing the venous side of the heart's entire blood output per minute. And all this is inside a sunken chest covered with hair, or a provocative one wearing a lacy bra!

To achieve this prodigious surface area in the relatively paltry volume of the chest, alveoli have to be very small and thin-walled. This means that bronchioles must be small too. They are: each semiglobular alveolus in a particular cluster is about 0.1 mm in diameter and one cell thick, and each bronchiole about 0.3 mm wide. And therein lies their weakness from a diving point of view. A scuba diver is risking exposing alveoli fractions of a millimetre in diameter and one cell thick to several atmospheres of pressure change. At only 10 msw the air pressure in the chest equals that inside a motor car tyre.

To tolerate this, pressure inside and outside the lungs must at all times be equal. A pressure difference of only 0.1 ATA may be enough to rupture the lungs, meaning that if a scuba diver lying at the bottom of the shallow end of a swimming pool inhales fully and then stands up, his or her lungs may burst.

Gas Exchange

The need for a huge thin-walled surface area, exposed to air on one side and a massive network of blood on the other, lies in gas exchange. The ultimate function of the lungs is oxygen absorption and carbon dioxide exhalation. Both are fluid/gas operations — oxygen from air to blood, and carbon dioxide from blood to air. The exchange occurs across a single layer of cells lining millions of air-filled alveoli and a single layer of cells lining the giant network of blood-filled pulmonary capillaries. So blood and air are necessary. This may be obvious, but it is not that simple. An efficient blood supply is essential — this is called *perfusion*. A good air supply is needed — this is called *ventilation*. And a rapid transfer of gas between air and blood is required — this is called *diffusion*.

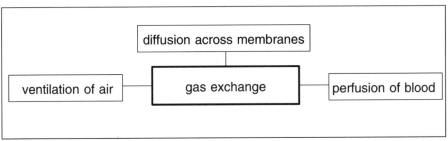

Perfusion, ventilation and diffusion are what lungs are about and they must all be normal and balanced for efficient gas exchange. If any one of them fails, gas exchange is impaired. A failure of perfusion of normally ventilating lungs will achieve no gas exchange. Good perfusion of non-ventilating alveoli will achieve no gas exchange. Good perfusion and ventilation of non-diffusing alveoli will achieve no gas exchange. Balance is essential.

Pulmonary Assessment in Scuba Divers

A full assessment of lung function would entail measuring all three aspects of pulmonary activity — ventilation, perfusion and diffusion. As the avoidance of pulmonary barotrauma is the only reason for doing lung function testing in an apparently normal scuba diver, only ventilation is directly assessed.

There are three aspects to assessing ventilation:
— clinical assessment by a doctor,
— chest X-ray,
— lung function test.

The clinical assessment forms part of any routine checkup and confirms the absence of any obvious disease. The history of the diver's health is investigated and the presence of normal air entry and exhalation listened for.

An X-ray provides an idea of the gross anatomy of the chest, and demonstrates heart size and shape, the major vessels and bronchi, the presence of overinflation or underinflation of lungs, scarring and tumours, diaphragm movement on inhalation and exhalation and, very importantly, air-trapping in bullae – pathological blister-like areas in the lung or on its surface. These are usually totally asymptomatic on land and the person is completely unaware of their presence until a spontaneous pneumothorax suddenly occurs. But under diving conditions and filled with air under pressure at depth, bullae easily burst on ascent with potential collapse of the lung, tearing of lung tissue, haemorrhage into the chest, and arterial gas embolism. Air-trapping, unless enormous, is not detectable clinically or on lung function testing. An X-ray is essential and should comprise both inspiratory and immediate expiratory chest views to assess diaphragm movement and detect bullae.

A full lung function test assesses all lung volumes and flow rates. It directly measures air volumes moving into and from the lungs, rates of flow achieved, and rates of change of flow. It computes residual volumes of airways, and detects any restriction to inspiration and any obstruction to exhalation under resting and forced respiratory conditions. Changes in the elasticity of the lungs, their compliance in moving readily with inspiration and expiration, and resistance to flow in airways are assessed. Conditions such as asthma and emphysema are readily detected.

As pulmonary barotrauma is a result of failure of exhalation of compressed air, to reduce costs in sport diver evaluation, a minimum basic assessment of lung function measures volumes and flow rates during exhalation only. At least three parameters must be measured:

FVC

The *Forced Vital Capacity* is the volume of air exhaled between a full inhalation and a maximal forced exhalation. It is the maximum volume of air a diver can move into or out of the lungs. It varies with age, sex, height, weight and population group. Standard tables or computerised machines are used to predict the volume in each person tested. The FVC normally lies between 3.0 and 7.0 litres in adults. Asthmatics often have a normal FVC. The minimal FVC acceptable for diving is 75 per cent of predicted FVC.

FEV1

The Forced Expiratory Volume in 1 second is the volume of air exhaled in the first second of a maximal exhalation. It is the first second of the FVC and indicates any airway resistance. The higher the resistance to exhalation, the lower will be the volume of air exhaled in the first second. The FEV1 is always reduced with any obstructive airways disease, including asthma.

FEV1%

As both the FVC and FEV1 vary with height, weight, age, sex and population group, their volumes in litres mean little unless a standard table or computer are at hand. So a ratio is used which is independent of all the variables. The volume of air exhaled in the first second is calculated as a percentage of total air exhaled.

$$\text{FEV1/FVC} \times 100 = \text{FEV1\%}$$

A diver with normal lung function will be able to exhale about 80 per cent of his FVC in one second. The minimum FEV1% acceptable varies between authorities; in Britain and Norway the lowest accepted is 70-75 per cent. As asthmatics always have a low FEV1 they will also have a low FEV1%.

Many doctors still use peak flow meters to measure the peak flow rate (PFR) as a test for respiratory efficiency in divers. The peak flow meter has no place in diving medicine. A very high flow rate, sustained for a fraction of a second only, is possible for people with severe obstructive airways disease. The peak flow meter will provide a favourable reading while the person then completes expiration with a six-seconds-long wheeze. Spitting or tonguing the mouthpiece will also provide normal results. The peak flow meter is useful only in assessing response to treatment of obstructive pulmonary disease.

There is one lung volume people cannot use or change − the air volume remaining after maximal exhalation. It is the volume of the tubular airways inside the lungs − the bronchi and bronchioles. It is called the *residual volume* (RV). Its importance relates to the maximum depth that can safely be reached by a breathhold diver. An average total lung volume (TLV) is about 6 litres. It is the sum of FVC and RV (TLV = FVC + RV). An average residual volume is about 1.2 litres. One can now ask, how deep can one breathhold dive, assuming average lung volumes?

On descent the surrounding water pressure compresses the air in one's chest. One can therefore descend until total lung air has been compressed to equal surface residual volume. With a TLV of 6 litres and a RV of 1.2 litres (one fifth), one can therefore dive to 5 ATA or 40 msw. At this point, lung air volume will be one fifth of that at the surface (Boyle's Law). Descending below this depth results in blood pooling in the great veins of the chest to equalise further decreasing air volume. Then chest wall crushing and internal tissue and vein rupture occur with massive intrathoracic haemorrhage.

Despite the theoretical safe average maximum of 40 msw, free dives to below 100 msw have been done. These would require extraordinarily flexible chest walls and lung volumes with relatively very small RVs and immense venous pooling capability. It is doubtful whether breathhold dives to these depths can be done without causing some pathology.

Divers who have a breathing source under water do not undergo these volume changes as the pressure of the inhaled air is set to ambient surrounding pressure at all times. The total lung volume is the same at the surface and at depth. What does vary is the density of the gas mix with pressure, as well as the partial pressures of the components in the mix (Dalton's Law).

Breathhold Diving

A breathhold diver is deliberately risking asphyxiation. During breath-holding the body continues to use oxygen and produce carbon dioxide. So the partial pressure of oxygen in the blood will drop (hypoxia) and the partial pressure of carbon dioxide will rise (hypercapnia – eventually leading to carbon dioxide narcosis). Either effect can cause unconsciousness and together they form a very dangerous pair.

Breathhold diving, especially with prior hyperventilation, is a classic exercise in diving physics. At the surface of the water, hyperventilating flushes out alveolar carbon dioxide. Following Henry's Law, arterial blood carbon dioxide levels drop too (hypocapnia). Alveolar oxygen and nitrogen pressures increase, obeying Dalton's Law, to compensate for the low carbon dioxide. During descent, water pressure increases and Boyle's Law reduces lung air volume. Dalton's Law continues to operate with a proportional rise in the partial pressure of alveolar oxygen. Henry's Law now drives this oxygen into pulmonary capillary blood, and pulmonary arterial carbon dioxide into alveolar gas. Alveolar oxygen drops and carbon dioxide rises.*

It is the high arterial partial pressure of carbon dioxide that is the stimulus for the overwhelming desire to breathe that ends the dive and forces a diver to surface. This will normally occur while the partial pressure of oxygen is still sufficient for body requirements. Should the arterial oxygen level drop below a critical level of 4 kilopascals (kPa), unconsciousness under water may occur without any warning. The same may happen if the carbon dioxide level rises above 6 kPa.

At the same time, other profound physiological changes are occurring in the diver. Lung ventilation has stopped. Diffusion and perfusion are still occurring. At a depth of 10 msw the early effects of chest squeeze are occurring. Lung air volume has halved, lung tissue is compressed, and alveolar architecture is distorted. Interference with normal perfusion threatens as the lungs become 'stiff' and engorged with blood.

Spear fishermen are breathhold divers and are very competitive. They want to stay under water for as long as possible. So:
- they train – this increases circulatory efficiency;
- they acclimatise to a raised carbon dioxide level in the blood. Many divers who dive regularly have their 'carbon dioxide threshold' or stimulus to breathe set higher than non-divers;
- they move as little as possible under water to conserve oxygen and reduce carbon dioxide production;
- they *hyperventilate* before the dive. This is the dangerous one. Let's look at two examples:
- Nick promised his wife some crayfish. Using a snorkel, he dives to 10 msw (2 ATA). At this depth, his lung air volume has halved (Boyle's Law), and the partial pressure of oxygen in his alveoli has doubled

---

* Pieter Landsberg has found that after vigorous hyperventilating these alveolar changes are not invariable and do not reliably reflect the blood gas status. At the end of the dive alveolar carbon dioxide may be very high or low, with low or moderate oxygen.

(Dalton's Law). This is beneficial in that more oxygen is now available. After 45 seconds, the high partial pressure of carbon dioxide forces him to surface, waving a crayfish. All is well, as his oxygen level is still adequate.

- Jeff is a competitive spear fisherman. He hyperventilates at the surface, breathing in and out as deeply as possible, until he feels dizzy. What he has done is to flush his lungs and alveoli so that the partial pressure of carbon dioxide in his alveoli has dropped to 2.7 kPa (normal alveolar carbon dioxide at sea-level is just over 5 kPa). This gives him a 'start', as the time required to build up the carbon dioxide to trigger levels will be longer. He has also increased his alveolar oxygen, the lost carbon dioxide being replaced by air. He now dives to 20 msw (3 ATA). The oxygen concentration in his lungs triples, giving him even more duration. He waits and waits for his fish, and just when he feels he must ascend, he gets his chance and spends a further 10 seconds spearing it. The desire to breathe is now very strong and he ascends rapidly. As he does so, the water pressure drops, but so does the partial pressure of oxygen in his alveoli. At 5 msw his alveolar oxygen drops too much and he loses consciousness. Luckily, a buddy is at hand to bring him to the surface and resuscitate him.

This is the classic description of *blackout of ascent* which has been the cause of death by drowning in many healthy breathhold divers. It is caused by a deadly sequence of events. The increased ambient pressure at depth decreases lung air volume and increases alveolar partial pressure of oxygen, so causing a higher gradient of oxygen into the blood from the lungs. Hyperventilating before the dive drops the baseline carbon dioxide level in the lungs and arterial blood and increases the time before a high arterial carbon dioxide stimulus forces the diver to surface. Oxygen is steadily removed from alveolar air during the dive but at the bottom the level is adequate, even at the end of the dive. Ascent, especially fast ascent, causes the oxygen level in the lungs to fall sharply with a rapid drop in the gradient of oxygen into the blood, severe arterial hypoxia and blackout.

The safety of the dive depends on:
1. *Ventilation* — a large FVC with relatively small RV will provide a greater oxygen reserve. This ratio is reduced with any respiratory ailment.
2. *Diffusion* — an efficient alveolar/capillary junction is needed for rapid transfer of oxygen and carbon dioxide. This is reduced by factors such as smoking and respiratory infections.
3. *Perfusion* — a good alveolar blood supply is needed for efficient degassing and upgassing. Any illness affecting lung blood supply will reduce perfusion.
4. *Fitness* — this improves muscle oxygen utilisation for a given exercise load. Oxygen consumption and carbon dioxide production during the exercise of hyperventilating will affect the safe duration of the dive. So will oxygen consumption and carbon dioxide production during the dive.

5. *Blood carbon dioxide load between dives* — inadequate time for breathing and carbon dioxide unloading at the surface between breathhold dives will cause rapid hypercapnia and even carbon dioxide narcosis and syncope at the bottom with the next dive.
6. *Dive depth* — the deeper the dive, the greater the chances of chest squeeze; the higher the oxygen gradient into blood at the bottom; and the steeper the hypoxia on ascent.
7. *Dive duration* — dives over 80 or 90 seconds place the diver in extreme jeopardy.
8. *Rate of ascent* — very rapid ascents cause a rapid drop in alveolar oxygen delivery and result in hypoxia.
9. *Patent foramen ovale* — a flap-valve between the right and left upper chambers of the heart is present in up to 25-37 per cent of people. If right-to-left shunts such as a PFO are present, this author believes that they may operate with the increased water pressure on the chest with breathhold diving and be an important cause of death in breathhold diving.

As the breathhold diver descends the water pressure around him or her increases. The chest and lungs become compressed. The right side of the heart, a very low pressure system, meets increased resistance to its attempts to pump blood into lung blood vessels. The pressure in the right atrium rises and the PFO opens. Venous blood, high in carbon dioxide and very low in oxygen, is shunted into the left side of the heart and back into the general circulation. Less blood reaches the lungs. This results in a decreased transfer of blood carbon dioxide into alveoli, plus a reduced draw on available alveolar oxygen during the dive. Arterial blood oxygen drops dramatically and carbon dioxide rises sharply. Analysing the gas in the alveoli at this point would show a relatively low carbon dioxide level and ample oxygen! Bottom syncope may then occur due to profound arterial hypoxia and carbon dioxide narcosis. Or a rapid ascent could beat diffusion of oxygen from, and carbon dioxide into, expanding alveoli and result in blackout of ascent.

Note
- Deep dives to below 30 msw without hyperventilating may also cause blackout of ascent as the alveolar oxygen partial pressure will increase at least four times, with very rapid absorption followed by an equivalently rapid drop on ascent.
- The same laws also apply to nitrogen. At depth, the nitrogen partial pressure in the alveoli will also increase. This is equivalent to breathing air at depth. Repetitive deep dives on a snorkel may cause excessive amounts of nitrogen to be absorbed, and bends on breathhold dives have been described.
- Oxygen utilisation by the tissues does not increase with depth. It increases with work. A diver at 10 msw and a diver at 100 msw will use the same amount of oxygen (when expressed in surface volumes) for the same work, ignoring the work of breathing a denser mix. This is why a

two per cent oxygen mix is safe at 90 msw and 20 per cent is required at the surface. Their partial pressures are the same (0.2 ATA) under these conditions.

● Similarly, the body does not produce more carbon dioxide at depth than at the surface. Metabolic requirements do not change — only pressures do.

Metabolism

The gases oxygen and carbon dioxide have been mentioned again and again. The questions arise:
— Why do we need oxygen?
— What is it used for?
— Where does the carbon dioxide come from?
The fine details are very complex and totally out of the scope of diving. The basic essentials are easily explained with an analogy. Take the case of a petrol engine. The fuel is octane. Octane consists of 8 atoms of carbon and 18 atoms of hydrogen linked in a straight chain (C_8H_{18}).

Inside the cylinders, the octane is mixed with air (i.e. oxygen), pressurised and sparked. The octane combines with the oxygen and explodes. If conditions were perfect, the end-products would be carbon dioxide (CO_2) and water (H_2O).

Octane + oxygen = carbon dioxide + water + energy + heat

As conditions are never perfect, some of the octane is incompletely combusted and carbon monoxide (CO) forms. Complete combustion yields carbon dioxide only.

The tissue cells are our engines, billions of them. Our fuel is glucose from our diet. Glucose is combined with oxygen to produce carbon dioxide, water, energy, and heat.

Glucose + oxygen = carbon dioxide + water + energy + heat

Obviously we do not explode oxygen and glucose under pressure. The overall reaction is broken down stepwise into many littler reactions, each releasing some of the energy and heat, and all strictly controlled. Our body heat is the result of this process. The carbon dioxide we breathe out is the end-product, together with some water vapour. The rest of the water formed is handled by the kidneys.

For every molecule of oxygen used, a molecule of carbon dioxide is formed.

At rest, about 0.25 litres of oxygen per minute are used. With *hard swimming*, up to four litres per minute are used. Note that this is oxygen used, not air consumption. Not all the oxygen breathed in is used. Inspired air contains about 21 per cent oxygen and exhaled air approximately 16 per cent oxygen.

How is oxygen carried to the tissues?

Within the blood are trillions of red blood cells, or erythrocytes. Within these cells is an iron-containing pigment called haemoglobin. Haemoglobin gives the blood its red colour. In plants, the equivalent pigment is chlorophyll, which gives them a green colour. Haemoglobin traps oxygen under conditions of high oxygen partial pressure (i.e. in the lung capillaries) and releases it under conditions of low oxygen partial pressure and high carbon dioxide partial pressure (i.e. in the tissues). Most of the oxygen is carried bound to haemoglobin. Only a small percentage is dissolved free in plasma, the straw-coloured liquid portion of blood when all the blood cells are removed.

What controls breathing?

Since breathing is an automatic process not requiring any conscious attention, there obviously must be a control mechanism. The respiratory centre controlling breathing is located in the brain. It receives its information regarding breathing rate and depth from the following (among others):

1. *Carbon dioxide partial pressure*. The partial pressure of carbon dioxide in the blood is the most powerful stimulus to breathe. A rise in the carbon dioxide level in the blood stimulates ventilation.
2. *Oxygen partial pressure*. This is a much weaker stimulus to breathe. A low partial pressure of oxygen does stimulate inspiration.
3. *Heat*. A rise in body temperature stimulates inspiration and a fall in temperature depresses breathing.
4. *Acidity*. Lactic acid is formed when the oxygen supply of actively exercising muscles falls. This increase in acidity stimulates ventilation to increase oxygen uptake.
5. *Joint movement*. Active movement of a joint triggers nerve reflexes to the respiratory centre in the brain and stimulates ventilation.

Under normal conditions the circulating carbon dioxide level is the main controlling force. But the body is beautifully coordinated. An increase in ventilation is linked to an increase in perfusion in order to maintain balance. All of the above respiratory-stimulating factors also stimulate heart output with increased perfusion of the lungs in order to take full advantage of the increased ventilation.

Diving Implications of Respiratory Disease

Normal breathing is essential for safe diving. The lungs are exposed to more potential danger than any other organ during a dive. If a diver has a history of any recent significant respiratory problem, a repeat medical, X-ray chest with inspiratory and expiratory views, and a full lung function test are imperative. Any condition that can affect the efficiency of the bellows system — its ventilation, perfusion or diffusion — must temporarily or permanently bar a diver from the sport.

Abnormalities of Ventilation

Ventilation of the lungs requires efficient inspiration and expiration. There are a number of conditions that can impair either one, the other, or both. Some are acute and temporary, such as bronchitis and pneumonia, and diving may continue after full recovery and clinical reassessment. Others are acute and cause permanent suspension from diving, such as a spontaneous pneumothorax. Many are ongoing and therefore automatically preclude diving, such as asthma, emphysema and lung damage due to chronic dust inhalation (pneumoconiosis).

Disorders of inspiration (restrictive pulmonary disease)

Failure of easy inspiration occurs when the normal compliance of the lungs is lost. They lose their elasticity and can no longer inflate normally to follow the expansion of the chest wall during inspiration. This occurs most commonly in quarry and mine workers, the cause depending on the dust involved. It may be coal, silicon, asbestos or cement, and diffuse intense scarring of the lungs can occur. Pulmonary fibrosis may also follow congenital cystic disease of the lung, lung infections, or abnormalities of the immune system of the body. The diagnosis is readily made on X-ray chest and impaired inspiratory results on lung function testing. The risk of pulmonary barotrauma with diving is enormous and diving is prohibited.

Inspiration and expiration are impaired with emphysema, most commonly caused by smoking, where overinflation of the lungs occurs due to breakdown of alveoli with a drastic reduction of alveolar surface area. The chest becomes barrel-shaped with a greatly reduced movement of the chest wall between full inspiration and expiration. These people often purse their lips and blow during exhalation, unconsciously increasing the partial pressure in their lungs to drive oxygen from alveoli into blood. Obviously they may not dive.

A short-term reduction in inspiration occurs most commonly with rib injuries, pleurisy and chest shingles where pain limits adequate inhalation. All tests should be normal on recovery.

Disorders of expiration (obstructive pulmonary disease)

Disorders of expiration cause airway obstruction and increased resistance to exhalation. The above disorders that cause ongoing inspiratory impairment usually have an obstructive element too, with significantly increased bronchiolar resistance. The commonest chronic disorder of expiration is asthma and the most dangerous acute combined inspiratory and expiratory condition is a spontaneous pneumothorax, where the lung can neither fill nor empty normally. Benign and malignant tumours, tuberculosis and fungal infections of the lung may be obstructive and restrictive and all are prohibitive to diving.

Abnormalities of Perfusion and Diffusion

Interference with the normal blood supply of the lungs impairs diffusion of oxygen, carbon dioxide and nitrogen. This occurs with pulmonary embolism where a deep vein thrombosis in the calf muscle embolises to the main venous return to the heart and is then pumped into the pulmonary arteries. It can also happen following thrombosis of superficial leg veins. Sarcoidosis, a condition characterised by the formation of granulomatous lesions in the lung, affects the alveolar membranes and interferes with diffusion. All diffusion abnormalites must preclude diving.

Spontaneous Pneumothorax

If air is allowed to enter the pleural cavity between the surface of a lung and the chest wall, the lung bellows system instantly fails. The vacuum that forms in the pleural space on inspiration and forces the lung to inflate is eliminated. The lung collapses and ventilation and diffusion cease.

Factors that predispose to a spontaneous pneumothorax under non-diving conditions are lung blisters and bullae, lung cysts, and cavities due to diseases such as tuberculosis. In most cases the lung collapses without any warning, often when the person is straining to lift a heavy object, sneezing or vomiting. These suddenly increase the pressure inside the lungs with tearing through the area of weakness on the surface of the lung. Sudden one-sided chest pain occurs plus difficulty in breathing. If the torn area allows air flow in one direction only by acting as a flap valve, each successive breath pumps more air into the pleural cavity and progressively

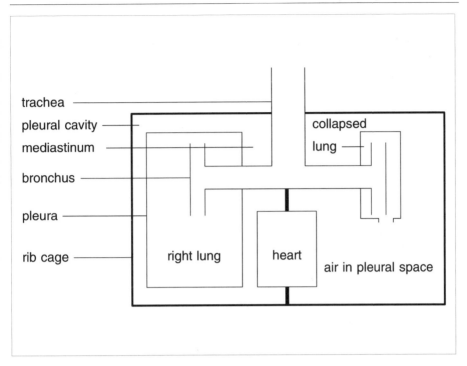

trachea

pleural cavity

mediastinum

collapsed

lung

bronchus

pleura

rib cage   right lung   heart

air in pleural space

Diagrammatic representation of a pneumothorax

compresses the affected lung. This is a *tension pneumothorax* and, if allowed to proceed, will steadily pressurise the chest, compressing the heart, mediastinum and the other lung into the opposite side of the thorax. Untreated, the person will die of cardiopulmonary failure.

The incidence of recurrence of a spontaneous pneumothorax is high, one-third of cases having another episode within five years of the first.

Under scuba diving conditions a pneumothorax may be precipitated by breathholding during ascent, coughing or vomiting under water, or blowing very hard while performing a Valsalva manoeuvre. Unless the leak is extremely small, the consequences are very grave. Air expanding inside the pleural cavity on ascent cannot escape and will pressurise the chest as with a tension pneumothorax and then drive the lungs up into the throat and beyond. If a tension pneumothorax develops at depth the diver will die under water. Ascent becomes impossible because of gas expansion, and remaining under water is impossible because of air supply limitations and progressive cardiopulmonary failure. A history of spontaneous pneumothorax must permanently preclude scuba diving.

But, and such is the enthusiasm of divers for their sport that there is always a but, some divers have continued diving after their pneumothorax by subjecting themselves to surgical stripping of the pleura of both lungs. The pleural cavity is eliminated, the lungs then healing by attaching themselves directly to the chest wall.

This procedure would seem a very drastic one for an otherwise healthy individual to undertake in order to scuba dive, and both lungs must be treated because surface blisters and blebs, if present, are most commonly found on both lungs. The question of lung scarring then predisposing to lung tissue tearing during diving with resultant arterial gas embolism must also be considered.

A pneumothorax can also occur following injury to the chest wall or open chest surgery for reasons such as coronary artery bypass procedures. It is important to exclude air-trapping by scarring and adhesions after surgery. A normal lung function test, X-ray chest, and uneventful chamber pressure test dive in an experienced diver could make requalification acceptable, provided that the underlying cause of the need for surgery does not persist.

Asthma

A survey report by Bove in *Skindiver* of December 1992 has indicated that 8.3 per cent of sport divers have or have had asthma, and that asthmatic divers have double or triple the risk of developing pulmonary barotrauma and arterial gas embolism. But seen in perspective, the overall occurrence is still small, being only about 1 in 200 000 dives.

Asthma is a condition associated with increased resistance to easy air flow out of the small tubular airways within the lungs. For some reason people are unwilling to accept a simple name for a common condition and prefer clinical elaboration or euphemisms or even resent or deny that their airways are anything less than perfect. So asthma is known by many other names, such as bronchial asthma, hyper-irritable airways, allergic asthma, atopic asthma, exercise-induced asthma, allergic bronchospasm, occasional tightness, a bit wheezy sometimes, mostly fine, and only when there is a cat around.

The basic problem, whatever the name chosen, is spasm of the tiny muscles surrounding bronchioles. This spasm constricts these tubules causing them to narrow, making breathing, especially breathing out, difficult.

This spasm is commonly relieved by the use of inhalant sprays such as salbutamol, and cortisone sprays such as beclomethasone. These alone usually provide rapid and easy control of wheezing and breathing difficulty, so that the user is able to participate in almost all activities requiring rapid and deep breathing — marathon running, swimming, athletics, mountain climbing, skydiving, snorkelling, etc.

Unfortunately, they do not protect the user from extreme possible danger while scuba diving. Air under pressure is proportionately denser. At a depth of 10 msw, air at 2 ATA pressure is twice as dense as surface air, so any difficulty with exhalation at the surface will be aggravated under water with this denser, heavier air. At 30 msw the air inhaled is four times denser than surface air so even more work is required to breathe. This increased effort, combined with the activity of swimming under water, may precipitate or aggravate an attack of asthma under water. The problem does not end here, however.

During ascent, the air inhaled at depth will expand. From a depth of 10 metres, the volume of air in the lungs will double at the surface. From 30 metres, the air in the lungs will quadruple in volume at the surface. Obviously, the lungs cannot double or quadruple in volume — they will burst, with fatal results. The solution is to exhale the expanding air during ascent. With restriction in airflow, as in asthma, the rate of flow of air out of the lungs may not be fast enough during ascent. Rupture of the lungs will then occur, with bleeding into the chest followed by bubbles entering torn vessels into the bloodstream and arterial gas embolism to the brain or heart, with fatal or crippling results.

Using a spray before the dive is not a guaranteed solution. The inhaled medication does not reach every single tubule within the lungs. Any remaining tubule still in spasm is liable to result in lung rupture. Any mucous plugs in any tubule will prevent access of the spray to the area in spasm. The duration of action of the spray is unpredictable. It may wear off during the dive. The general effects of absorption of these sprays into the body under conditions of high pressure are also unpredictable — a sudden racing of the heart rate with irregular beats and dangerous abnormal rhythms may occur; severe blinding headaches may strike; nausea and vomiting under water may happen. All of these are potentially life-threatening in themselves, exposing the diver to the sudden hazard of drowning. Couple them to a diver struggling to reach the surface quickly and being unable to exhale expanding gas and you have a deadly situation. Promising to do shallow dives only is also no answer. The major effects of pressure/volume changes occur above 10 msw.

Asthmatic divers expose their buddy divers to increased risks. Buddy divers rely on each other for help in an emergency — it is the prime reason for always diving in pairs. Expecting buddies to stand by in case of breathing difficulties under water is totally foolhardy — there is absolutely nothing they can do. They cannot exhale for their asthmatic partners. Not telling them of the problem is worse. Should they require urgent help during a dive with an assisted ascent, their lives may be threatened by their asthmatic partners being unable to vent exhaled air adequately. Double disaster then threatens.

However, statistics seem to indicate only a very remote chance of an asthmatic diver developing serious complications, and the question of people with 'mild' asthma diving has been a bone of contention between divers and doctors for years. The problem is that the doctor has to decide whether a particular diver's lungs can exhale dense expanding gas. In a doctor/patient relationship statistics don't help too much. No doctor wants a statistic as an ex-patient, not to mention the legal implications of approving fitness to die.

A past history of asthma is acceptable to some diving physicians provided the last episode was more than two years previously; the diver is on no medication to control bronchospasm; and the asthma is not cold induced or exercise induced because these are normal diving conditions.

The problem of asthma and diving rages on. As further figures become available perhaps a qualified and not totally exclusive approach may be possible for asthmatic divers. At the present time asthmatic divers must understand that a chance of fatal barotrauma does exist, and that they dive at their own risk.

Smoking and Diving

Smoking is a disease that was introduced into Europe by Christopher Columbus who caught it from a North American Indian. The weed *Nicotiana tabacum*, a relative of the deadly nightshade, was then named after the French ambassador at Lisbon, Jean Nicot, who sent the seeds to the queen of France, Catherine de Médicis. She subsequently died at Blois on 5 January 1589.

Smoking and diving don't mix. Tobacco smoke contains a number of chemicals including nicotine, carbon monoxide, assorted tars, and sulphur-cyanides. The harmful effects of smoking are both short-term and long-term, local and general.

Local effects

1. Irritation of the lining of the nose, mouth, throat, bronchi and alveoli occurs. This leads to chronic swelling of these membranes with catarrhal mucus production and mucus plugs. These cause obstruction of Eustachian tube function and difficulty in equalising the middle ears on descent plus reverse squeeze on ascent; obstruction of sinus outlets leading to sinus squeeze and reverse squeeze; obstruction of bronchioles predisposing to chronic cough, air-trapping and pulmonary barotrauma of ascent.
2. Decreased permeability of alveolar walls reduces gas diffusion with inefficient oxygen uptake and carbon dioxide and nitrogen degassing.
3. Decreased elasticity and compliance of the lungs to chest wall movement occurs. Lung function tests show increased airways resistance to breathing. With time, breakdown of alveoli occurs, resulting in progressive and irreversible lung damage and emphysema.
4. Reduced resistance to infection of the nose, sinuses, throat, bronchi and lungs predisposes to rhinitis, sinusitis, pharyngitis, bronchitis and pneumonia.
5. Chronic irritation disposes to malignant change and cancer of the respiratory tree anywhere from mouth and nose to lungs.

General effects

1. Smoking increases blood viscosity and stimulates spasm of arterioles. Both cause increased resistance to blood flow and high blood pressure. This then predisposes to cerebral haemorrhage or thrombosis of cerebral arteries and stroke.

2. Stimulation of heart rate occurs with irregular beats and rhythms. Simultaneous spasm of the coronary arteries may lead to a heart attack.

3. Absorption of cancer-producing chemicals occurs with an increased incidence of cancer of the stomach, bowel, bladder, prostate, thyroid and liver.

4. Damage to the cardiovascular and respiratory systems causes irreversible loss of general health, physical fitness and endurance.

Neurological Requirements of Scuba Diving

The ultimate reason for venturing under water is sensory input to the brain. A scuba diver trains, spends money and risks life and limb to satisfy the demands of the large grey-white organ in his or her skull. Whether a study of marine life, salvaging a wreck, fondling a moray eel, underwater photography, or sheer wonder of Nature is the objective, it is the brain that motivates and appreciates all.

The Brain

The brain serves and dominates everything in the body. It has millions of nerve fibres extending to every single organ and tissue. It receives masses of incoming sensory information regarding the external environment and the internal operation of every body organ system, then simultaneously and continuously transmits millions of motor impulses to coordinate and react to all this information. But, important as they are, sensory and motor activity are just the homework the brain does to enable it to bring to bear its highest faculties, such as understanding, appreciation, ambition, creativity, humour, hope and passion.

In the diving situation a healthy brain and nervous system form the third great medical requirement. Healthy cardiovascular and respiratory systems are the other two prime demands that together handle the gas needs that make it possible for the brain to appreciate the underwater environment. A heavy nitrogen overload in or out of solution, failure of oxygen supply, or carbon dioxide build-up, rapidly and fatally affect the extremely vulnerable brain.

The highest brain faculties such as self-awareness, thought, speech, reading and writing are centred in the grey matter of the two large convoluted hemispheres of the cerebral cortex. There too are based primary control of voluntary movement and ultimate awareness of sensation — sight, sound, taste, smell, fine and coarse touch, pressure, hot and cold appreciation, body position, vibration sense, and pain sensitivity. The cerebral cortex correlates all these higher faculties and sensory inputs and then directs appropriate movements in response. Below the base of the back of the brain lies a large motor subcentre, the cerebellum, which automatically coordinates and fine-tunes all required movement and proper balance of the body.

The control centres of unconscious vital bodily functions, such as breathing, heart rate, blood pressure and temperature regulation, are found in the brain stem, the most primitive part of the brain, situated between the cerebral cortex and the spinal cord.

The Spinal Cord

At the joint between the skull and the first cervical vertebra of the neck, the brain stem emerges as the spinal cord and descends into the spinal canal of the vertebral column. Between each vertebra spinal nerves emerge and, level by level, systematically supply the entire body with sensory fibres to detect every modality of sensation, and motor fibres to control every voluntary and involuntary movement.

Peripheral Nerves

The peripheral nerves are composed of both sensory and motor fibres carrying information to and from the brain via the spinal cord. This information is transmitted very rapidly because nerve conduction is electrical. In addition to the sensory and motor fibres controlling voluntary movement, involuntary nerves belonging to the *autonomic nervous system* also exist. These relay information controlling unconscious vital functions, such as digestion, circulatory control, breathing, and gall bladder filling with bile.

Neurological Assessment in Scuba Divers

Confirmation of the normal working of the nervous system is essential before diving. The three major aspects required for normal brain function must be assessed.

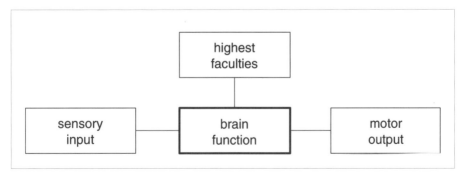

Any condition that predisposes to failure or impairment of any of the highest faculties of the brain, such as self-awareness and orientation to place and time, must be immediately disqualifying. Should a history of previous unconsciousness, due to injury for example, be present, even with no residual defects at all, special investigations such as an electroence-phalogram (EEG) are essential to exclude latent problems that may present under diving conditions. Hyperventilation and breathing hyperbaric oxygen can precipitate a seizure. The EEG must therefore include a tracing of the electrical activity of the brain during hyperventilation.

Conditions affecting the spinal cord and peripheral nerves may or may not preclude diving depending on their type, severity, and the ability and willingness of the diver and his buddy or buddies to adapt safely. On a one-on-one buddy system the diver must have normal vision (excluding minor short-sightedness, far-sightedness and colour-blindness), hearing, sensation, muscle power, gait, balance and coordination. Balance is often tested by asking the subject to stand with the feet together and eyes closed. Excessive swaying (positive Rhomberg test) indicates a cerebellar problem. Tendon reflexes (e.g. the knee jerk) should be normal. Scratching the sole of the foot with a blunt object should result in the toes curling downwards. Should the big toe extend upwards and the other toes fan out (Babinski response) serious neurological impairment may be inferred and diving must be prohibited.

Diving Implications of Neurological Disease

Normal higher faculties are the prime neurological essentials for safe diving. Compromise may be possible in sport divers with sensory defects such as blindness in one eye or deafness, or even defects of the motor system such as poliomyelitis or paraplegia, but conditions causing even momentary aberrations of diver awareness and insight must disqualify any diving. These include both physical and psychological impairments.

Physical Conditions Impairing Higher Faculties

Epilepsy

Epilepsy is a condition characterised by sudden and unheralded loss of consciousness. There are several types, the most dramatic being *grand mal* epilepsy where unconsciousness is associated with breathholding, prolonged convulsive spasms of body muscles, and a period of confusion and memory loss after the attack. *Petit mal* epilepsy, while also striking without warning, causes only a momentary lapse of consciousness with none of the profound motor disturbances of major seizures. The conversation or activity continues after a few seconds as if nothing had happened. Modern medication usually provides excellent control of epilepsy, enabling people with the condition to live absolutely normal lives.

The cause is unknown in most sufferers, but epilepsy can be the presenting feature of a cyst or tumour inside the brain; or follow a head injury with bleeding under the skull or scar tissue formation in injured brain tissue. Whatever the cause and no matter how effective treatment may be in controlling episodes, persons with epilepsy must not dive. The risk of even momentary unconsciousness under water is unacceptable.

Fever convulsions during infancy are not included in the ban provided they do not recur after the age of three. In some cases epilepsy occurring during childhood and stopping after puberty may not totally bar diving, provided no anti-seizure medication whatsoever has been taken for at least five years, and an EEG with hyperventilation and flickering light stimulation is completely normal.

Fainting attack (syncope)

The term *fainting attack* or *syncope* covers a number of conditions that can cause partial or complete loss of consciousness. It is very important not to be lulled into a false sense of security by assuming that the episodes are due to 'heat' or 'low blood sugar' or 'low blood pressure' and are therefore insignificant from a diving point of view. All cases of syncope must be investigated before any further diving can be considered.

Having excluded illnesses such as epilepsy, cerebral tumour, diabetes, heart problems and stroke, the possibilities of heat aesthenia, low blood pressure, low blood sugar, and anxiety can be assessed. Provided they can be reasonably explained, the latter possibilities do not generally exclude further diving unless they can cause syncope under water.

Heat aesthenia. This occurs in stuffy, crowded and poorly ventilated places. Although body temperature usually remains normal, people sensitive to these environmental conditions may faint. Unlike epilepsy, heat aesthenia does not occur without warning. The victim feels faint and dizzy, and is often sweaty and very pale. He or she feels ill before losing consciousness. Lying down or sitting with the head between the knees in a well-ventilated or cool place usually relieves the episode before syncope occurs. It passes rapidly in any event and no confusional state occurs afterwards.

Low blood pressure (hypotension). Many young people, especially young women, have blood pressures ranging around the 100/60 mark. After standing for some time, especially in hot conditions, or during their menses or pregnancies, gravity-pooling of blood in the veins of the lower body may occur. This reduces blood pressure even further and the supply of blood to the head may become inadequate. It can also follow sudden standing after sitting or lying down, and is especially common when getting up from a hot bath. Features similar to those of heat aesthenia appear, ranging from dizziness to temporary unconsciousness, but pass quickly after lying down for a while.

Syncope due to heat aesthenia or low blood pressure is extremely unlikely under sport scuba diving conditions. The water is invariably much cooler than body temperature and gravity-pooling of blood cannot occur under the gravity-free conditions of total submersion with neutral buoyancy.

Low blood sugar (hypoglycaemia). A drop in blood glucose is potentially hazardous under water. In the absence of other disorders affecting glucose levels, such as diabetes mellitus, hypoglycaemia is usually the result of an excessively restricted diet, anorexia or bulimia. It is much more common in females than males, probably because women are much more figure-conscious than men, especially when they are going to expose their bodies on a beach or a boat on a diving holiday.

People on crash or very restricted diets must ensure a reasonable carbohydrate intake a few hours before diving. This enables both liver and muscle tissue to recharge their reserves of glycogen, the storage form of glucose in the body. Under exercise conditions this glycogen is broken down into glucose and provides the extra energy source needed for increased metabolic demands while ensuring that blood glucose is adequate for brain needs. The normal blood glucose a few hours after eating is about 4-6 mmols/litre. Should the blood glucose level drop much below 3 mmols/litre, the picture closely resembles heat aesthenia and low blood pressure, with faintness, dizziness, pallor and profound sweating. The danger is that hypoglycaemic syncope may persist until sugar is administered. Under water this is patently impossible and pallor and sweating will not be noticed. Sudden unconsciousness may be the first sign.

Anorexics and bulimics must not dive. They are pathologically reticent about telling the truth about their eating habits and are unable to control their obsession about being fat, even when clearly emaciated. Their carbohydrate energy reserves are very limited, their strength greatly reduced, and their liability to develop a severe drop in blood sugar with exercise under water greatly increased. In bulimics this is compounded by induced vomiting, with fluid loss, relative dehydration and an increased likelihood of bends.

Anxiety and low blood calcium (hypocalcaemia). Although in itself not a physical impairment, acute anxiety can result in grossly impaired changes in body chemistry. Aside from the increased tendency of very anxious people to panic given a stress challenge under water, hyperventilation is an additional risk. But this is very different to the controlled deep hyperventilation of breathhold divers intent on reducing their arterial carbon dioxide levels. Anxiety-induced hyperventilation is rapid, shallow and ongoing and can achieve profound hypocapnia with a sharp rise in the alkalinity of blood, a steep fall in ionised calcium, intense spasm of the hands and feet, and syncope. On land, syncope is curative for intensely agitated hyperventilators, as they stop their rapid breathing while unconscious and spontaneously recover when blood chemistry restores itself. Under water, uncontrolled anxiety is very dangerous.

Cerebrovascular accident (stroke)

Sudden unconsciousness can occur with interruption of the normal circulation to the brain. This may be due to *thrombosis* with a clot obstructing a cerebral artery, *haemorrhage* due to rupture of a blood vessel or an aneurysm in the brain, or *embolism* of a blood clot to the brain. Recovery or residual paralysis, weakness, numbness, loss of speech, etc., will depend on the exact site and extent of the damage, but any history of cerebral vascular disease (even if unconsciousness is very transient with full recovery) must permanently disqualify diving.

Acute cerebral decompression illness

A history of previous cerebral injury due to arterial gas embolism (AGE) or brain tissue nitrogen bubbling must be very carefully assessed. Any residual deficit must exclude further diving. This can be very difficult to detect as it may involve only subtle changes in dexterity, mental acuity or personality. British Naval policy requires confirmation by an approved doctor with a minimum of seven days off diving. The US Navy stipulates a four-week lay-off from diving. Many diving physicians will not permit any further diving even with apparent full recovery. The situation therefore depends on the details of the diver's hyperbaric incident, the extent of recovery and the opinion of his medical adviser.

Head injury

Head injury at any time in the past resulting in even brief unconsciousness and no residual brain damage requires a full neurological assessment, including an EEG with a hyperventilation tracing. Any abnormality excludes diving.

Migraine

Migraine can be very problematic in sport diving and is a source of headache to the diving physician as well as the subject. Among commercial and navy divers migraine is usually grounds for disqualification from further diving. The difficulty relates to the time of onset and treatment. If a diver experiences a migraine before entering the water, the dive obviously must be aborted. Once under water the diver is subjected to cold, vascular changes and exercise demands. In addition, stress, nitrogen narcosis, and skip breathing with carbon dioxide build-up may occur. Any one of these may precipitate or aggravate a migraine leading to nausea, vomiting and vertigo under water in addition to the difficulty of coping with a violent headache. To complicate things, most cases of migraine have an *aura* before the headache starts. This may present as blurred vision, tunnel vision, flashing lights, ringing in the ears, etc. If these occur after a dive the question of distinguishing them from acute cerebral decompression illness including AGE is very problematic. When the diver then develops a blinding headache and begins to vomit, the dilemma worsens.

Painfully dilated blood vessels inside the confines of the skull bones, the underlying membranes, and the overlying scalp, are thought to be the cause of migraine. Treatment of migraine is directed at narrowing these dilated blood vessels, but giving medication aimed at constricting blood vessels can have unpredictable effects on blood pressure, heart rate and heart rhythm when coupled to the vascular changes of diving.

An estimation of the safety of scuba diving in known migraine sufferers must depend on the frequency, intensity and duration of past episodes. If severe, or while preventative treatments such as beta-blockers, clonidine, flunarizine or pizotifen are being used, diving must be forbidden. Trying to abort an acute attack with ergotamine or sumatriptan before diving is exceedingly perilous. It is only when migraine episodes are infrequent, and the usual precipitating causes, such as caffeine, cheese amines, wine, etc., have been identified by experience and eliminated to the best of the diver's ability, that diving should be considered in migraine.

Other brain conditions

Some illnesses primarily affect the brain tissue itself, causing compression of the brain inside the skull, interference with normal nerve pathways, or destruction of the fatty insulating myelin of nerve fibres. Impairment of the highest functions may be accompanied by changes in sensory and motor function. These illnesses include cysts and tumours, multiple sclerosis, brain syphilis and narcolepsy. Diving is forbidden. Scuba diving after acute inflammatory conditions of the brain such as encephalitis and meningitis depends on the completeness of recovery and the proven absence of any residual defects.

Psychological Conditions Impairing Higher Faculties

Panic

Don't just stand there – PANIC!

(Sign at the controls of Pentow Marine's vessel, the *Reunion*.)

Panic is sudden, unreasoning and overpowering fear, which overrides all reason and training and does not permit any logical or reasonable action. It is probably the greatest killer among young and inexperienced divers who are confronted by severe stress, namely a threat to life, whether real or imaginary. The onset of panic is a self-propagating, rapidly accelerating process, which takes the diver from anxiety regarding his situation, to uncontrolled, stark terror in which rational reaction to the predicament becomes impossible.

There are three dimensions to panic:
- the diver,
- the diving equipment, and
- the environment.

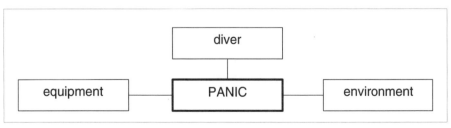

It is the interaction between these three that determines whether a diver has a pleasant and productive dive or dies.

The diver. The basic object of diving is the transport of the diver's awareness and individuality into the water. From there, he or she will enjoy a coral reef, a cave, work on a rig, or salvage a wreck. Personality and apprehensiveness will determine the response to any problem. Different divers react differently to the same problem. An example will illustrate the point.

A lone diver has just visited the cave at the bottom of Wondergat, a deep inland sinkhole. The dive was a night dive to 40 metres using a swim line tied to the bottom of a floating shot line. Forgetting to untie his swim line, he ascends up the shot line, not knowing that the swim line, loosely looped in the water, has entangled itself with his scuba cylinder. At 30 metres, he is abruptly brought to a halt as the rope tightens. It is pitch black around him and he does not know why he cannot ascend.

Responses:

- Martin Brown, under these conditions, stopped, thought and checked. Using his light, he confirmed that he was on the shot line and that there were no overhangs above him. He then checked his air supply and depth gauge. Looking around and then down by methodically beaming his light, he saw two strands of rope extending down from his back pack.

    Withdrawing his knife, he cut the strands and ascended safely, mentally kicking himself for forgetting to untie and coil his swim line and for diving without a buddy.

- Cuthbert Quiver, a novice diver who suffered from severe anxiety for which he took tranquillisers, stopped with his eyes bulging into his mask. He had not really wanted to dive but, egged on by his 'friends' over a few beers, he had capitulated. With the sudden halt, he was convinced that some monster was trying to trap him in the dark and, finning furiously, hyperventilating and waving his arms, he let go of his torch which floated to the surface. He than inflated his buoyancy compensator, which pulled him even tighter against the ropes. Screaming through his demand valve and thrashing violently with his limbs, he used up his air supply and drowned, tightly suspended 30 metres from the surface by his life jacket.

The first dimension, diver awareness and personality, is affected by:
Physical factors:
- training and planning,
- fitness and fatigue,
- experience,
- diving problems, e.g. seasickness, vomiting, barotrauma, vertigo, water inhalation,
- alcohol and drug abuse,
- underlying medical problems, e.g. epilepsy, asthma, diabetes.

Psychological factors:
— anxiety and emotional instability,
— phobias,
   visual limitation, e.g. night diving,
— disorientation due to weightlessness or diffused light.

The diving equipment. Diving advertisements and TV films have given female divers an ultra-glamorous and sensuous image and male divers mega-macho and super-stud appeal. What they really are, are poor souls wrapped in tight rubber; their vision limited by masks, with snorkels over their ears; mouths clamped over second-stage demand valves; backs suffering under the weight of heavy cylinders; their breathing made difficult by straps, buoyancy vests, wet suits and weight belts; pipes and gauges tangling around them; and liable to break their necks by stumbling over their fins. In addition, they have knives on their legs, torches and/or cameras in their hands, plus assorted ropes, tools and other paraphernalia.

  On entering the water, they have much greater mobility and less weight restriction, but all the above equipment can conspire to place them in peril. This is the second dimension to panic. A displaced mask, leaky demand valve, empty cylinder, restricting wet suit, very heavy weight belt or lost fin will all cause diver reaction, ranging from a rapid assessment and handling of the problem, to real distress and anxiety, to panic.

  Borrowed or unfamiliar equipment is also a source of danger. The reserve valve may be in an unaccustomed place, the weight belt may be too heavy or have a different clip, making it difficult to ditch, the mask may not fit properly and leak. New or borrowed fins may fall off or cause cramps. Experience, training and practice in the use of equipment are the only solutions to safe handling of equipment difficulties under water.

The environment. At this stage, we have a diver, either calm, tense or terrified, fully or inadequately geared up, with great or minimal expertise, about to jump into the sea, a sinkhole, a cave, a lake, an ice-hole, or into the surf. This is the third dimension to panic.

  The sea is vast and bountiful and beautiful. Man is the intruder, and it is he who calls the sea dangerous. Fish don't complain that the sea is dangerous. The sea has tides, currents, swells, surf, rocks, cold temperatures, poisonous and hungry inhabitants, clear and turbid areas, kelp, caves, boats with propellers, and wrecks (which have sharp edges, crannies and traps, unstable plating and sometimes explosives). If our air-breathing, rubber-wrapped diver knows these things and dives within their limits, the sea is rarely dangerous, it is only merciless to fools. It is invariably the first two dimensions (the diver and the equipment) that cause the problem. The water simply finishes the job. In fact, it is rarely the equipment that fails, but the diver's poor maintenance and lack of knowledge and training with his life-support system.

Alcohol

The use of alcohol instantly negates any safe dive plan and one does not have to be very drunk to be at risk. Being a socially acceptable custom and commonly enjoyed by divers at their clubs and on diving holidays, alcohol intake may range from occasional to regular to habitual; but the vast majority of regular alcohol users will deny excess. The question, 'When last did you take a drink?' if asked on a Tuesday morning at tea-time will often indicate the real situation.

'Yesterday,' usually points to a habitual daily intake. 'On Sunday,' suggests a weekend drinker; 'I'm not sure,' an occasional imbiber; and 'Today,' means a serious alcohol problem.

About 80 per cent of adults who drown took alcohol before entering the water. Alcohol, drugs and swimming *never* mix. Look at the reasons. Alcohol causes:
- overconfidence – risks are taken beyond training, fitness and ability;
- inability to react adequately to the situation resulting in panic;
- hypothermia due to skin flushing and rapid heat loss;
- increased likelihood of vomiting with inhalation of vomit and water;
- possible suicidal tendencies.

A realistic minimum time of abstinence from any alcohol before diving is 8 hours. If the alcohol intake was enough to cause slight tipsiness, 12 hours must be allowed. With reactions such as vomiting or a hangover, 24 hours should elapse before attempting to dive, and copious quantities of water and fruit juice should be taken during that period. Uncontrolled over-indulgence requires medical help and permission to dive must be refused until the problem has been overcome.

Psychological instability

Assessment of the psychiatric status of a diver is a vital, but the most intangible, aspect of a diving medical, and the most risky side of diving instruction. Emotional stability and mature judgement are fundamental to safe diving. A dive school can teach a student all he or she needs to understand to dive safely, but when the time comes for open water experience the undersea environment may expose sudden intense claustrophobia or anxiety and precipitate panic. Student divers may intimate early during their pool training that they are unhappy under water and their instructors should then pay particular attention to giving these students one-on-one guidance, even after hours if necessary, to promote confidence and improve underwater skills. Other students, too shy to mention their problem when the rest of the class is progressing with obvious enthusiasm, may not be forthcoming and the instructor must be on the lookout for them. They often take a long time to tog up, are always last in the queue to demonstrate the particular skill being taught, and have great difficulty in achieving neutral buoyancy because they involuntarily keep their lungs half-full at the surface – this increases buoyancy and, instead of exhaling precious air, they require excessively heavy weight belts in order to descend. They empty their air cylinders uncommonly quickly, and tend to perform frequent hasty free ascents from the deep end of the pool. They will appreciate kind and understanding attention from a discerning instructor and in most cases will become adequate scuba divers.

Neuroses and psychoses. The inherent perils of diving may aggravate manic states, or stimulate suicidal ideation in depressive divers with underlying marital, social or financial stress, or cause sudden psychotic or neurotic behaviour. As it is the diving buddy who may suddenly be faced with the problem of dangerously abnormal behaviour in his or her diving partner, diving buddies should be socially compatible and know each other well.

But social compatibility can cause problems too. Many divers, commonly women in the 30 to 45 age group, take up diving solely to satisfy the demands of their partners. They are secretly very unhappy about diving but decide to give it a try in order to appease mate insistence. There is really a double problem − the male need to prove mid-life virility with youthful enterprise, and the heavy apprehension of his spouse who is unwillingly training as his diving buddy. In most cases the disconsolate lady finds to her unbelieving delight that scuba diving is stupendous, and becomes an avid protagonist of the sport. In a minority, real insecurity and even secret terror persist, but so strong is her devotion to appease that she will continue to dive. Dive leaders and instructors should be aware of this in new students, and watch out for undue apprehension in qualified diver couples joining a dive trip. If excessive misgivings seem to be present, insist on an up-to-date diving medical with a diving physician. The uncontrollably anxious spouse will usually accept a failed medical with unconcealed relief.

Another socially based cause of potential diver difficulty is loneliness. A significant number of men and women decide to take up diving solely to increase the likelihood of meeting a soulmate. Diving is not the objective − parading in a wet suit and chatting to new acquaintances is the goal. They dive infrequently and have dubious skill once some time has passed.

Psychoactive medication. Millions of tranquillisers, antidepressants and sleeping pills are used every day around the world. Stress, even if minor, is often greeted with an obliging offer of a 'safe little something for your nerves'. Not a single one of any of these medications, no matter what anyone personally experienced in their use may say, is ever acceptable in safe diving. Diving requires emotional stability. These medications are taken precisely because such stability is impaired. They do not cure anything − they merely dull reaction to the underlying problem. Dulled reaction in an emotionally unstable diver is very dangerous under water.

The effects of psychoactive drugs under hyperbaric conditions are also unpredictable. Excessive drowsiness or sluggishness or susceptibility to nitrogen narcosis may suddenly occur. This also applies to illicit drugs including hallucinogens, opiates and marijuana. Diving and drugs don't mix.

Conditions Impairing Motor and Sensory Nerve Function

Whereas the loss or potential loss of any modality of the higher faculties is unacceptable for diving purposes, disability due to loss of motor or sensory function need not necessarily be totally disqualifying, except for conditions such as motor neurone disease and multiple sclerosis.

Motor neurone disease

This disorder of unknown cause results in patchy damage to motor nerve units in the brain and spinal cord which control muscle movement. Nerves supplying sensory information remain intact. Progressive weakness and then paralysis occur with loss of coordination and reflex activity. There is no known treatment and diving must be banned.

Multiple sclerosis

Multiple sclerosis affects the insulating fatty myelin layer of the white matter of the brain and spinal cord. The cause is unknown and it presents with initial transient weakness of one or more limbs, sudden loss of vision in one eye, numbness and tingling in a limb, or slowly progressive clumsiness. It is usually relapsing, with long periods of improvement in remission followed by acute episodes of worsening, alternating over 15 to 30 years. Eventually, terminal paralysis with uncontrollable spasms and incontinence occur. Because of the progressive and untreatable nature of the disease, and the unpredictable efficiency of degassing from already damaged areas of brain tissue, diving is not permitted even during the early stages or with remissions.

Poliomyelitis

Much less common nowadays because of national compulsory immunisation during infancy, poliomyelitis is a viral disease which attacks motor nerve cells in the spinal cord. This results in damage to the motor nerve supply of the limb muscles with resultant wasting and weakness. With certain provisos, diving may be taught to poliomyelitis victims. (See diving with a physical handicap pp 59-61.)

Paraplegia

Injury to the spinal cord occurs most commonly after motor vehicle accidents, or trauma from a fall while climbing, parachuting, or parasailing. There is usually fracturing of the bony spine resulting in crushing or cutting of the spinal cord. If complete, permanent paralysis and total anaesthesia of the body below the level of the spinal cord injury will result. Damage to the cord above the fourth cervical vertebra in the neck is invariably fatal as all the respiratory muscles, including the diaphragm, are then paralysed, making it impossible for the victim to breathe. Section of the spinal cord lower in the neck will cause *quadriplegia* with paralysis and anaesthesia of both arms and both legs and loss of control of bodily functions. Damage to the lumbar spinal cord causes paraplegia with paralysis and anaesthesia of the legs and loss of bowel and bladder control.

The problems related to the rehabilitation of paraplegics have received massive and world-wide attention because the majority of paraplegics are young people with normal and active brains and, aside from their lower body disability, a normal role to play in their society. If the level of transection of the spinal cord is low lumbar, diving after recovery from the acute trauma is often possible and can play an important role in rehabilitation.

Diving with a Physical Handicap

For many years hydrotherapy has been used in the treatment and rehabilitation of physically disabled people. The technique utilises the buoyant effect of water to negate gravity and facilitates retraining and exercising of weakened muscles and joints. Extending the concept raised the question, 'Is it safe for physically disabled people to dive?'

There are three primary major hazards in sport diving. The first two are post-dive tissue bubble formation following an inert gas load at depth, and arterial gas embolism following pulmonary barotrauma. Their prevention, in health terms, requires cardiovascular and pulmonary fitness. Drowning is the third hazard and its prevention requires clarity of higher faculties – consciousness and full awareness in the subaquatic environment. Any medical condition that predisposes to any of these three hazards must mean a failed diving medical.

But what about people who have had injuries to their limbs or spinal cord – such as amputees, poliomyelitis victims and paraplegics? Aside from their physical or functional loss of limbs, they may technically satisfy all three primary medical requirements for safe diving. All sport divers use fins, which after all are man-made contrivances, to assist swimming. Given the possibility that a suitable artifice could similarly be provided to assist a paraplegic with total paralysis of both legs, should he or she dive?

The answer is – it depends. The first absolute requirement is the absence of any significant medical problem in addition to the physical handicap. Circulatory disturbance in a paralysed limb will affect tissue degassing after a dive and predispose to bends. Bedsores or areas devitalised by the pressure of sitting or lying will do the same. Efficient breathing of dense air under hyperbaric conditions requires fully functional muscles of respiration. This sets the limit to the level of spinal cord injury in paraplegic divers. Aside from the diaphragm, which receives its nerve supply from the third and fourth cervical portions of the spinal cord in the neck, there are numerous secondary muscles of respiration in the chest and abdomen essential for effective breathing and coughing. These receive their nerve supply from the dorsal spinal cord (the portion of the cord between the neck and the first lumbar vertebra) and the upper portion of the lumbar spinal cord. Any paraplegic considering diving must therefore not have damage to the spinal cord higher than the second lumbar segment.

In the case of amputees, the reason for their amputation is important. Limb loss following an accident or injury is not as significant as amputation because of arterial disease or the complications of diabetes. Persons with the latter must never dive. Whereas suitable prosthetic devices can be constructed to compensate for the accidental loss of both legs, the loss of both arms is almost insurmountable. Should a demand valve become dislodged it would be impossible to replace it without assistance. Buoyancy compensation requiring manual control of venting and inflation requires buddy support. Yet people affected by the thalidomide tragedy, when pregnant mothers using the drug for morning sickness gave birth to babies with grossly underdeveloped or absent limbs, have dived and loved every minute of it. Under these circumstances two buddies, both dive masters or instructors, are required.

Approval to dive must be tightly qualified in the case of handicapped people. There are very few formal diving courses for the handicapped so the conditions under which they may dive must be individually discussed between the diving physician and the instructor at the particular diving school approached.

The first essential is the ability of the handicapped person to swim and maintain the head above water without any artificial aid whatsoever.

Details of the particular techniques to be used must be carefully considered. In the event of the functional loss of the lower limbs, as in paraplegia, or amputation of both legs, or loss of an arm and a leg, a trio buddy system must be used, allowing two divers to assist the handicapped person into and from the water, and to ensure that either non-handicapped buddy can also be assisted in an emergency.

Possible problems and modifications relating to every piece of diving gear must be foreseen and a little ingenuity applied to compensate for the physical defect. Regular harness straps may slip off weak or wasted shoulder muscles. Weight belts may slide off wasted hips. High or low limb amputations, the quality of limb stumps, and cost will determine the safety and advisability of using artificial limbs under water. The loss of one leg may be compensated for by using a fin with a large surface area on the normal leg, but practice exercise is then essential to avoid leg cramps because of the heavier resistance load. A dolphin kick may be needed to avoid swimming in a circle. Finned or webbed gloves may be considered for paraplegic divers. Buoyancy control must provide not only neutral buoyancy, but vertical and horizontal control. Wasted, artificial or amputated legs significantly alter the centre of balance of the body and predispose to swimming in a head-down position or, worse, ascending in that position. Weight must be distributed between weight belts and ankle or fin weights until neutral buoyancy and free axial mobility are achieved.

The question of depth limitation and embarking on decompression-stop dives must be fully discussed between the doctor, the handicapped diver and the instructor. The degree of disability will dictate limits. Wet suits must always be worn to avoid skin damage to trailing, anaesthetic and paralysed legs by contact with coral life. Swimming side-by-side with the handicapped diver between two alert buddies will help to avert such injury.

Diving after Brain Surgery

Most diving physicians would bar any diving after surgery involving the brain. The problem is that any surgery to the brain must in itself cause damage to nerve fibre tracts simply to reach the objective of the operation. There is a later risk of precipitating a convulsion under water with the higher partial pressure of inspired air oxygen, and any interference with the capillary circulation or venous drainage of the area could predispose to acute cerebral decompression illness.

Ear, Nose and Sinus Requirements of Scuba Diving

After healthy cardiovascular, pulmonary and nervous systems, the next priority for diving is the ability of a diver actively to increase the pressure in the middle ear and passively to compensate for pressure changes in the sinuses with depth.

The Ear

Extending from the cartilaginous external ear to the inner ear deeply buried in the bone of the skull, the ear serves two functions – hearing and orientation. Together they serve to provide awareness of sound and control of body position.

Anatomy

The ear has three compartments:
- external ear,
- middle ear, and
- inner ear.

The compartments are all very different, but they do have common features:
1. They are separated by thin but tough membranes.
2. Each compartment has a passage or tube leading to it.
3. All three compartments are in the bone of the skull and are therefore incompressible (i.e. they cannot change volume without violent objections from the diver).
4. The external and middle ears are normally air filled. The inner ear is always *fluid* filled, and its passage communicates with the cerebrospinal fluid around the brain.
5. Passage obstruction causes squeeze.

The hearing organ is the *cochlea* (Latin for snail-shell) and the balance organ is the *vestibular apparatus*. They are attached to each other at the *vestibule* (Latin for an entrance-court with rooms leading off it), and together they comprise the inner ear or *labyrinth*, so-called because of its complex shape. The vestibular apparatus and cochlea are fluid-filled, the

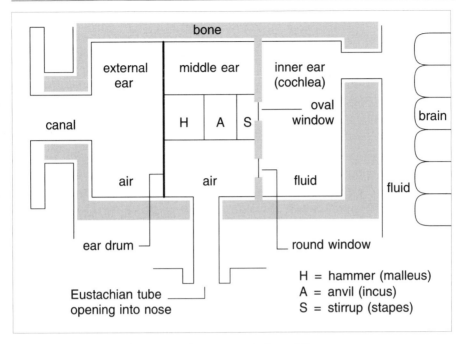

Diagrammatic representation of the ear

fluid in the cochlea communicating with the cerebrospinal fluid in and around the brain. The cochlea is a spiralled organ containing membranes and hair cells tuned to vibrate in sympathy with incoming tones. Different-pitched tones cause different hair cells to vibrate. Their vibration is then converted into electrochemical energy and transmitted to the brain as a nerve impulse in the auditory nerve. Being fluid-filled, the cochlea is normally *immune* to Boyle's Law and pressure changes.

Sound reaching the ear from outside passes into the external ear canal, an open pit in the side wall of the skull. This canal is closed off by a taut membrane at its inner end — the *tympanum* or ear drum. The function of the ear drum is to vibrate in air. Behind the ear drum is the middle ear, a small air-filled cavity whose canal, the Eustachian tube, opens to air on the back wall of the nasal cavity. The middle ear serves to transmit sound from the ear drum to the cochlea. As the cochlea is fluid-filled and the ear drum vibrates in air, a mechanical connecting system exists. It consists of three tiny bones or *ossicles* which form a miniature articulated hydraulic press. The *malleus* or hammer is attached by its handle to the inside of the ear drum. The head of the hammer has a tiny joint with the anvil-shaped *incus*, which in turn is joined to the *stapes* or stirrup. The stirrup is the smallest bone of the three and weighs just over one milligram. But it is the most important of the three bones because its oval-shaped footplate seals the *oval window*, a hole in the fluid-filled inner ear.

The system is ingenious and works as follows: The tiny vibrations of the ear drum are transmitted to the hammer handle. The head of the hammer thrusts the anvil against the stirrup which rams like a piston against the fluid behind the oval window, setting up pressure waves in the fluid of the inner ear. These pressure waves are then detected by the hair cells of the cochlea. The lever system of the ossicles plus the mechanical advantage of a relatively large-diameter ear drum driving against a tiny footplate magnifies the movement of the eardrum 22 times at the footplate. As fluid is incompressible and the cochlea is embedded in the hardest bone of the body the system could not work unless there was a weak spot that could give and move a little with the thrusting of the footplate against liquid. There is − the *round window*, a membrane between the cochlea and the middle ear. It bulges as the stirrup shoves. From a diving point of view the round window is very important. It can rupture with an excessively violent attempt to equalise on descent, resulting in cochlear fluid and then brain fluid leaking into the middle ear and, via the Eustachian tube, out through the nose. This effect is covered under ear barotrauma.

Hearing in air

Nothing designed by man can even nearly compare with the astounding sensitivity and selectivity of the ear. The maximum sensitivity is just short of consciously hearing random movement of air nitrogen and oxygen molecules hitting the ear drum. At the same time the ear can tolerate the volume of electronic guitars loud enough to make the entire body quiver. It can then selectively hear the normal-volume speech of one person in a roomful of people and dismiss the babble of surrounding conversation plus the amplified music of a band in the background. Or it can discriminate and identify the source of a single faulty note from one instrument in an entire orchestra.

Hearing begins with vibration of the ear drum, but vibration is really too coarse a word. What does one call ear drum movement of one millionth of a millimetre − one tenth of the diameter of a hydrogen atom − at high sound frequencies? Even more incredible are the membranes in the inner ear. The movement of these membranes vibrating to convert sound energy into electrochemical nerve impulses is about one ten-billionth of a millimetre!

But the wonder of hearing does not end here. The ear is capable of distinguishing direction of sound. This may initially seem a simple task but its complexity is apparent when one considers that while a sound in a room directly reaches the ear, the sound is also being reflected off the walls, floor, ceiling and furniture towards the ear. The point is that the ear is able to disregard all sounds except the first one that reaches it, and unerringly direct its attention to the source.

The range of normal adult human hearing is about 100 to 12 000 cycles per second (cps). In childhood the upper range may be as high as 40 000 cps. The ear is much less sensitive to very deep bass tones which is just as well otherwise the vibrations of the body would be heard. Moving the head on the spine would sound like a lumber saw, chewing would be a thunderous experience, and the bedlam of exercise would deter any sporting activity.

The ear also hears by bone conduction, but this is a subjective experience. If one chews potato crisps the loud crunching noise is due to sound being transmitted to the ears by the bones of the jaw. Someone nearby will not hear the munching because it is not being transmitted through air (unless the chewer really crunches!). When one speaks, the sound the speaker hears is heard by air conduction and bone conduction. The audience hears by air conduction alone. Many of the low tones produced by the vocal cords are lost during air conduction, and are heard by bone conduction only by the speaker, who firmly believes his or her voice is full and rich and cannot believe the tinny whine when it is heard on a high-tech recording!

Hearing under water

Under diving conditions sound is heard by bone conduction only. The minute vibrations of the ear drum are completely damped by flooding the ear with water. In air, the relatively slow speed of sound permits its direction to be judged, but under water its speed is too fast. Both ears receive the sound virtually simultaneously and the ear's ability to distinguish sound direction is completely lost. It is heard quite clearly, but a look-around is needed to find the source.

The speed of sound in air is about 335 m/sec. In fresh water, it is about 1 400 m/sec; and in sea water, 1 550 m/sec. This means that sound waves travel faster and better the denser the medium, and in water, the speed of sound is about four times that in air. Water is a better transmitter of sound than air, so sound travels further under water. We have all seen those war movies where the submarine crew sits very quietly, with engines off, while the destroyer above listens for her. Low-pitched sounds carry *better* than high-pitched ones under water.

Transmission of sound in water is further enhanced by reflection off the surface and off the bottom, especially if the sea-bed is rocky. Reflection from the surface is very efficient − 99.999 per cent of the sound reaching the surface is reflected back into the water. As a result, transmission of sound from water to air, or from air to water, is very poor. This principle of reflection is also involved in underwater explosions and pressure waves. (See Underwater Explosions.)

Hearing in a decompression chamber

Pressurised air in a chamber or bell causes speech distortion. The voice becomes more and more tinny as the pressure increases. The speed of sound increases with the increased gas density and it is thought that more of the voice is transmitted directly through the wall of the throat and less by transmission through the mouth.

In a helium-oxygen environment, the helium produces a characteristic distortion of speech, called the 'Donald Duck' effect. It is attributed to an increased frequency of resonance in heliox mixtures. At great depths, the voice is so distorted as to be unintelligible, and electronic descramblers must be used to adjust the frequency to an understandable form.

Orientation

At the vestibule of the inner ear the footplate of the stirrup plugs into the oval window. To one side is the cochlea, only concerned with hearing. To the other is the vestibular apparatus which informs the brain about the orientation of the head in space. It continuously provides information about movement – forwards, backwards, up, down or sideways. It maintains equilibrium and, if conditions are confusing, induces disorientation or vertigo.

The vestibular apparatus consists of three *semicircular canals*, half-circular fluid-filled tubes all entering a common cistern, the *utricle* (Latin for a little leather bag), and the *saccule* (Latin for a small sac or cyst).

The semicircular canals detect movements of the head. They are sensitive to *kinetic* changes, that is, sudden changes in the direction of the head – up, down or sideways, and inform the brain and cerebellum via delicate and specific nerve impulses as to the exact position of the head. The semicircular canals are able to do this because they are orientated in all three dimensional planes. One is sensitive to vertical movement, the second to sideways movement, and the third to forwards and backwards movement.

They operate by inertia, similar to crashing through the windscreen of a car when the brakes are suddenly applied. No movement of the head is possible without causing some ripple disturbance in the fluid within the semicircular canals. As with hearing, hair cells are involved. Each canal has a mound of hair cells projecting into a small cup of gelatinous material. Any movement in a particular plane or combination of planes affects these hair cells. Nerve impulses are immediately generated to inform the brain of the current situation.

The utricle and saccule are *static* sensors. They detect continuous forward or sideways movement. So going for a walk without moving the head will trigger the hair cells of the utricle, informing the brain that forward progression is proceeding. Should one then decide to move sideways without moving the head, the hair cells of the saccule will fire. Diving forwards, downwards and turning to one side will trigger all three semicircular canals, the utricle and the saccule.

The information received by the brain from the vestibular apparatus about the position of the head and its orientation and movement in space elicits a response. It affects the incredibly complex process of balance. The brain receives information from the cochlea regarding the sonic state of the environment. It receives information from the vestibular apparatus about the position and movement of the head. The eyes provide information about the visible conditions, and the skin and joints provide information about the current posture of the body. Within milliseconds the brain then correlates and processes all this information, adjusts the tone of every muscle in the body, decides on an appropriate response and coordinates hitting a speeding cricket ball for six or a baseball for a home run.

Under diving conditions, many of these sources of information are absent. The effect of gravity on joints and the 'feel' of up and down disappear. With poor visibility or night diving the eyes provide no useful information. The direction of any sound source is indistinguishable. The diver then relies solely for orientation on the vestibular apparatus in the inner ear.

The Sinuses

The sinuses are a complex maze of air-filled spaces in the bones around the nose. Every sinus has an opening into the nose, allowing movement of air between the nose and the sinus. They are named after the bones in which they exist. Above the nose and the eyes the *frontal* sinuses are found in the frontal bone of the skull. The roof of the nose, directly under the brain, is formed by the ethmoid bone and in it are the *ethmoid* sinuses. Right at the back of the nose, and above the openings of the Eustachian tubes, is the *sphenoid* sinus in the sphenoid bone. To each side of the nose, in the maxillary bones of the cheeks, are the *maxillary* sinuses.

Function of the sinuses

Together with the nose, the four groups of sinuses form a complicated array of air spaces in the upper face and floor of the brain. Their exact function is obscure. Their openings into the wall of the nose are too small to assist effectively with nasal humidification of inhaled air. It has been suggested that they serve to lessen the weight of the skull, but as the total weight loss would be much less than the weight of a small fez, this author is sceptical of this explanation. Imparting resonance to the voice has been mooted, but this resonance would be a subjective one, the sound being heard only by the speaker by bone conduction and quite inaudible to the listener who hears by air conduction only.

An interesting theory is that the sinuses are developmental accidents and have no function at all. During growth of the face, for example, most of the growth is downwards and sideways as the cheek bones develop to provide support for the teeth. The lining of the nose then simply follows the growth of the enlarging cheek bone cavity formed. As the face develops, the outer layer of the bones of the forehead grow more rapidly to conform to the facial bones and draw up nasal lining to form the frontal sinuses. This explanation would mean that the sinuses are important only as sites of possible disease, such as allergy, sinusitis and, for a diver, sinus squeeze.

Diving Implications of Ear, Nose, Throat and Sinus Disease

Difficulty in equalising pressure in the air spaces of the skull is by far the commonest complaint of divers. These air spaces comprise the sinuses, the external and middle ears, and the cavities in decaying teeth. They are peculiar in that they are all rigidly confined in bone (or tooth) and each has a canal that opens to the atmosphere. Being rigid spaces they cannot respond to pressure changes by varying their volume so they are all vulnerable to Boyle's Law. Any obstruction to their canals while diving will challenge this vulnerability. Being connected to the atmosphere exposes them to bacteria, dusts and pollens, and the combination of infection, allergy and canal obstruction is the cause of the overwhelming majority of diver difficulties.

Disorders of the External Ear

Swimmer's ear (otitis externa)

The external ear, be it small, large, shell-like or bat is the Achilles' heel of *Homo scubiens*. The external ear canal is a three-centimetre-long tube which conducts sound waves in the air to the ear drum. It is an unfortunate fact of sport diving that of all the numerous orifices possessed by divers, the external ear canal is the only one that cannot be protected or discreetly covered. It *must* be totally exposed to the sea. Boyle's Law, unforgiving and ever threatening the delicate middle ear with squeeze, demands that the external ear canal be flooded when a sport diver dives. This means exposure to the polluted, bacteria-rich water of the sea or an unclean dam or lake.

Causes of swimmer's ear. Only two barriers protect the external ear from bacterial attack by the diving environment – wax and the membrane lining of the external ear canal. But many divers do their best to destroy both by sticking things into their ear canals and having a good scratch around.

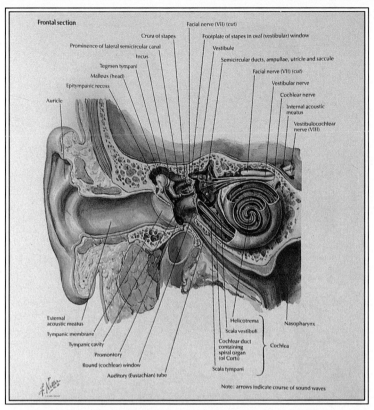

Frontal section

Facial nerve (VII) (cut)
Crura of stapes
Footplate of stapes in oval (vestibular) window
Prominence of lateral semicircular canal
Vestibule
Incus
Semicircular ducts, ampullae, utricle and saccule
Tegmen tympani
Facial nerve (VII) (cut)
Malleus (head)
Vestibular nerve
Epitympanic recess
Cochlear nerve
Internal acoustic meatus
Auricle
Vestibulocochlear nerve (VIII)

External acoustic meatus
Tympanic membrane
Helicotrema
Scala vestibuli
Nasopharynx
Tympanic cavity
Cochlear duct containing spiral organ (of Corti)
Promontory
Cochlea
Round (cochlear) window
Scala tympani
Auditory (Eustachian) tube

Note: arrows indicate course of sound waves

Pathway of sound reception.

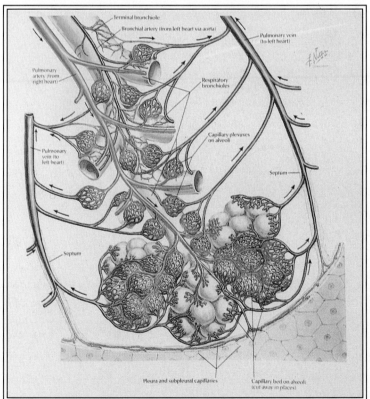

Terminal bronchiole
Bronchial artery (from left heart via aorta)
Pulmonary vein (to left heart)
Pulmonary artery (from right heart)
Respiratory bronchioles
Capillary plexuses on alveoli
Pulmonary vein (to left heart)
Septum
Septum
Pleura and subpleural capillaries
Capillary bed on alveoli (cut away in places)

Intrapulmonary blood circulation.

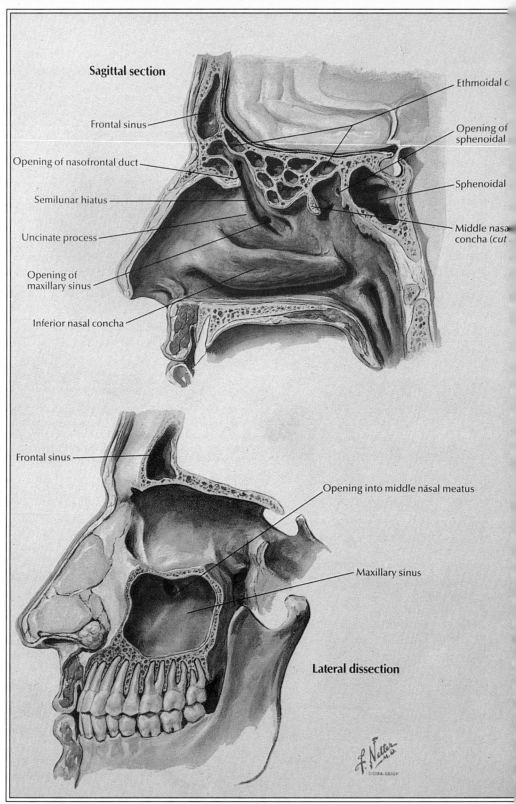

Sagittal section

Frontal sinus

Opening of nasofrontal duct

Semilunar hiatus

Uncinate process

Opening of maxillary sinus

Inferior nasal concha

Ethmoidal c

Opening of sphenoidal

Sphenoidal

Middle nasa concha (cut

Frontal sinus

Opening into middle nasal meatus

Maxillary sinus

Lateral dissection

The paranasal sinuses.

Wax removal. Wax, or cerumen, is produced in the external ear canal. Contrary to popular belief, wax is good stuff. It is not an excretory product of the ear. It is a protective non-wettable substance covering the delicate membrane lining of the canal and preventing it from becoming water-logged. A soggy membrane is the first step to infection — otitis externa or swimmer's ear.

Wax in the external ear canal should be removed only when build-up threatens to obstruct the canal, prevent free drainage of water from the ear after a dive, and predispose to external ear squeeze. This is usually heralded by the sudden onset of a deaf feeling in the ear. The ingenious methods of wax mining used by divers include the use of pens, pencils, hairpins, toothpicks, matchsticks, fingernails and the pointed tool of a Swiss knife that is good for removing stones from horses' hoofs. The ubiquitous cotton bud is especially popular. Here is a maxim. *Never put anything smaller than your elbow in your ear.* Cotton buds have no place in an ear. They simply plough up the wax and scratch open the membrane, leaving the canal wide open to invasion by aquatic bacteria. Use a cloth to clean away any socially abhorrent wax lurking at the opening of an ear. If deeper wax must be removed, let a doctor do it and then wait a few days before diving to enable a wax covering to develop again. Divers who dive regularly have very little wax build-up in any event. Frequent immersion rinses most of it away.

Dandruff. People with dandruff often suffer from maddeningly itchy ears. The need to obtain relief by ear gouging can be almost intolerable and the incidence of chronic external ear canal inflammation is accordingly high in these individuals. Treatment is available and should be sought. The use of shampoos containing coal and pine tar solutions, or medicated with zinc pyrithione or selenium sulphide will help control the dandruff. Topical antibiotic applications, with or without cortisone, are available for ear canal infections and the treatment of ear canal eczema.

Exostoses. Long-term exposure and irritation of the ears by water can lead to the development of bony thickenings called exostoses in the bony wall of the external ear canal. These can result in partial or complete obstruction of the external ear canal, leading to occlusion by wax or preventing proper drainage of water from the ear after a dive. The stage is then set for swimmer's ear to develop. Under these circumstances surgical removal of the exostoses may become necessary.

Management of swimmer's ear. Swimmer's ear differs from the commonly found mixed infections of the ear canal in non-divers in that a particularly virulent bacterium, *Pseudomonas aeruginosa*, is often the causative organism in divers. *Pseudomonas* is a water-loving bacterium and is found in all lakes, dams and even the drinking water of most cities. A scratched, moist and boggy ear canal is an open invitation to an intensely painful infection. The organism is highly resistant to all oral antibiotics and the condition requires daily injections or even hospitalisation for infusions of very expensive and potentially toxic drugs such as gentamycin, plus the topical use of antibiotics such as polymixin B, chloramphenicol and neomycin.

Prevention
1. Do not attempt to remove wax by using cotton buds or other foreign bodies. Have wax build-up assessed during a diving medical and even when attending a doctor for an unrelated complaint — it only takes a moment. If wax accumulation is significant, let a doctor remove it.
2. Keep a plastic bottle of 3 per cent saline in your dive bag. Using a clean dropper, rinse the ears with the solution to remove debris and organic contaminants after diving.
3. Instil protective drops into both ear canals. These drops either remove water (are astringent) or repel water (are hydrophobic) and include dilute acetates, oil, or alcohols as their base. They maintain a dry, slightly acidic ear canal and are readily available at most pharmacies. Several are effective, depending on sensitivity and availability, such as:
   - olive oil drops prior to diving to maintain a water-repellent surface in the canal;
   - 2 per cent acetic acid in aluminium acetate after diving;
   - 5 per cent glacial acetic acid in propylene glycol after diving;
   - 5 per cent aluminium acetate in water after diving.

Treatment. When swimmer's ear has developed, medical help is necessary. Inflammation of the external ear canal presents with pain. Deafness may also be a feature due to swelling of the membrane lining. If the diver is in a remote area with *no doctor available* then, depending on pain and sensitivity, daily packing of the ear with a cotton wick impregnated with one of the following is useful:
- Neomycin and polymixin in a vaseline-lanolin base.
- Neomycin, polymixin and hydrocortisone in aqueous solution.
- Gentamycin, betamethasone, tolnaftate, and iodochlorhydroquinone in an emulsified base.
- If earache is severe, benzocaine ear drops may be tried. The drops should be warmed by immersing the closed bottle in warm water taking care not to allow any water into the bottle. Instil 5-10 drops two-hourly and plug the ear with cotton wool.

These medications all require a prescription for their use. If the diving destination is remote, a doctor must be consulted before the trip to discuss the management of possible common ailments and obtain advice and advance permission to use these medications if needed.

If the condition remains unresponsive to treatment or is recurrent, a culture of the causative organism should be taken to identify the bacteria and determine which oral, injectable and topical antibiotics will be effective.

Once swimmer's ear has developed all diving and swimming must stop to avoid further wetting of the ear canal and flushing out of medication. Only when the canal has healed may diving be continued.

Disorders of the Middle Ear

The middle ear is the mechanical amplifier of the hearing process. Anything that threatens the integrity of sound conduction in the middle ear must temporarily or permanently prohibit diving.

Middle ear infection (otitis media)

Bacteria can reach the middle ear in two ways:
— via the Eustachian tube from the nose;
— via a perforated ear drum.
The first may occur following attempts at equalising during an episode of upper respiratory infection. Equalising drives the infection into the middle ear. The second usually occurs after barotrauma. The middle ear becomes filled with blood, mucus and water and bacterial growth begins. The acute pain and vertigo with ear drum perforation usually subside quickly during the dive to be replaced by a deaf feeling after surfacing. Bleeding from the nose or ear is often noticed. Several hours to one day later, the throbbing pain of otitis media begins.

Management of otitis media
Prevention. Do not dive with an upper respiratory infection. It commonly causes difficulty with equalisation, making middle ear barotrauma a real possibility. The use of decongestants, either orally or nasally, is not wise either. They may facilitate equalising, but will also assist in driving bacteria into the middle ear. In addition, they may wear off during the dive with reverse block on ascent.

Treatment (see also p 112)
1. Broad-spectrum antibiotics are indicated, especially after ear drum rupture due to barotrauma. The risk of otitis media is high.
2. WARNING! Ear drops may only be used if no history of barotrauma is present and there is no discharge from the ear. With a perforated ear drum, the use of most antibiotic drops may lead to permanent deafness. Drops containing antibiotics such as polymixin B, neomycin and chloramphenicol, with or without hydrocortisone to relieve inflammation, are available. Once again — they can cause permanent deafness if the ear drum is perforated.
3. If the ear drum is intact but pus formation in the middle ear occurs, the surgical introduction of a grommet to assist drainage may be necessary.

Do not dive with otitis media, a perforated ear drum or if a grommet is in place. A perforated ear drum takes an average of two to four weeks to heal and this must be confirmed by a doctor. A grommet must first be removed and the drum allowed to heal. The only exception could be dry chamber dives where one of the necessary personnel has a perforation. Chronic infections of the middle ear permanently bar diving.

Middle ear barotrauma (Squeeze) (see p 107)

Mild squeeze relieved by ascent and successful equalising should be allowed eight hours before diving again. Even mild squeeze does cause some swelling of tissues in the middle ear and invariably results in equalising difficulty with repetitive dives. Each episode of difficulty compounds the problem. Severe squeeze with bleeding from the nose and a blocked feeling in the ear should bar diving for four weeks, and medical opinion must be sought to exclude a perforation (see p 112).

Middle ear surgery

Surgery to the middle ear includes skin grafting to repair a perforated ear drum, work on the bony chain, and replacement of the stirrup. Any procedure that involves the stirrup or the oval window permanently excludes diving. The risk of forceful equalising damaging the oval or round windows becomes too high. Any diving after other surgery to the bones of the middle ear must be discussed between the diver, the diving physician and the ear surgeon who did the work.

Disorders of the Inner Ear

Abnormalities of the inner ear affect hearing or balance. Any abnormality of vestibular function is immediately disqualifying. Vertigo and disorientation under water are perilous.

Deafness

Hearing standards vary in different countries and also depend on the type of diving being done. Commercial and military divers have minimum hearing standards which must be met and should be repeated annually. Among sport divers lower standards are usually acceptable, provided the diver can equalise very easily. The risk of compounding partial inner ear deafness with middle ear damage would make diving unacceptable.

A conservative standard would be the ability to hear sounds at 30 dB at frequencies between 500 and 8 000 cps. With totally deaf people, sport diving may be approved on condition that very strict provision is made for a meaningful buddy system, for example, a signal line and a normal-hearing buddy trained to read signing.

Labyrinthitis

An acute viral infection of the vestibular apparatus induces profound vertigo with extreme disorientation, nausea and vomiting. Full recovery must be confirmed by a diving physician before recommencing diving.

Ménière's disease

This condition affects both the cochlea and the vestibular apparatus and is characterised by recurrent episodes of vertigo, ringing in the ears (tinnitus) and slowly progressive loss of hearing. Its cause is unclear but all diving is permanently barred.

Seasickness

There are very few divers who have not, at one time or another, suffered from seasickness. The only people who are immune under any sea conditions are those with totally non-functional inner ears — they are stone deaf and have no inner ear balance mechanism. The inner ear is the organ responsible for inducing seasickness.

Normal balance depends on harmony between all the sources of positional information received by the brain. When a diver is sitting on a beach and looking straight out to sea:
— nerve pressure sensors under the skin inform the brain that the ground is under the diver;
— the eyes inform the brain of the surrounding view and confirm that the ground is downwards;
— the static receptors in the inner ear inform the brain that the diver is sitting still;
— the semicircular canals inform the brain that the head is being held erect.

If the diver now sits in a boat rolling and yawing from side to side and pitching from fore to aft, the situation is very different. The skin sensors and eyes inform the brain that the diver is assuredly sitting still in a boat, but the inner ear relays that the diver is moving up and down and backwards and forwards and from side to side at the same time. Conflicting information causes motion sickness. The brain does adapt within two or three days of ongoing exposure, or after short periods of regular exposure, but these can be the most miserable days of a diver's life. Adaptation is often heralded by a gentle rocking feeling when back on land. This memory of movement ('sea legs') is at the same frequency as that of the sea conditions recently experienced.

Development of seasickness
1. *Proceeding out to sea.* Maximum pitching of the dive boat occurs when moving out to sea as the boat has to plunge through waves and bobs over crests and troughs of oncoming swells. The first feelings of being ill at ease appear. Odours such as diesel, petrol and raw fish become very

noticeable and nauseating. The diver becomes pale and restless and tries to find a place to be alone. Going below deck makes things worse, as does any heat from the engines. Fine beads of perspiration appear on the upper lip and forehead. Saliva production increases, and exaggerated swallowing and yawning occur. Then nausea and vomiting occur, which may be short-lived with full recovery from seasickness, or become ongoing to the point of dehydration and collapse.

2. *Moored on site*. The pitching of the bows decreases on site, but rolling, yawing and moving up and down begin. This may precipitate seasickness and will aggravate an already sick diver's condition.

3. *Under water*. Early symptoms of seasickness usually disappear rapidly once the diver is below the surface. The cold water is refreshing and inner ear confusion stops, but haste to enter the sea can cause trouble under water if an inadequate or too hurried predive check-list was done. There may be no air in the cylinder, the cylinder valve may still be closed, the regulator may not even be connected to the pillar valve, etc. During the ascent, problems can recur if variable reference points are reintroduced, such as in-water decompression stops on a separate floating shot line or a line attached to the boat. Holding on to this line will ensure a correct and constant decompression-stop depth as the buoy or boat moves up and down on the surface swell, but the bottom, if visible, will approach and recede with the movement. The solution is simple and also applies to heights: don't look down.

4. *Returning to shore*. Once back on the boat and returning to shore, the seasick diver invariably recovers. No longer does the boat pitch and roll, and the smooth passage between suddenly gentle swells restores hope that survival is not only possible, but probable.

If the diver has suffered from prolonged vomiting during a day at sea, he or she may become incapacitated as a result of fluid loss and exhaustion and a doctor must be consulted. Dehydration and electrolyte loss can be very substantial and intravenous fluid replacement and other therapy may be necessary.

Predisposing factors to seasickness

1. *Alcohol*. From ruefully remembered personal experience, alcohol the night before is an extremely potent factor in promoting seasickness the next morning.

2. *Food*. Divers must eat frugally and intelligently. Overindulgence (which usually includes alcohol abuse) results in a bleary-eyed, flatulent diver braving the morning seas when the best place would be in bed, asleep.

3. *Age*. Older divers are less susceptible to seasickness than young divers. This probably relates more to decreased sensitivity of the inner ear to changes in motion than innate resistance.

4. *Sex*. Seasickness is commoner in women. It is very unlikely that this observation has any truth in real physical terms. It is most probable

that women simply expose themselves less to exploits that require acclimatisation, such as fishing.

5. *Sensory confusion.* Sitting in the bows or stern of a dive boat causes maximum disturbance of the inner ear. Pitching and yawing are most marked in these places, which pivot around the central, relatively motionless, middle of the boat.

6. *Psychological factors.* It is often said that seasickness is 'all in the mind'. Anatomically, this may be correct, but seasick infants belie such a simple explanation. Fear of becoming seasick is definitely relevant, and once one diver begins vomiting, others will follow his or her example. Nervous expectancy and preparedness for seasickness would be closer to the truth.

Prevention of seasickness

1. Eat lightly and do not drink alcohol the night before diving.

2. Ensure that all your equipment is placed in a logical and orderly fashion next to you on the dive boat. Do not leave your mask in one place, fins in another, and your cylinder in a third. Sorting out equipment in a rocking boat will guarantee vomiting if one is predisposed to seasickness.

3. Concentrate on factors that will assist the brain in orientating acceptably. The eyes and body should actively fix on steady bearings:
   — keep the head upright and steady,
   — stare at the horizon,
   — do not look down at the deck or water,
   — do not try to read — this removes eye reference and makes things worse.

4. Anti-seasickness drugs generally act by preventing seasickness rather than treating it, so it is logical that they be taken before seasickness starts. It is pointless to tell sport divers not to take anti-seasickness medication because the drugs may cause drowsiness. They will not listen. The fear of uncontrolled vomiting while sitting in a hot wet suit in a rocking boat under a blazing sun makes drowsiness a pleasure, not a side-effect. As the main dangers of drowsiness are sluggish reactions and nitrogen narcosis at shallower than usual depths, a practical compromise is necessary. *A maximum depth of 30 msw must not be exceeded if any anti-seasickness medication is used.* A seasick diver has no business at 30 msw in any event.

   The choice of drug depends on local availability and the duration of exposure to the sea. The drug should be taken one to two hours before going to sea.

   (a) *Hyoscine (scopolamine).* This drug blocks the passage of nerve impulses from the balance organs in the inner ear to the vomiting centre in the brain. It is intended for severe sea conditions and useful for trips to sea lasting less than six hours. It must not be used more than once a day as blurred vision, a very dry mouth and drowsiness then make it dangerous. The dose is 0.3 to 0.6 mg by mouth. It must not be taken in combination form with other stimulants or antihistamines if diving is intended. Hyoscine combinations are absolutely contraindicated. In South Africa uncombined hyoscine is only available as a skin patch (Scopaderm TTS) which slowly releases the drug through the skin over 72 hours.

(b) *Dimenhydrinate (dramamine)*. Dramamine has been used without reported untoward effects at depths to 50 msw. The dose is 50 mg six-hourly. It is intended for moderate seasickness and is available without prescription.

(c) *Cyclizine*. Available without prescription, cyclizine assists with prevention of mild seasickness. The dose is 50 mg four-hourly.

(d) *Metoclopramide*. Metoclopramide is useful in mild cases of motion illness. The dose is 10 mg three times a day. A prescription is required.

(e) *Cinnarizine and domperidone*. A combination of the two drugs cinnarizine 25 mg and domperidone 10 mg is useful in preventing all but severe seasickness. The two tablets are taken together at six-hourly intervals. It is suggested that medication begin 24 hours before diving starts in order to assess individual susceptibility to drowsiness and allow time for acclimatisation to these effects. In this author's experience, divers actively working at 30 msw for prolonged periods reported no adverse drowsiness under water. A prescription from a doctor is required for both drugs.

Once violent seasickness starts, the diver must forget about any diving that day.

Disorders of the Nose and Throat

Nasal allergy and irritation

The commonest ailment among sport divers is nasal allergy and irritation. The combined incidence of all other diving problems becomes almost insignificant when compared with the incidence of grey-blue swelling of the membranes in the human nose.

As the nose is the first organ to sample the air in the breathing process it is exposed to more dust, pollen, fumes and smoke than any other tissue. This is aggravated by the fact that the lining of the nose is designed to humidify air. It is thick, corrugated to provide a large surface area, and covered with mucus-producing cells. Air streaming through the nose rapidly absorbs moisture from mucus and just as readily deposits its burden of pollution on to the sticky film.

In some people, frank allergy or chemically induced swelling results, with severe hayfever or nasal stuffiness. In most cases the person is unaware of any membrane swelling in his or her nose until the patency of the Eustachian tubes is challenged. This challenge requires a pressure differential and commonly occurs when driving down a mountain pass or descending in an aircraft. The atmospheric pressure (in millibars) outside the ear increases while that in the middle ear remains low. Discomfort or frank pain occur, which may be relieved by chewing, swallowing or performing a Valsalva manoeuvre. Under diving conditions the pressure differentials are measured in bars, not millibars, so the problem is vastly worse.

Inability to equalise pressure in the middle ear due to nasal congestion is by far the commonest complaint of divers.

Management of nasal congestion
Prevention. Without quitting one's job, selling up and moving to a pollution-free island, the avoidance of industrial pollution, dusts and pollens is impossible. The one nasal irritant that can be avoided is smoking. Stopping smoking often cures equalising problems.

A deviated nasal septum is often associated with equalising difficulties. When the thin plate dividing the two nostrils is deviated to one side, the interference with air flow through the nose commonly results in membrane swelling. Surgical straightening of the septum restores normal air flow.

Treatment. To a large degree, treatment of nasal congestion depends on need, diving frequency and the willingness of the diver to comply with long-term treatment. There is no total cure. In a few cases, an underlying allergy can be pinned down to one or two specific causes, such as cats or pollen only. Desensitisation by regular injections of gradually increasing strengths of solutions prepared from cat fur or pollen mix may then help. In most cases the choice lies between decongestants, antihistamines, and nasal cortisone and anti-allergy sprays. Many of these are dangerous under diving conditions.

Decongestants
1. Oral decongestants almost invariably contain pseudoephedrine, a drug that mimics adrenaline in action. It shrinks the nasal lining, and improves nasal function and equalising ability. As adrenaline is a powerful natural hormone, mimicking its action can cause side-effects including an increased heart rate, palpitations, high blood pressure, hallucinations, psychotic states, muscular weakness, difficulty in passing urine, sweating, thirst, tremors, dry mouth, breathlessness, disturbances in glucose metabolism, blurred vision, and cardiac arrest. Pseudoephedrine should preferably not be taken before a dive to assist equalising.
2. Nasal decongestants usually rely for their action on the drugs oxymetazoline and phenylephrine. Their side-effects are not as dramatic as oral decongestants and include local stinging in the nose, headache, a rapid heart rate, and high blood pressure. They have two main disadvantages:
    (a) *Rebound congestion occurs.* The drugs act by producing intense

spasm of the blood vessels in the nasal mucous membrane. This shrinks the lining and stops mucus production. Relief of congestion occurs. The nasal membrane, deprived of its normally rich blood supply, dries out and becomes devitalised. As the effects of the drug wear off the membrane swells again, but this time due to both allergy and drug injury. The swelling is worse than before and results in a totally blocked nose. Repeated sprays cause an ever-worsening cycle of blocking and unblocking, the user becoming virtually addicted to the spray for shorter and shorter periods of temporary relief. At this point the spray must be stopped despite intensely uncomfortable nasal congestion and a doctor must be consulted.

(b) *The effects may wear off during the dive.* Nasal sprays are very commonly used by divers and probably contribute to the fact that middle ear barotrauma is by far and away the commonest diver injury. *A drug-assisted descent does not mean a safe ascent.* As the effects wear off, rebound congestion occurs, made even worse by the extreme dryness of the compressed air breathed by scuba divers. The stage is set for reverse block. Air expanding in the middle ear on ascent cannot easily escape through the Eustachian tube and into the nose. The ear drum begins to balloon outwards. It becomes very taut, causing sharp pain. With further ascent the expanding air either rushes with a high-pitched squeal through the Eustachian tube, or the ear drum simply bursts outwards.

Antihistamines. Instead of shrinking swollen membranes by squeezing off their blood supply, antihistamines act by preventing the production or effects of histamine. In the allergic process histamine and a number of other compounds are produced by allergic tissues. If histamine production is inhibited, allergic swelling decreases or stops. The problem is that histamine is also used by the brain as one of the normal chemical transmitters in nerve conduction, so the use of antihistamines affects cerebral function too. Drowsiness, blurred vision, heaviness of the limbs, weakness and ringing in the ears can occur (among numerous other side-effects). These make the classical antihistamines such as chlorphenira-mine, promethazine and mepyramine unsuitable for diving.

Newer antihistamines have been manufactured, which do not cross the membrane barrier between cerebral capillaries and brain cells and exert their effect primarily on nasal mucous membranes. These drugs include loratidine, cetirizine and astemizole. As they cannot reach the brain they should in theory be safe, but drug effects on land cannot be presumed to be the same under water. If these antihistamines do cross into brain cells with the increased pressure of diving, their effects would be unpredictable. In this author's experience, over 200 sport divers have dived to 18 metres using these products without experiencing any noticeable subjective side-effects.

Nasal cortisones. Steroid hormones are normally produced by the adrenal glands in the body. Cortisone is an immensely powerful antihistamine and anti-inflammatory, and these properties are taken advantage of when cortisone therapy is used. But its side-effects when used orally for prolonged periods are profound, including decalcification of bone, thinning and weakening of connective tissue, and duodenal ulceration. To avoid these, in nasal preparations microgram doses only are sprayed directly where required — on to the nasal membranes. Absorption into the body is limited to minute amounts, but care must be taken with prolonged use.

The cortisone sprays include betamethasone, budesonide, and beclomethasone, and the more powerful fluorinated cortisones, flunisolide and fluticasone. These products take time to exert their effect so regular use in strictly controlled dosages over several months is needed.

Management of equalising difficulties before a diving trip. Most sport divers dive relatively infrequently and do not suffer any particular nasal or equalising difficulty when on land, except perhaps for occasional sneezing when the pollen count is high. They are understandably loath to undertake continuous treatment of their nasal congestion just in case they may want to dive. They want a regime of treatment to help them when they dive.

The following management is useful, provided it is approved and prescribed by a doctor to ensure no contraindications in a particular diver. If possible, it should be begun one month before diving and is recommended for adults only.
1. Douche both nostrils with a mixture of ½ teaspoon salt and ½ teaspoon bicarbonate of soda dissolved in 200 ml warm water three times a day and just before bed. Glass or plastic nasal douches are available and are more efficient than sniffing up the liquid from a cupped hand. Douching washes away sticky mucus, clears the nose of particles of pollen, dust, etc., and provides better exposure of the membranes to nasal medication. Douche the nose just before using a nasal spray.
2. Use two sprays of fluticasone in each nostril once a day; or two sprays of budesonide in each nostril twice a day; or two sprays of flunisolide in each nostril twice a day.
3. Take one 10 mg tablet of loratidine, cetirizine or astemizole once a day as a single evening dose.
4. One week before the trip add pseudoephedrine (available in tablet combination with the above or as separate tablets) in two to three divided doses. The total dose per day should be 180-240 mg.
5. Stop *all* tablets the day before diving begins.
6. Continue regular nasal douching and steroid sprays during the holiday.

Nose bleeds (epistaxis)

Chronic nasal allergy, abuse of nasal decongestant sprays and drying of nasal membranes by the inert propellant in steroid sprays can cause recurrent nose bleeds. If these become regular, diving must stop until the problem has been attended to. Equalising increases the pressure in one's head and can easily precipitate a severe bleed under water with accumulation of blood in the mask, forced swallowing of blood, anxiety and panic. High blood pressure must also be excluded as a possible cause. Most cases of recurrent nose bleeds require cautery of the bleeding site by a doctor.

Management of acute nose bleeds. Most nose bleeds occur from the blood vessels near the front of the nose. The majority are self-limiting and require little assistance. Severe nose bleeds require packing by a doctor. In intermediate cases the following usually suffices:

1. Have the person sit erect and with the head tilted forward on to the chest. This increases venous back pressure on the bleeding vessel and assists clot formation. It also stops blood from running into the throat.
2. Compress the nostrils between two fingers for ten minutes.
3. If bleeding persists, plug the nose. Nasal gauze strip or even cotton wool drawn into a cylinder may be used. Moistening cotton wool with water makes it easier to insert. Feed the plug straight back *parallel* to the roof of the mouth. Do not try to push it upwards into the nose. This is acutely painful and the plug will jam against the internal curled bones on the side wall of the nose. Try to ensure that the nostril is packed as firmly as possible. Continue nasal compression between two fingers.
4. Nasal plugs made of compressed oxidised cellulose are easy to insert and should be included in a diver emergency medical kit. These plugs swell to many times their compressed dry volume when wetted with blood and are effective. Insert them parallel to the roof of the mouth.
5. Keep the nose plugged for 12 hours. Remove the plug slowly and gently to avoid causing sneezing which may restart the bleeding. Dab away any blood and mucus from the nostrils. Do not blow the nose!

Disorders of the Sinuses

In diving mechanical terms, the sinuses are no different from the middle ear. They are rigid air spaces connected by an opening into the nose and are subject to the same problems as the middle ear. The only difference is that any pressure differential in sinuses cannot be voluntarily equalised. Their openings into the nose are either patent or blocked. Blockage causes squeeze.

Sinus allergy

Being only extensions of the nasal cavity, sinuses are also affected by allergy and inhaled irritants. These cause diver problems when membrane swelling occurs near or at the openings of the sinuses into the nose. Air flow through the openings may be obstructed. Polyps may be present. These are localised areas of membrane growth resembling wet grapes hanging from a stalk. They may act as a ball valve while diving. Polyps obstructing a sinus opening in the nose cause squeeze on descent. Polyps obstructing a sinus opening in the sinuses cause reverse block. Polyps may have to be surgically removed — a looped wire snare is slipped over them and their narrow stalks snipped off. Treatment of sinus allergy is the same as nasal allergy and diving restrictions are identical.

Sinusitis

Infection of the sinuses presents with acute pain over the involved sinuses. In severe cases an accumulation of pus may occur. This is seen on X-ray as a fluid level of liquid topped by air. The management of sinusitis follows the principles of nasal infection but pus formation requires surgical drainage.

Disorders of the Mouth and Throat

Infection occurs more commonly in the mouth and throat than anywhere else in the body. Upper respiratory infections include tonsillitis, pharyngitis and laryngitis. They are all relatively easily treated and are important from a diving point of view only because they bar diving while they are present. The reason is mainly related to mouth breathing of very dry air while exercising under water. The effects are very similar to those experienced by runners who exercise with an upper respiratory infection. Mouth breathing dries and further devitalises membranes already damaged by infection and inflammation. Deep breathing also draws the infection deeper into the airways and a simple sore throat can progress to bronchitis or pneumonia. Infections of the mouth and gums are similarly aggravated by drying and will get worse.

Divers must care for their teeth. Dental caries is a potential cause of violent diver pain. If the opening to a dental cavity is obstructed by food or a swollen gum, the tooth may collapse on descent. If obstruction occurs on ascent, expanding air in the cavity can explode the tooth.

The absence of teeth is important too. A dental bridge must fit firmly and properly. If dislodged under water it may be inhaled with disastrous results. People with dentures should dive only if they can firmly retain the rubber mouthpiece between their lips and gums. Diving with dentures is like diving with a marble in the cheek. An accidental bump or being hit on the face by a fellow diver's fin may dislodge the mouthpiece and the dentures and result in sudden respiratory obstruction under water.

Visual Requirements
of Scuba Diving

Vision Under Water

Divers are observant souls and when they enter the sea, they use their eyes. They notice three things — things are darker, colours are different, and things look bigger.

Things are darker

In the clearest ocean water, such as that around the British Virgin Islands or the Maldives, only 20 per cent of the surface light reaches 10 metres, and one per cent reaches 85 metres. This means that the bright illumination of the sunny day above is very reduced. The harsh clear shadows of the surface recede, making contrast between objects much less.

Colours are different

Sunlight or white light includes a spectrum of visible light from red to violet. Clean water has a maximum transparency to blue wavelengths of light and absorbs the other colours. Coastal waters allow the yellow-greens through. The other colours are absorbed by suspended material such as plankton and pollution. Reds and oranges are absorbed first. To see *true colours*, even at 10 metres, underwater lights are needed.

This absorption and scattering of light by suspended particles limits vision and diffuses illumination, and with poor visibility the light intensity appears the same in all directions. On descent or ascent the surface and sea-bed disappear and a diver may feel suspended in a featureless green, blue or grey watery sphere. This may cause loss of orientation with up, down and sideways all having the same light intensity. Only a dangling pressure gauge or the direction of ascending bubbles show down and up.

Things look bigger

When a beam of light passes through transparent substances of different optical densities it is bent at the interface between them. Light reaching the surface of the eye (the cornea) is bent or refracted into the eye. It is an air/tissue interface, the cornea being optically denser than air. Having passed through the cornea, light is then fine-focused by the lens on to the retina at the back of the eye. The air/cornea interface is the main site of focusing. Most of the necessary bending of light waves occurs here. Within the eye the lens is surrounded by liquid with only minute differences in optical density and very limited refracting ability. A normal cornea is essential to clear vision.

Should a diver decide to snorkel down to check an anchor without using a mask, his or her eye would not be able to focus, as a water/cornea interface would be present. Their optical densities are too similar and no effective refraction can occur. Everything would be blurred. This is the reason for using a mask while diving, as well as protecting the eye from harmful denizens of the sea.

A mask does enable focusing, but why should things appear larger?

The reason is the introduction of a water/glass interface. Light passes from water into glass and then from glass into the air inside the mask. The light is bent at each interface so that the mask acts like a pair of low-power binoculars. An apparent image is formed, which is closer and larger than the real image — about 25 per cent closer and 30 per cent larger.

But wearing a mask or helmet does cause problems:

Limited field of vision. The field of vision is limited by the size of the mask and its distance from the face. The further from the face (the eye) the glass is, the narrower will be the field of vision. It is rather like looking through a tunnel. The longer the tunnel, the smaller the field.

If a diver wears a mask above the surface of the water, there would be air outside the mask and air within. This cancels any refraction by glass, just as things are not magnified when looking through a window. The field of vision is limited only by the size of the mask as no effective refraction occurs.

Under water, refraction between the water outside and the air inside the mask reduces the field of vision. There is a limit to the degree that light can be bent. Beyond a certain point, any light reaching the surface of the mask from one side will be reflected off the surface of the glass. None will reach the eye. This limit is an angle of 48.6 degrees on each side, making a total visual field of 97.2 degrees. Beyond this, all the light is reflected back into the water. A magnified image is paid for with a narrower field of vision.

Mask squeeze. A mask contains an air space, which must obey Boyle's Law. As pressure increases with depth, mask volume decreases. This has the novel effect of attempting to suck out the diver's eyes and is called mask squeeze. For this reason, all diving masks include the nose so that air can be vented through the nostrils to compensate the pressure increase without a decrease in mask volume.

Short-sighted Divers

Using a mask and depending on the water/glass/air interface to enable one to see under water is fine, provided one has normally curved corneas. But what about those thousands of frustrated divers who have very curved corneas and are short-sighted? Their visual images are focused in front of their retinas making a beautiful red fern coral a gaudy blob and a stone fish a brown glob until a poisonous spine is virtually up a nostril. What options are open to them?

Management of short-sightedness (myopia)
Five thousand years ago, the Chinese tried to cure myopia by sleeping with sand bags on their eyes. They understood that their corneas were too curved and were trying to flatten them. Nowadays there are three possibilities open to divers:
1.   the use of prescription lenses,
2.   the use of soft contact lenses,
3.   undergoing corneal surgery − a procedure called radial keratotomy.

1.   *Prescription lenses.* These are the simplest means of correcting submarine myopia. Lenses specifically ground and polished to the user's needs are fixed to the glass of the mask. These adjust the angle of light waves reaching the over-curved cornea of a myopic eye, making it possible for a great white shark to be focused very nicely on to the retina. The mask should be a good one, fitting the user's face comfortably and easily as it will become a 'designer model', suited to one person only.

2.   *Soft contact lenses.* At the present time, these are probably the most convenient means of correction for divers. Errors of refraction are corrected at the surface of the eye, making a specially modified mask unnecessary. Aside from avoiding the owl-like appearance of prescription lenses they do have some real disadvantages, however. They have to be sterilised and cleaned, sensitive eyes will not tolerate them, and eye irritation and infection are always potential complications.

Having one's mask inadvertently dislodged or kicked off during a dive will eliminate the surface tension needed to retain contact lenses in place. They may float off, to be lost for ever in the sea. Disposable, cheap, soft contact lenses are available and are currently the ultimate in diving optical accessories.

The cornea has no blood supply. It receives its oxygen by direct absorption from the air to which it is exposed. During decompression after hyperbaric conditions, the excess nitrogen absorbed diffuses directly from cornea to atmosphere. Being permeable to nitrogen and oxygen, soft contact lenses allow these interchanges of gases to occur. Hard glass contact lenses do not permit speedy nitrogen diffusion with decompression, and corneal swelling or even bubbling is a potential hazard. Hard impermeable lenses are not safe for diving.

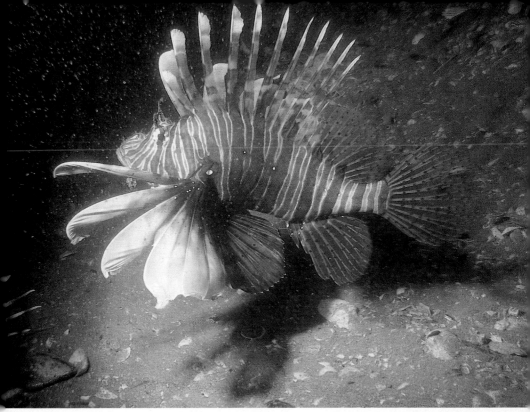

Lionfish photographed at Sodwana.

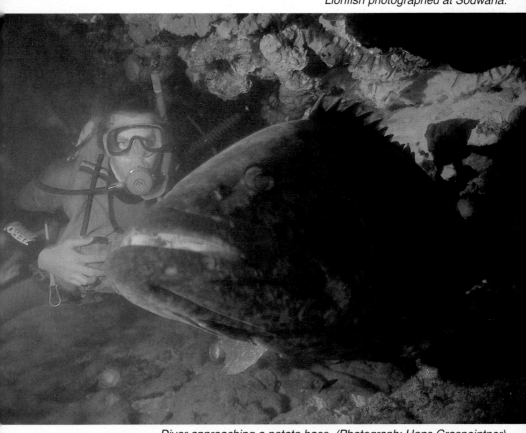

Diver approaching a potato bass. (Photograph: Hans Graspointner)

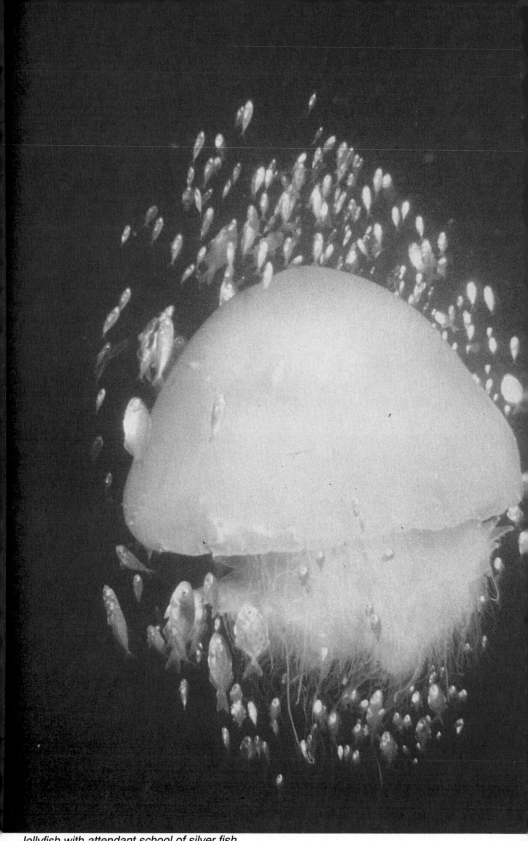

Jellyfish with attendant school of silver fish.
(Photograph: Hans Graspointner)

3. *Radial keratotomy.* In 1939, Dr Tsutomu Sato, a Japanese ophthalmologist, began experimenting with surgery as a treatment for myopia. He tried to reduce the sharp curvature of the cornea by making tiny, radial, spoke-like cuts on the outer edge of the cornea. Initial great success faded as many patients started slowly to go blind. The Russians took up the challenge about thirty years later. They had better instruments, more advanced technology and could predict more accurately the probable results of radial keratotomy. Nowadays, the procedure has become so commonplace in Russia that patients literally queue for surgery by a string of doctors. The initial trials were watched with great interest by Sweden and America. The Swedish authorities urged caution, stressing the possible complications and unknown long-term results. The Americans began radial keratotomy in 1978 and in 1985 the National Eye Institute laid down guidelines for the selection of patients for radial keratotomy.

Who are suitable candidates for radial keratotomy? Not all myopics can be helped. Healthy corneas are essential. The subject must not be too short-sighted. Refractive errors are measured in dioptres (a unit of measurement of the refractive power of a lens equal to the reciprocal of the focal length in metres). A normal cornea requires a zero dioptre correction. A myopic cornea requires positive correction, but a maximum of six dioptres is generally acceptable for surgical intervention. Only adults should be operated on — myopia is usually maximal at about twenty-plus years. The candidate must be realistic in his or her hopes. The operation may provide only partial correction, not eliminating the need for lower prescription glasses.

What does the operation involve? A myopic cornea focuses light in front of the retina. Radial keratotomy flattens the curve of the cornea so that refracted light can be focused accurately on the retina. A series of tiny incisions are made with a diamond knife in a radial pattern round the edge of the cornea. These fine cuts weaken the periphery of the cornea. This weakened zone then bulges outward because of the internal pressure of the eye, pulling on and flattening the central corneal area. The result is a cornea with a central shallow curvature and a peripheral sharp curvature. As the central area of the cornea over the iris is used for vision, the refracted image then falls closer to or on the retina.

The procedure obviously is a delicate one. The incisions must extend through about 95 per cent of the wall of the cornea (a thickness of half a millimetre). They must not penetrate the cornea or the inner layer of endothelial cells will die, and they cannot be repaired or replaced by the eye. The number of incisions depends on the degree of myopia. The more short-sighted the person, the more cuts are required. Between four and thirty-two incisions are usually made. They must not extend over the central zone, or they will interfere with vision.

Should the patient also have astigmatism, the delicacy increases. An astigmatic cornea has an irregular curvature, being more curved in one plane and less curved in another. This can cause a doubling or ghosting of vision. The surgeon must then calculate the number, angles and sites of the cuts to ensure that both myopia and astigmatism are corrected.

The procedure takes about twenty minutes and is done on one eye at a time so that the patient can be ambulant and at home in one day, with a patch over one eye and using the other eye. It also avoids disaster should something go wrong. Either local or general anaesthesia is used, depending on the patient's state of health and his courage – he will see the diamond scalpel approaching his eye!

What can go wrong? About half of the patients are delighted with the results. Just over ten per cent are unhappy. The rest are so-so. There are a number of possible complications – excessive light or glare sensitivity, infection, inability to drive at night due to oncoming headlights refracting in the scars causing starbursts, and fluctuations in focus, sometimes within hours, requiring the use of glasses on one day and not on another. The cornea may be overcorrected, causing the image to be focused behind the retina, the exact opposite of myopia. The patient is back to glasses, this time for long-sightedness. Blindness or serious loss of vision are very uncommon.

Should divers undergo radial keratotomy? The long-term results and complications of radial keratotomy are unknown. The degree of correction is not totally predictable and visual aids may still be necessary.

It would be rash for a diver to undergo the operation just to improve his focus under water. For those divers who have already undergone the procedure, the awkward questions arise of nitrogen uptake and degassing in corneal scars. Increased pressure at depth should not be a problem, provided mask equalising is meticulously done. But beware of mask squeeze! The effect of a relative vacuum on the distorted and weakened curvature of a keratotomised cornea could be much more severe than that on the even curvature of a normal (albeit myopic) cornea. Pressure distortion could have unpredictable consequences after radial keratotomy.

Visual Standards for Divers

The minimum visual requirements for diving are surprisingly lax. Only enough is required to ensure an accurate buddy system, the ability to react to danger, safety around boats, and the capacity to read clearly pressure gauges and a timing device on the arm. So both far and near vision are required.

Far vision is commonly measured by the diver's ability to read letters on a distant chart. The Snellen chart has varying-sized rows of letters. A normal eye can read the line designated 6/6 or 20/20 from a distance of 6 metres or 20 feet. The largest letter is designated 6/60 (20/200) meaning a normal (or a far-sighted) eye can see it from a distance of 60 metres (200 feet). Short-sighted people are unable to read the 6/6 line, but can make out one of the larger lines (6/9, 6/12, 6/18, 6/24, 6/36, 6/60). Using their glasses or contact lenses provides correction. If fully corrected they can then read the 6/6 line. Being unable to visualise the 6/60 letter, even with corrective lenses, represents legal blindness as it means a loss of visual acuity of more than 80 per cent. Military and commercial standards vary, but for sport divers at least one eye should be correctable to 6/9 (20/30).

Near vision is measured by the ability to read simple print such as a newspaper. Here normal and short-sighted people cope, but far-sighted people need corrective lenses. Far-sightedness *(hypermetropia)* is just the reverse of short-sightedness. The curve of the corneal surface is too shallow and the visual image is focused *behind* the retina. But far-sighted divers cannot use contact lenses because they would then only be able to read their gauges — everything else, including their buddy or a coral reef, would be blurred. Far-sightedness, unless severe, is not generally corrected under water as bifocal mask lenses would be needed. These divers must ensure that the dials on their gauges and timing devices are large and luminous enough to be read under gloomy subsurface conditions.

As one ages, the lens of the eye stiffens and its ability to fine-focus the image from the cornea on to the retina decreases. This usually becomes apparent after forty. Things close by become blurred and written material has to be held further and further away until the print becomes too small to read anyway. This is called *presbyopia* (Greek for old man's eyes). Although the cornea is curved normally, the effect of lens stiffening is identical to far-sightedness. Magnifying corrective lenses have to be used for reading on land, and underwater readouts must be large and bright. The good news for short-sighted divers is that as they reach forty-plus their 'old man's eyes' will tend to correct their short-sightedness and improve their vision under water. Perhaps the only known advantage of ageing!

Colour vision is the ability of the eye to distinguish between red and green when tones of these colours are presented in complex patterns. The Ishihara test uses coloured dots. Dotted numbers are seen against differently coloured dotted backgrounds. Inability to see these numbers is called *colour blindness* and is an inherited trait. Colour vision is completely irrelevant as far as scuba diving is concerned. The reason is simple — starting with red, colours are absorbed by water and disappear anyway as soon as one is more than a few metres deep. Below about 10 msw the sea is brown and green and blue. Above water, colour vision is necessary if selecting colour-coded gas cylinders, or if navigation is required.

Diving Implications of Musculoskeletal Disease

The musculoskeletal system comprises the bony skeleton and the muscles that move articulating bones. Diving requires coordinated muscle action, and strength and ease of joint movement. Conditions that would absolutely preclude diving are those that predispose to lumbar spine disorders, bone death (osteonecrosis), and ailments that may mimic, mask or provoke acute limb or joint decompression illness.

Lumbar Spine Disorders

Man is the only creature on earth who always stands erect on two feet, maintaining a vertical spine against the unrelenting drag of gravity. Man is also the only creature on earth who suffers from chronic backache. No one is immune and over 80 per cent of people will suffer from low backache at one time or another in their lives. Of all the possible causes for permanent disability claims in the insurance industry, the commonest by far is back pain. It affects people of all sizes and shapes and in every occupational group – labourers and academics, fat and thin, muscular and scrawny, short and tall, male and female.

The spine is a stack of 26 bony vertebrae, each separated from the next by a fibrocartilaginous pad or disc. The discs act as elastic spacers, keeping the vertebrae apart and providing the spinal nerve roots, arising directly from the spinal cord, room to pass between vertebrae and out of the spine. Discs also allow tilting of one vertebra on another. Each individual tilt is small but the sum is forwards, backwards or sideways movement of the spine. In the vertical position each disc supports the mass of the body above it, so the lowest discs, in the lumbar spine, bear the brunt in terms of compression force. Should compression on a lumbar disc become excessive, the disc tears and ruptures, with extrusion of the soft centre of the disc. The space between the two vertebrae decreases and the spinal nerves between them become pinched. And once a disc tears it stays torn. Cartilage does not heal and repair itself like bone, muscle or skin. Any damage to a disc is permanent. But things can get worse: the spinal cord lies directly behind each disc and if extrusion of the disc pulp is backwards, the spinal cord itself becomes compressed and a bed in an orthopaedic ward is guaranteed.

The problem is, aside from crawling to keep the lumbar spine horizontal or living under zero-gravity conditions, there is little one can do about an inherent situation. If one is tall, there is more leverage and strain on the lower back. If one is brawny with big shoulders, it's even worse. If one is fat or has a comfortable belly, the same applies. The ideal vertical person is a petite pygmy.

From a back point of view, diving is good and bad. It's good because neutral buoyancy is as close as anyone can get to zero-gravity conditions and absolute freedom from spinal strain. It's bad because divers have to lift, lug, haul and shove before they can achieve the luxury of weightlessness.

A little understanding of the mechanics of the lumbar spine will help prevent undue stresses and avoid unnecessary damage. The lumbar spine is most stable in extension and least stable in flexion, so prevention of damage is obvious — *don't bend forward and lift*. Unfolding the normal inward curve of the lumbar spine by leaning forward to pick up a bar of soap in a shower, or to tie a straggling shoelace, is a very common cause of acute lumbar disc damage and recurring backache for life. If supporting the weight of the upper body by an unstable flexed lumbar spine is enough to rupture a disc, attempting to lift a heavy cylinder, compressor or dive bag while bending over is lumbomechanical Russian roulette.

Use your head and then your legs. Face the object squarely. Get close to it, spread your feet and bend your knees. Keep your back straight and your upper body vertical to the ground. Hold the object firmly with both hands and straighten your knees, using the power of your thigh muscles and being careful not to lean forward. Use the same technique in putting the object down. If you can't easily lift the object by squatting and using your legs, it's too heavy for you and you are going to get a hernia because squatting opens the hernial canals and straining to lift completes the job.

Watch your posture. Don't slouch when sitting. Walk tall and exercise your back. Strong back muscles do assist by providing muscular support and stabilising the lumbar spine. Brisk walking and extension exercises are best. Deadlifts are worst and are well-named because bending over with straight legs and jerking up a heavy weight will crush your discs stone dead.

Ensure an adequate intake of calcium in the diet. One gram a day will help to avoid osteoporosis, the condition characterised by progressive vertebral decalcification and softening of bone. If your diet is restricted by choice or design, speak to your doctor about your calcium and vitamin intake and, if you are female and fiftyish, about the advisability of female hormone replacement.

The human spine is extremely prone to flexion injury. Divers carry heavy objects and are very liable to develop lumbar problems. Divers voluntarily equalise pressure changes in their middle ears. They must also learn to equalise pressure stresses on their lower backs.

Dysbaric Osteonecrosis
(Aseptic Bone Necrosis; Bone Rot)

Dysbaric osteonecrosis (DON) is an area of bone death and was first described in compressed-air workers in caissons in the early 1900s. The connection between a history of joint bends and subsequent X-ray signs of death (necrosis) in bone was first made by Bassoe in 1913. Exposure to hyperbaric conditions does not have to be deep. The disease has occurred following caisson work at only 11 metres. Exposure does not even have to be repetitive. It occurred in three of five men who escaped from the submarine *Poseidon* in 1931, after being trapped at 38 msw for nearly three hours. The condition occurs very rarely in sport divers who dive up to 50 msw and follow recommended sport diving tables and ascent rates.

Predisposing factors

DON occurs most frequently among older male commercial divers with long diving experience. The incidence increases with depth and dive time, being least common with short, shallow air dives, and most common with deep helium saturation dives, especially if a history of joint bends exists. Other predisposing factors are high blood fats, obesity, diabetes, peripheral vascular disease, haemoglobin disorders, alcoholism, and the use of cortisone.

Causes of dysbaric osteonecrosis

DON is a disease of long bones — that is, arms and legs. Anyone who has eaten a marrow bone knows that there is a lot of fat in bone marrow. A lot of fat means a lot of possible nitrogen uptake with diving. Marrow bones are limb bones. Ribs, skull, pelvis and spinal bones have very little fat and less nitrogen storage capacity. Marrow could explain the reason for the condition in arms and legs. Food for thought?

If one looks for common factors to try to explain DON in divers, three factors emerge:
1. fat metabolism is involved;
2. adequate blood supply and oxygen carriage by blood is important;
3. conditions causing bone decalcification are relevant.

Interference with the blood supply causes death of bone, fat and marrow cells supplied by the blood vessels involved. Breakdown of fat results in the liberation of free fatty acids. These acids attack calcium in bone and form dense soaps in the dead area. After some weeks, new blood vessels grow into the area from nearby normal bone and healing begins.

There is a definite relationship between DON and exposure to inadequate decompression, missed decompression, acute decompression illness, and experimental diving. As a diver's breathing mixture consists of an inert gas and oxygen, both have been blamed, that is:
- inert gas bubbles,
- oxygen toxicity.

Inert gas bubbles. Bubbles may appear in arteries, capillaries or veins inside a bone, impairing the available blood supply (oxygen supply) to the bone after a dive. Bubbles may also occur in the bone marrow, *outside* blood vessels. On ascent, pressure drops and volume increases. The enlarging bubbles then compress the blood vessels from without but within a rigid bone and produce the same effect – interference with oxygen supply and hypoxia of bone. Inadequate release of inert gas inside bone may occur after a dive even without a very heavy gas load. If lung degassing is impaired due to disorders of ventilation, perfusion and diffusion, bubbling can result. Decompressing after a dive with the limbs in a very flexed position, such as sitting on folded or crossed legs, kinks knee and hip veins and prevents easy venous transport of inert gas to the lungs for exhalation.

Oxygen toxicity. A high partial pressure of oxygen to the brain causes reflex constriction of blood vessels. People who breathe hyperbaric oxygen become pale. Reflex constriction of vessels in bone, if intense, could lead to the same effect as obstruction with bubbles – the tissues beyond the spastic vessels become hypoxic. Famine in the midst of plenty. In addition, a too-high oxygen partial pressure may interfere with local metabolism in bone, disrupting glucose utilisation and the essential energy supply of bone and marrow cells. High oxygen concentrations and pressures can cause the formation of free oxygen radicals. In its normal form oxygen exists as two oxygen atoms linked together with no residual electrical charge. At a high partial pressure this link may break, resulting in positively and negatively charged oxygen ions. These are intensely chemically active and may damage bony fibrous tissue (collagen) and fat and marrow cells in bone. Tissue damage then causes swelling within the tight confines of a bone and interferes with circulation, nitrogen release and bone nutrition.

Vasoactive substances. Damage to fat cells may result in the release of vasoactive substances – chemical triggers that can result in clotting of blood inside the blood vessels in the area and further bone damage.

Classification of DON

DON only affects long bones and, as the diagnosis is made after viewing an X-ray of a bone, the disease is classified according to its X-ray appearance. It can affect the extreme end of a bone (the metaphysis) just below the joint surface. As a result the joint surface may gradually collapse with pressure of use. Loss of the smooth curved articular surface and subsequent arthritis occur. These are called Type A lesions and occur most commonly at the large joints of the shoulder, hip and knee. DON can also occur in the head, neck or shaft of a bone behind the metaphysis. These are called medullary or Type B lesions, and rarely cause too much trouble, as healing usually occurs as with a fracture of a limb.

The difference between DON and a fracture is that in DON the diver may be totally unaware of all this activity in his bones, as it is usually a painless procedure until joint distortion occurs. X-ray changes are *late* signs of DON. They may take three or more months or longer to develop. To detect DON before gross joint collapse occurs, computerised scanning techniques are used. A tracer dose of radioactive technetium 99 (Tc 99) is injected, and scanning detects 'hot spots' in damaged bone; but practical considerations and cost limit the usefulness of isotope studies to symptomatic cases.

Whether long bones should be routinely X-rayed in divers has been a hotly debated point. In the UK it is recommended that commercial divers working below 12 msw have X-rays of long bones before any hyperbaric exposure, and then again every two years, as well as immediately and four months after any joint bend. Divers are understandably loath to undergo repeated irradiation and they argue that debilitating DON is rare. The incidence varies greatly from country to country. In a UK survey of more than 4 000 divers, the UK Medical Research Council Decompression Sickness Central Registry reported a six per cent incidence of bone necrosis. Of these, the vast majority had shaft or only suspected joint involvement. Only one per cent of commercial divers had definite joint involvement, and of the one per cent, very few had actual gross damage to the joint surface.

So in the UK series, DON with serious joint damage or disability was rare. Chinese commercial divers, on the other hand, have reported an 80 per cent incidence – which only goes to show how fiendish Oriental nitrogen can be!

Diving after DON. Once Type A DON with joint involvement has occurred, diving must be stopped. Type B involvement of the head or shaft will heal and diving may continue after healing. Unexplained DON is a problem because it may indicate susceptibility to DON. If it occurs in a diver who always dived within the rules, future scuba diving should be limited to no-decompression-stop diving to a maximum depth of 18 msw.

Conditions that Mimic or Mask Acute Limb Decompression Illness

A number of disorders can present with joint pain and be confused with acute limb decompression illness after diving. The problem is compounded because any pre-existing inflammation or swelling of a joint will interfere with capillary circulation, diffusion and inert gas transport after a dive, and predispose to a bend in that joint. The diver will then assure everybody that the pain is due to an old sports injury and is old-hat and of no particular diving significance. While he or she swallows an anti-inflammatory tablet or a pain-killer, joint DON begins, never to be recognised as such because the subsequent destruction will be attributed to ongoing or repeated inflammation and only-to-be-expected arthritis.

Gout

Acute gout is caused by an elevated uric acid level in the body and presents with exquisitely painful swelling and redness over a joint. The smaller joints of the hands and feet are usually involved but major limb joints can be affected. It is barely conceivable that anyone experiencing an acute gouty attack would want to dive, but it is very important that the diver waits for all swelling to subside once the acute pain has been treated and ensures that the blood uric acid level is properly controlled.

Rheumatoid arthritis

This illness belongs to the auto-immune group of diseases where the body produces antibodies against its own tissues and then responds with inflammation to the resulting damage. It is a process of autodestruction and may result in severe deformity and crippling of joints. It usually first involves the small joints of the fingers but can affect any joint or connective tissue. Like gout, the inflammatory process in rheumatoid arthritis can mimic or predispose to acute decompression illness. Unlike gout, rheumatoid arthritis is usually progressive and treatment involves ongoing use of drugs such as anti-inflammatories, gold salts and cortisone. These alone bar diving and the risk of DON in diseased joints is unacceptable.

Venereal diseases

Syphilis, gonorrhoea and non-specific urethritis (NSU) are not simply diseases of the reproductive organs. Their effects can be generalised and arthritis is not uncommon. Once again, bends and DON are hazards and diving must wait until treatment is complete and any joint swelling has subsided. Chronic or tertiary syphilis may produce gross joint destruction and diving is then permanently disallowed.

Bone injuries

Diving is not permitted during healing of any bony fracture. Healing of bone and associated blood vessels must be complete, and the time will depend on the severity of the injury and the presence of any complications such as infection. A conservative approach is usually taken with fractures of limb bones, especially the weight-bearing bones of the legs, because of the possibility of acute limb decompression illness and DON at an incompletely healed fracture site. If no complications occur:
– femur: 6 to 12 months
– tibia: 6 months
– fibula: 6 to 10 weeks
– humerus: 6 to 10 weeks
– radius or ulna: 6 weeks
X-ray confirmation of healing must be done with limb bones and all swelling must have subsided.

Fractures of the sinuses bear mention in that the thin bones of the maxillary, ethmoid and frontal sinuses are also the walls of the eye socket. It depends on how you look at the injury. Is a fracture of a paper-thin bone, separating an eye from a sinus cavity, a fracture of the eye socket or a fracture of a sinus? In any event a Valsalva manoeuvre or reverse block on ascent can drive air in a sinus into the tissue around the eyeball (orbital surgical emphysema).

Bone infections

Infection in bone usually follows an injury, with or without a fracture, that breaks the skin and exposes underlying bone. Disrupting the integrity of the skin provides a route for bacterial invasion and if a bone is injured too, the likelihood of bone and bone marrow infection (osteomyelitis) is high and may become chronic. Any infection must be completely cured before diving as the risk of DON is real.

Soft tissue injuries

Any significant bruise, sprain or strain that causes swelling or pain on movement should be allowed to heal before diving is recommenced as interference with degassing may occur. This may require only a few days, or several months in the case of severe tearing of the ligaments of an ankle or knee. Painless full function must first be restored.

Muscular disorders

There are a number of relatively uncommon muscle disorders, most of which are familial, which present with insidious and progressive muscle weakness with or without obvious wasting. Some present during childhood and others during adult life. They are collectively known as the *muscular dystrophies*. In some cases the degree of wasting and weakness is very slight. In others the patient may be wasted, deformed and bedridden. The different types are characterised by the muscle groups first affected; for example, the calves or the shoulder girdle muscles. As a general rule, people with muscular dystrophy must not dive, but if the degree of disability and weakness is slight, the decision to dive and the restrictions required must be made after discussion between the diving physician and the muscle specialist involved in the case.

Another rare disorder which causes weakness and easy fatigability of muscle is *myasthenia gravis*. It usually affects the muscles of the face and throat as well as the muscles of respiration. The primary defect is a chemical abnormality at the precise site where nerve impulses are transmitted to muscle fibres. Nerve signals from the brain ordering a particular group of muscles to contract are blocked and the muscles do not respond. As the disease may affect muscles of the respiratory system, one of the vital systems needed in diving, people with myasthenia gravis may not dive.

Diving Implications of Gastrointestinal Disease

Aside from being the site of alcohol absorption, the gastrointestinal system is important from a diver's point of view because it is subject to common ailments such as diarrhoea and vomiting, and pain in the abdomen may mimic acute decompression illness. Being open to the air via the mouth it is also subject to barotrauma. Diving should be stopped if any abdominal symptom is present. Abdominal pain under water can be incapacitating; vomiting can result in water inhalation and, together with diarrhoea, predispose to dehydration and acute decompression illness.

Some conditions temporarily exclude safe diving until treated. All ongoing or intermittent chronic diseases of the gastrointestinal system causing pain, vomiting, diarrhoea, and fluid or blood loss permanently bar scuba diving.

Peptic Ulcers

Gastric ulcers affect the stomach, and duodenal ulcers involve the duodenum which drains the stomach via the pyloric valve. Collectively they are called peptic ulcers. They are erosions in the inner membrane lining of the stomach or duodenum and can deeply penetrate or even perforate the underlying smooth muscle wall of the gut. Their cause has been attributed to a number of factors including stress, excessive hydrochloric acid production by the stomach, inadequate acid production, abnormalities of the immune system, and side-effects of medicines such as aspirin, cortisone and non-steroidal anti-inflammatory drugs (NSAIDs). An interesting, relatively recent finding is the presence of the bacterium *Helicobacter pylori* in the floor of duodenal ulcers, adding an infective agent to the list of causes.

Scuba diving is contraindicated with active acute or chronic gastric or duodenal ulceration. Pain may mask acute abdominal decompression illness, and spasm of the muscles of the stomach may predispose to gas trapping and stomach barotrauma of ascent. Healing should be complete and proven by direct optical examination of the stomach and duodenum by gastroscopy.

Gallstones

Bile is produced in the liver and stored in the gall bladder. It contains bile salts which emulsify fats during digestion, and bile pigments which are the breakdown products of haemoglobin released during normal red blood cell replacement in the body. Bile also serves as a route for excreting many end-products of metabolism and ridding the body of drugs, toxins and medicines. During a meal the gall bladder contracts, sending a flow of bile into the duodenum to assist digestion.

Gallstones occur when bile pigments in the gall bladder come out of solution in bile. This is often preceded by an episode of gall bladder inflammation (cholecystitis). The initial deposit of inflammatory cells and pigment slowly grows by accumulating further layers of pigment. There may be only a few or hundreds of stones present but the individual is usually unaware of the growing stone crop until one of them jams in the duct leading from the gall bladder to the duodenum. The chances of this happening are about two per cent each year. Violently painful biliary colic results and the invariable outcome is the surgical removal of the gall bladder.

Diving may be permitted with silent gallstones, as most cases are diagnosed incidentally while X-raying or scanning the abdomen for an unrelated complaint. Many divers with gallstones will not even know they have them in any event. Once an attack of acute inflammation of the gall bladder occurs, or a stone makes its presence felt, diving should stop until the gall bladder has been removed and all symptoms have disappeared. In commercial diving six months off diving work after surgery is recommended. Among sport divers, any earlier clearance to dive must be obtained from a diving physician.

Spastic Colon

Also called the irritable bowel syndrome, the main feature of this condition is colicky abdominal pain. Although diarrhoea or constipation may also be present, all investigations are essentially normal. Pain is attributed to incoordinate contractions and spasm of the muscle in the bowel wall. There is usually a strong history of emotional, financial or work stress.

Divers with a history of spastic colon must exert great caution during an acute attack or if they are on medication. Although most antispasmodics are considered safe by many diving physicians, disturbances in vision and blood pressure control, as well as drowsiness, can occur. Because of a strong emotional overlay, many people with spastic colons are also using tranquillisers or antidepressants and these are totally unacceptable while diving.

Gastroenteritis

Viral infection of the gastrointestinal tract is extremely common. Occurring most frequently during spring and early summer, it almost vies in frequency with winter colds and coughs. Nausea, vomiting, abdominal cramps and diarrhoea, in any combination, occur.

A common bacterial variety is a 24-hour episode of diarrhoea and vomiting due to coliform bacteria following stool contamination of food. It is invariably self-limiting. The importance of these symptoms from a diver's point of view is threefold:

1. Cramps can cause underwater incapacity, and fluid loss predisposes to acute decompression illness.
2. The condition can occur while on holiday in a remote area and the diver must be able to cope alone with the situation.
3. The diver must be aware of the problem, obtain a prescription, and discuss the safe use of any of the following medications with his or her doctor before embarking on a diving trip to a remote destination.

Management of gastroenteritis

1. Stop all diving.
2. Stop any dairy product intake or fatty food consumption. All food should be bland, and boiled, baked or lightly grilled. Boiled chicken, fish, rice, pumpkin and potatoes, and thin soup are examples of suitable foods.
3. Encourage fluid intake. Replacement of lost body fluids is the cornerstone of treatment. Water, weak black tea, soda, and fruit juice diluted 1:1 with water are examples.
4. If nausea or vomiting persist, antiemetics are required. Many are available and include dimenhydrinate, metoclopramide, domperidone, cyclizine and prochlorperazine. If vomiting is the major feature, oral use of these drugs may be ineffective as they will be rejected almost as soon as they are swallowed. Rectal suppositories of cyclizine or prochlorperazine may then help. If frequent diarrhoea makes this impractical, an intramuscular injection by a doctor of an antiemetic such as cyclizine or prochlorperazine may be required.
5. Abdominal cramps are commonly handled by the use of antispasmodics such as hyoscine and atropine sulphate.
6. Diarrhoea can usually be controlled by dietary restriction and adequate fluid intake. If persistent, loperamide or diphenoxylate with atropine sulphate are usually effective. Binding agents containing the clay kaolin, apple pectin and milk of bismuth may also help.
7. In severe cases hospitalisation is required for intravenous replacement of fluid and electrolytes such as Ringer's lactate plus added potassium chloride to combat dehydration and electrolyte loss.

Salmonella and Shigella Enteritis

These bacterial diarrhoeas are most commonly spread by the stool/oral route – eating food contaminated by flies or prepared by infected food handlers with poor personal hygiene. In divers contamination can also occur after entering sewage-contaminated water. Enteric fever is caused by the *Salmonella* species. The *Shigella* species causes bacterial dysentery and, if water-spread, *Shigella* can survive up to three days in sea water. Diarrhoea may be profuse and mucus and blood may be present, with severe cramping pain and fever. Nausea and vomiting are common.

Management of bacterial diarrhoeas

Prevention
1. Try to determine whether any particular bacterial dysentery is currently prevalent in the area before embarking on the trip.
2. Speak to your doctor about the advisability of taking suitable antibiotic therapy, such as norfloxacin, with you on the trip.
3. Avoid eating dubious foods, possibly contaminated fruits and vegetables, and drinking local water in areas with primitive sanitation.
4. Ensure an adequate supply of bottled water or boil all water before drinking.
5. Avoid diving in areas contaminated by sewage.

Treatment
1. General management is on the same lines as gastroenteritis.
2. If fever becomes a persistent feature, or mucus and blood appear in the stool, medical assistance is necessary as the different bacteria have different sensitivities to antibiotics.
3. If medical help is unavailable, oral norfloxacin 400 mg twice a day for three days generally provides cover against all *Salmonella* and *Shigella* dysenteries. Previous discussion with and permission from a doctor is necessary, and norfloxacin must not be used before puberty.

Hiatus Hernia

The term hernia refers to the protrusion of any portion of the gut through a defect in any part of the wall of the abdomen. A hiatus hernia occurs when a segment of the stomach, near or at the entry of the foodpipe into the stomach, slides or rolls through a weakness in the diaphragm and into the chest cavity. This weakness exists where the foodpipe penetrates through the diaphragm to reach the stomach. It presents with a feeling of fullness in the upper abdomen, or frank heartburn, and commonly occurs at night in bed. Sitting up helps, as gravity then causes the herniated part of the stomach to fall back.

The importance of a hiatus hernia in divers relates to gear. Tight suits, straps, weight belts and buoyancy jackets may press on the abdomen and encourage herniation. Divers who equalise by air swallowing (aerophagia) may also develop difficulty if air trapping occurs at depth in a roll of herniated stomach. Acute pain due to expanding air on ascent may occur. Divers with hiatus hernias should ensure a comfortable fit of their gear, and divers who develop upper abdominal or low chest pain with diving or after diving should contact their doctors *re* the possibility of a hiatus hernia. In most cases dietary care, losing excess weight and occasional antispasmodics and antacids control the hernia. Only rarely is it so severe that surgery is required.

Other Hernias

There are several other potentially weak sites in the front of the abdominal wall through which bowel can herniate. The commonest places are the groins, the navel and the mid-abdomen after childbirth when the exertions of labour strain the vertical rectus muscles straddling the middle of the abdomen, leaving a gap between them.

Commercial divers may not dive with a hernia as their work demands heavy lifting. Sport divers are exposed to lifting of compressors and cylinders and should have their hernias repaired. The wound must be fully healed before diving begins again (three to six months, depending on the amount of boat handling, lugging and lifting done). The same would apply to any abdominal surgery.

Colostomies

Some diseases of the bowel, such as cancer, are of such a severe nature that the bowel or rectum has to be removed. The lower end of the remaining bowel is then brought through the front wall of the abdomen and joined to the surface of the skin. Emptying of the colon is done into a special bag placed over the opening.

Diving is not a problem, but care must be taken not to injure the delicate site of anastomosis by straps or a weight belt.

Ulcerative Colitis

This disease of unknown cause manifests as ulceration of the inner lining of the bowel and presents with diarrhoea, blood in the stool, abdominal pain, weakness and weight loss. It is treated symptomatically with drugs such as salazopyrine and cortisone. In some cases the colon has to be removed. It is a relapsing condition with periods of relative normalcy followed by episodes of acute recurrent bloody diarrhoea. Diving is generally prohibited.

Crohn's Disease

Also a disease of unknown cause, Crohn's disease results in patchy inflammation of the gut with thickening and scarring. It interferes with normal bowel motility and presents with pain. It may proceed to malignancy. Removal of affected bowel sections is commonly required. Diving is generally prohibited.

Pancreatitis

The commonest cause of an inflammation of the pancreas is long-term alcohol abuse, although a single episode of excessive alcohol abuse can also lead to irreparable damage to the pancreas. The pancreas produces digestive enzymes and damage results in abnormalities of digestion and food absorption. Liver damage due to alcohol is usually present too. Diving is prohibited. Pancreatitis may follow penetration of a peptic ulcer through the back wall of the stomach or duodenum into the pancreas behind. It can also occur if a gallstone blocks a common bile and pancreatic duct. Further diving would then depend on treatment and healing of the ulcer or gall bladder problem and the return of normal pancreatic function.

Hepatitis

Acute viral infections of the liver are not unusual and usually proceed to complete healing and recovery and subsequent life-long immunity. The commonest viruses causing the condition are Type A and Type B hepatitis viruses, although Types C, D and E also occur. The disease presents with jaundice, the staining of tissues including the skin and whites of the eyes with bile pigment as a result of obstruction of the normal bile flow from the liver and spillover of bile pigment into the blood. Hepatitis A is spread by direct contact with infected persons, and hepatitis B by blood contact, contaminated needles and syringes, and sexual contact. A vaccine immunising one against hepatitis B is readily available. Three injections, given over a few months, are required to ensure permanent immunity. It is highly recommended that every diver be immunised against hepatitis B. The chances of contamination by infected blood during a diver rescue or resuscitation attempt are very real.

Hepatitis is a considerable insult to the liver and diving should only be renewed six months after liver function tests have completely returned to normal. Hepatitis B may progress to chronic hepatitis, the person being apparently well but being an active carrier and capable of spreading the disease. Diving is then permanently prohibited. In severe cases of acute hepatitis of either type, permanent damage to the architecture of the liver may result, leading to scarring and cirrhosis of the liver. With chronic liver disease, obstruction to normal venous flow occurs with opening of venous shunts. Multiple arterio-venous shunts predispose to venous bubble spillover into the arterial system and arterial gas embolism. Diving is again permanently prohibited.

Diving Implications of Genitourinary Disease

Aside from chronic renal failure, kidney transplants and AIDS, disorders of the genitourinary system do not permanently bar sport diving.

Pregnant women should wait until the child is born before continuing diving. The reasons have been considered on pp 11-13. Kidney stones and urinary tract infections and obstructions should be properly investigated and treated before diving is continued.

Venereal diseases must be treated before diving again. This includes syphilis, gonorrhoea and herpes genitalis. AIDS poses special problems, and because of its growing threat to divers will be considered here in more detail.

AIDS

During the mid-1970s a killer virus spread silently and unnoticed to all five continents. Between 1981 and 1985 the virus was identified and the news of a brand-new, incurable and lethal sexually transmitted disease reached an unbelieving world. The Acquired Immune Deficiency Syndrome (AIDS) now threatens to be the greatest and most frightening epidemic the world has ever known. The disease is caused by the Human Immunodeficiency Virus (HIV) and two types of HIV disease have been found:

HIV-1

HIV-2

The HIV-2 epidemic originated and is still concentrated in West Africa, but has spread beyond its borders following emigration of HIV-2-afflicted locals or tourist sexual contact with infected West Africans. The HIV-1 epidemic was at first most prevalent among the homosexual population and intravenous drug abusers of North America, Brazil, Western Europe, Australia and New Zealand. A second pattern of spread from bisexuals to the heterosexual population occurred in sub-Saharan Africa, South America (particularly in Brazil), and in the Caribbean. A third, more recent spread, occurred through North Africa, the Middle East, Eastern Europe, Asia and the Pacific.

By mid-1992 the World Health Organisation (WHO) estimated 10 to 12 million people throughout the world were HIV-positive. Most, if not all, are doomed to die. And the incidence is increasing rapidly. The overwhelming majority (about 60 per cent of the world total) of cases are in sub-Saharan Africa, where much of the spread has been attributed to infected prostitutes passing the disease on to transport drivers working the Central African to South African routes. The highest incidence of HIV is found in Kenya, Zaire, Uganda, Tanzania, Zambia, Malawi, Mozambique and Zimbabwe where the disease is spreading at a horrific rate, with some estimated figures approaching well over half of the sexually active population in some areas of these countries. In South Africa the incidence is highest in the Natal-Zululand area, and lowest in the Western Cape. The disease has long since crossed the threshold into the heterosexual population and the initial factors of homosexuality and syringe-sharing among drug abusers have been overwhelmed and superseded by heterosexual promiscuity.

Methods of spread

1. Vaginal, anal or oral sexual contact with an infected partner.
2. Sharing contaminated needles among drug abusers.
3. Blood transfusions with HIV-infected blood.
4. Infection of the newborn by an HIV-positive mother.
5. Tattoos, acupuncture etc., with contaminated needles.
6. Needle-stick or scalpel injury in medical staff working with HIV-positive patients.
7. Giving CPR to an HIV-positive victim with blood in the airways.

The disease is only spread by infected blood or sexual contact. Mosquitoes have not been shown to carry the HIV virus. Kissing or saliva contact does not cause infection, unless blood is in the saliva, and nor do sweat or urine contact. Touching, sneezing, coughing, working together, sharing food utensils, towels and combs etc., cannot cause the spread of AIDS.

The disease process

There are several types of white blood cells in the body. Some act as scavengers, actively ingesting and destroying foreign bacteria and viruses. Others, such as the lymphocytes, are involved in the immune system. There are two main groups of lymphocytes – the T lymphocytes and the B lymphocytes. The HIV virus, once in a new host, invades a particular type of T lymphocyte – the T4 helper lymphocyte. These normally function by inducing B lymphocytes to produce antibodies, and other specialised cells to release substances toxic to invading organisms. Inside the T4 cell the HIV virus invades the cell genes and incorporates itself right into the DNA genetic material of the T4 cell. The cell loses its helper function and is reprogrammed into an HIV factory.

During the initial few months following infection with the disease, proliferation of the HIV virus is explosive, with the takeover of trillions and trillions of T4 cells. At this time there is no way of detecting the virus. The diagnosis depends on the detection of antibodies produced by the body in response to HIV invasion, and the virus attacks the very heart of antibody production – the T4 helper lymphocyte. The virus itself is not detectable, only the antibody response to its presence. This initial period of HIV negativity is called the *window period*. The person will test HIV-negative because antibodies are below detectable levels, but will be enormously infective to others because of the prodigious duplication of HIV virus that occurs during the window period.

Only after three to six months will the person convert to HIV positivity on testing a sample of blood, urine or saliva. It must be clearly understood that the test measures antibodies produced by the victim. It does not test for the virus itself, and only blood is infective. At this point the profound replication of the virus diminishes and may appear dormant for many years, but incidental infections demanding antibody production may reactivate HIV proliferation for a while. Finally the immune system fails and full-blown AIDS appears. It does not present as a disease in itself. It allows other infections to manifest. Diseases such as previous tuberculosis, long dormant and safely encapsulated in the body, may be reactivated or acquired for the first time. Other opportunistic diseases, which virtually never gain a lethal foothold in a healthy individual, appear. These include certain parasitic, bacterial, viral and fungal infections as well as some tumours.

Management

This is preventative only. There is no cure. Once HIV positivity becomes full-blown AIDS, the death rate is 100 per cent. HIV infection is due to escalate at a phenomenal pace now that it is well entrenched around the world, and sexual promiscuity has become a lethal game. Condoms, previously used to prevent pregnancy, must now be used to prevent death.

Diving and AIDS

HIV-positive persons should probably not dive, at least not without informing their buddies of the situation. There is a moral obligation because a rescuer may have to resuscitate a bleeding HIV victim. Ideally, this should also mean wearing a medic-alert necklace informing an unknowing rescuer that the victim is HIV-positive and precautions are necessary, but the ethical, personal and social ramifications of having HIV disease are still raging in most countries. Non-contact non-return mouth-to-mouth airways are available, but the problem with CPR is its urgency. A suitable airway would have to be immediately on hand at all times – on the dive boat, at the shore base, and perhaps even in the buddy's BC pocket. Suitable gloves, plastic aprons and goggles are also necessary to avoid inadvertent blood contact through existing skin injuries or via the eyes, should the victim be coughing or spluttering blood. The problem is a truly dreadful one, because an emergency can occur at any time on land or sea, and unwitting rescuers have already paid with their lives for saving an HIV-positive victim.

Once full-blown AIDS is present, diving must be totally barred.

Diving Implications of Endocrine Disease

Endocrine diseases involve the hormone-producing glands of the body — the pituitary, adrenal, thyroid, parathyroid, pancreas, testes and ovaries. Frank endocrine disease presents with serious symptoms and signs and results in immediate unfitness to dive. The one condition which is common and, like asthma, has been a bone of contention between divers and doctors for years is diabetes mellitus.

Diabetes mellitus

This disease is caused by failure of the beta cells of the islets of Langerhans in the pancreas to produce enough insulin, the primary glucose-controlling hormone. Diabetes occurs in two distinct forms:

1. Juvenile diabetes, which occurs in children and young adults and requires regular injections of insulin for control.
2. Maturity-onset diabetes which begins later in life and can usually be controlled by dietary restriction alone, or added oral therapy.

The difficulty with juvenile diabetes is that the sufferer is poised on a balance with coma on either side. Inadequate insulin can lead to coma due to an excessively high blood sugar level (hyperglycaemia). Excess insulin results in a very low glucose level (hypoglycaemia) which also causes coma. In the past, juvenile diabetes has been an absolute contraindication to diving. Control of diabetes has now become very sophisticated and most diabetics achieve excellent control by strict attention to diet, insulin injections and exercise. Most diving doctors still refuse permission to dive because of the risk of coma and the exercise and cold stresses of diving. Some diving physicians do permit well-controlled, fit and responsible insulin-dependent diabetics to dive, provided certain precautions are taken. It is almost invariably a low blood sugar that causes coma, the diver having had a dose of insulin and then omitting to eat. The blood sugar plunges and no glucose from food is available to restore the level. Coma and even death can result. The buddy must be educated about diabetes and be able to render assistance and glucose if needed. A supply of glucose must always be available on the boat. The diver must be under the care of a specialist in diabetic management and the situation and required precautions discussed between that specialist, the diving physician and the diver. Even then, the diver must realise that a significant risk is present and the responsibility remains his alone.

As the insulin-dependent diabetic ages, the secondary effects of diabetes may appear — hardening of arteries and kidney damage, among others. Diving must then be prohibited.

Maturity-onset diabetes presents with different problems. Coma is not usually a feature, but obesity and concurrent arterial disease often take its place. The latter two predispose to acute decompression illness. The safety of oral medications under diving conditions is another difficulty. If diet alone controls blood sugar levels and the patient is trim and fit, many doctors would permit diving.

Other endocrine disorders

Pituitary and adrenal gland diseases are immediately disqualifying for diving. These glands are involved in every vital function and diving becomes very dangerous. Thyroid disease has to be considered carefully. An underactive thyroid predisposes to very rapid hypothermia and all its complications, and drastically reduces a diver's ability to cope with exercise stress. An overactive thyroid predisposes to uncontrollable abnormalities of heart rate and rhythm under water. If the thyroid derangement is mild and well controlled, diving may be considered.

Barotrauma

Barotrauma refers to pressure damage to tissues. It results in forced volume changes in closed air spaces and occurs when air spaces cannot otherwise comply with pressure changes in accordance with Boyle's Law. There are two possibilities:
- increased pressure causes descent barotrauma,
- decreased pressure causes ascent barotrauma.

Descent Barotrauma

As a diver descends, the pressure around him increases. If this increase cannot be equalised in an air space its volume must decrease. If the air volume cannot decrease (for example, an air space in bone, a face mask, or a diving helmet), swelling of tissues and bursting of blood vessels occur to accommodate the required air volume decrease and equalise the pressure. This is called *squeeze*.

Ascent Barotrauma

This is the reverse problem. On ascent, an increase in volume occurs with the drop in pressure. If escape of the expanding gas cannot occur, explosive destruction of tissue can result.

An air space must be present for pressure/volume effects to occur. Such spaces occur in:
- the ear,
- the sinuses,
- the lungs,
- decayed teeth,
- the gut, and
- diving equipment.

Ear Barotrauma

A real understanding of ear barotrauma requires knowledge of the anatomy and working of the ear. This has been presented on pp 62-64.

External ear barotrauma of descent (External ear squeeze)

While diving, the external ear floods with water up to the ear drum. If water cannot enter the external ear due to wax lumps, ear plugs, or a tight hood or mask straps, a relative vacuum forms between the obstruction and the ear drum, and external ear squeeze occurs on descent.

Example
*   Flora has an ear completely blocked by a hard lump of wax. As she descends to 4 msw she develops sharp pain in the ear which is not relieved by equalising. She becomes very agitated and ascends noisily.

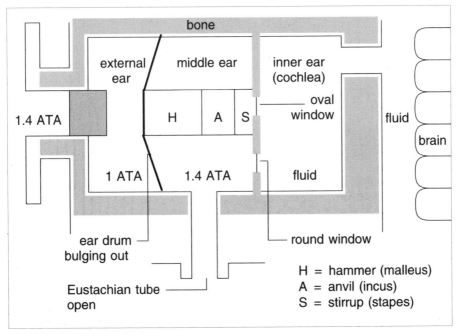

External ear squeeze

At 4 msw the pressure is 1.4 ATA. The pressure in Flora's external ear is still 1 ATA. Her ear drum bulges outwards to accommodate the decrease in volume, causing pain. A similar experience occurs with ear plugs, which must never be used in diving. Hoods should fit easily and admit water.

Middle ear barotrauma of descent (Middle ear squeeze)

The middle ear contains the three tiny bones (hammer, anvil and stirrup) involved in hearing; is always air filled; and communicates with the air in the back of the nose via the Eustachian tube.

The Eustachian tube allows air into and from the middle ear. At the surface it functions continuously, because oxygen in the air of the middle ear is constantly being absorbed by the membranes of the middle ear, creating a vacuum that the Eustachian tube corrects.

On descent, the Eustachian tube tends to block, and the increased pressure in the water-filled external ear pushes the ear drum inwards.

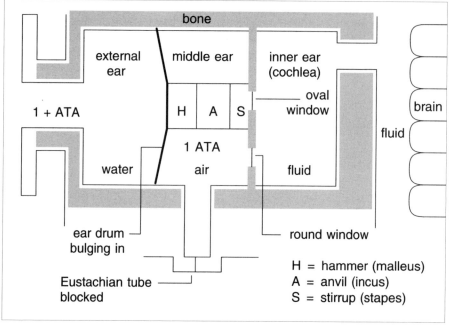

Middle ear squeeze

Air must be introduced into the middle ear to equalise the pressure. This can be done by swallowing, moving the jaws, or a Valsalva or Toynbee manoeuvre. These have the effect of opening the valve-like mouth of the Eustachian tube and letting air into the middle ear. This must be done continuously during descent, and especially frequently (at least once per breath) during the first 10 msw where volume changes are greatest.

If equalisation is omitted or delayed, the pressure in the nose presses the lips of the Eustachian tube together, blocking and then locking them. Equalisation is then impossible and the diver must ascend until equalisation is possible.

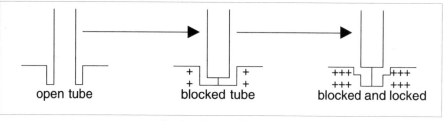

Omitted equalisation

If equalisation is not done: At 2 msw (1.2 ATA), the volume in the middle ear decreases by one-sixth; at 5 msw (1.5 ATA), by one-third, etc. This causes pain, due to inward bulging of the ear drum, swelling of the membranes lining the middle ear, and, if continued, bleeding into the cavity. This is middle ear squeeze (barotrauma of descent). Any bleeding in the middle ear commonly drains out of the Eustachian tube and presents as a trickle of blood from the nose after the dive.

Ear pain on descent followed by a nose bleed on ascent means that significant middle ear descent barotrauma has occurred. Repetitive dives will aggravate any damage and bleeding can easily recur. The diver may even find that equalising becomes easier with repetitive dives but this is because there is blood, tissue swelling, or both, in the middle ear. This reduces the air volume in the middle ear and causes apparent improvement and ease of equalising ability.

But after each dive the ear will feel blocked or deaf because of liquid interference with the middle ear's 22-times amplification system. This deafness may seemingly disappear during the next dive, but this is only because hearing by bone conduction operates under water. The middle ear is damped when the external ear canal is full of water. On surfacing and returning to hearing by air conduction, deafness will recur.

If the diver persists in descent without equalising, the ear drum may rupture. Pain and a loud noise herald the event then, as cold water enters the middle ear, pressure is equalised and pain disappears. Sudden vertigo and nausea may occur from the abrupt temperature drop in the middle ear, but this is usually temporary as the water in the ear quickly warms.

Causes of a blocked Eustachian tube
1. Failure to attempt equalising.
2. Upper respiratory infection e.g. a cold.
3. Nasal allergies e.g. hayfever.
4. Smoking.
5. Nasal polyps.
6. Use of oral isotretinoin in acne treatment.

Example
• Flora has her ears syringed and decides to try diving again. Unfortunately, she is allergic to her buddy Jimmy's aftershave *Sweaty Passion* and begins sneezing as her nose congests and blocks. Back at 4 msw, she cannot equalise, gets ear pain once again and surfaces very loudly. She has exchanged external ear squeeze for middle ear squeeze.

Squeeze may also be experienced in aircraft, especially unpressurised ones. On descent, the air pressure increases and air must enter the middle ear to equalise the pressure. This can be assisted by chewing during descent, swallowing, or holding one's nose and blowing. Only very rarely is pain experienced during ascent in an aircraft. In this case, the air pressure is decreasing, and the middle ear vents through the Eustachian tube. Any obstruction causes barotrauma of ascent as described below.

Note
Diving mammals such as whales and seals cannot and do not need voluntarily to equalise their middle ears on diving. They are protected against squeeze because they have large veins in their middle ears which simply distend with blood on descent to compensate air volume drop. Their round windows are buttressed with fibrous bands which give great strength.

Middle ear barotrauma of ascent

On ascent, the gas in the middle ear expands and the excess vents through the Eustachian tube. If the tube blocks, this escape cannot occur. Obstruction is usually caused by a plug of mucus or blood from a previous squeeze.

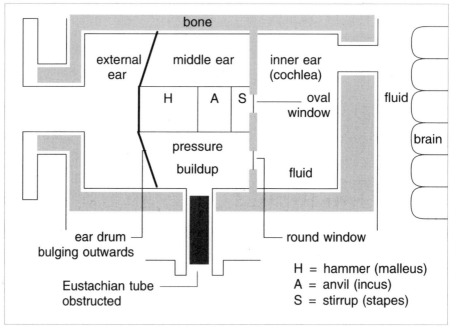

Middle ear barotrauma of ascent

Inner ear barotrauma of descent

The inner ear is the organ of hearing and balance. It is a fluid-filled space with its passage communicating with the fluid bathing the brain. As such, it is normally immune to pressure and volume changes, because no air spaces are involved.

Inner ear barotrauma occurs only with descent when the diver attempts to equalise with excessive force. Any increase in the pressure within the skull is transmitted to the fluid in the inner ear. The round window is the flexible membrane between the inner and middle ear that permits effective cochlear fluid movement with stirrup vibration in the oval window. (See Hearing in air p 64.) If the pressure of an equalising attempt becomes too high the round window bulges and bursts into the middle ear.

Example
- Poor Flora has been persuaded by Jimmy to try once again. At her favourite 4 metres, she still cannot equalise because Jimmy is still using *Sweaty Passion*, and her nasal lining is grossly swollen. Bravely, she endeavours pneumatically to blow her head off with an enormous equalising attempt. The pressure in her head builds up with the force of her blowing. This is transmitted through the fluid around her brain to the inner ear. The round window bulges, then bursts into the middle ear. Flora experiences immediate severe pain, vertigo and ringing in her ear (tinnitus). Clawing her way to the surface, she finds she is totally deaf in the ear and, screaming at Jimmy, she gives up diving and her allergy.

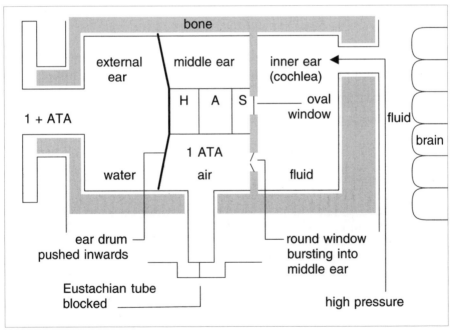

Inner ear barotrauma of descent

Round window rupture is a medical emergency. Cerebrospinal fluid in and around the brain will leak through the hole in the inner ear into the middle ear and then drain into the Eustachian tube. From there it reaches the nose and presents as a drip of clear brain fluid from a nostril. The nose is not sterile and the possibility of infection spreading from the nose to the inner ear to the brain is very high. Meningitis is an extreme hazard.

The sudden development of a clear nasal drip accompanied by deafness and vertigo after a maximal equalising attempt must be regarded as inner ear barotrauma. Immediate medical help must be sought. Do not blow the nose! Do not attempt any equalisation! Do not fly in an aircraft!

In the event of inner ear barotrauma occurring, surgery is necessary to repair the ruptured round window. Diving is then permanently prohibited.

Management of ear barotrauma

Prevention
1. Ear barotrauma, especially middle ear squeeze, is very common among novice divers. They are too concerned about monitoring depth, cylinder pressure and buoyancy to think about ears. Pain is the signal to equalise, but their Eustachian tubes are already blocked or locked. They ascend a few metres to relieve the pressure, equalise, then descend to their next pain level in a yo-yo descent to the bottom. Equalisation must be a constant process from the surface. If properly done with every exhalation the diver has no sensation of pain with increasing depth − only a reassuring clicking of the ear drums.
2. Don't dive if equalisation cannot be done at the surface because of a cold, nasal allergy or smoking. Have these treated and stop smoking. (See Management of nasal congestion p 77 and Management of equalising difficulties before a diving trip p 79.)
3. Wax lumps should be removed by a doctor before a diving trip. Do not use ear buds for cleaning ears. They damage the delicate membranes of the canals and open the way for infection.

Treatment. Any combination of deafness, a persistently blocked ear, tinnitus, vertigo and earache following equalising difficulty under water indicates ear barotrauma. Inner ear barotrauma must be suspected if partial or complete deafness, vertigo, nausea or vomiting, and loss of balance occur. Medical help is essential to establish the exact problem and treat the damage.
1. *Stop further diving.*
2. *Do not* use anaesthetic or antibiotic ear drops. It is essential first to exclude ear drum rupture. If the ear drum has been perforated the antibiotics used in most ear drops can cause permanent deafness. A doctor must be consulted.
3. Oral pain-killers may be used to alleviate earache.
4. Local heat, such as a warm bottle, may be soothing.
5. Take one 60 mg tablet of pseudoephedrine three times a day for five days.
6. Spray one puff of oxymetazoline nasal spray into each nostril three times a day, or instil three drops of oxymetazoline nasal drops into each nostril three times a day, for five days.

7. Oral antibiotics must be used after ear drum or round window rupture.

Sinus Barotrauma

Like the middle ear, the sinuses are air spaces in the bone of the skull with openings to the nose. Blockage of these openings occurs for the same reasons (see Disorders of the sinuses, p 80):

1. Upper respiratory infection e.g. a cold.
2. Nasal allergies e.g. hayfever.
3. Smoking.
4. Nasal polyps.

The sinuses do not have the valve system of the Eustachian tube, so active equalising is not possible. Exactly as with the middle ear, there can be sinus barotrauma of descent and ascent.

Example

•   Jimmy is trying to impress his new love, Philomina. *Sweaty Passion* has given him nasal congestion too, so at 6 msw he develops a tearing pain in the forehead above his nose. Equalising his mask gives a little relief, and he takes Philomina down to 12 msw to watch the sea cucumbers play. On ascent, the pain improves, and on surfacing, he smiles at his love, not knowing that his mask has a fluid level of green mucus and blood.

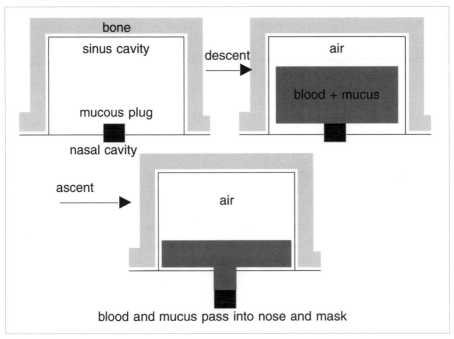

Sinus barotrauma of descent

Jimmy has had a frontal sinus squeeze (sinus barotrauma of descent). As with middle ear reverse block, sinus barotrauma of ascent can occur.

Dental Barotrauma

Teeth are incompressible, so the presence of gas pockets within them will cause problems with diving. This air can only arise from dental decay or with fillings that have trapped air in the tooth.

Dental squeeze

On descent, the pressure on the tooth increases. If the enamel over the cavity is thin, the tooth can implode.

Dental barotrauma of ascent

Gas that has entered a cavity in a tooth at depth may become trapped by a fold of gum tissue. On ascent, pressure decreases, volume increases, and the tooth can explode.

Management of dental barotrauma
Prevention
1. Divers must take care of their teeth. All fillings must be firm and healthy.
2. Inform your dentist that you scuba dive. He will then pay particular attention to potential trouble.

Treatment. This is directed at pain relief before seeing a dentist.
1. Oral pain-killers should be used.
2. If pain is very severe pressing a small wad of cotton wool soaked with alcohol on the tooth may help. This could be whisky or other spirits.
3. Oil of cloves is also useful. Grip a small wad of cotton wool soaked in the oil between the jaws at the site of the affected tooth.
4. If available, lignocaine spray (two sprays every three hours) on to the tooth will provide some relief.

Equipment Barotrauma

Any piece of diving equipment containing an air space is a potential cause of diver barotrauma. Most are minor injuries only, but some can kill.

Mask squeeze

Mask squeeze occurs for two main reasons:
— the diver fails to equalise his or her mask;
— the mask is too large.
It is interesting that divers who struggle to equalise their middle ears very rarely get mask squeeze; and divers who do develop mask squeeze

generally do so because they can equalise their middle ears *too* easily – for example, by a small movement of the jaw from side to side. This is enough to open their Eustachian tubes and allow air under pressure to enter the middle ears. But it allows no air to pass through the nose into the mask because the rubber nose piece is firmly pressed by water pressure against the openings of the nostrils. Voluntary snorting or blowing is required to push air past the nose seal and into the mask. Divers with middle ear equalising problems snort vast amounts of air into their masks as they hold their noses and strenuously blow. A puff of nasal air always occurs on releasing the nose while blowing to equalise.

Large masks are unnecessary and ill-advised. They are unnecessary because refraction of light at a water/glass/air interface limits the angle of view to 97.2 degrees anyway. (See Underwater vision p 82.) A large mask protruding further from the face will only reduce this angle of view by providing a small tunnel to peer through. The ill-advisedness lies in the large volume of air required to equalise pressure changes on descent. This becomes even more apparent on a breathhold dive when the amount of air available for mask equalisation is both limited and shrinking with every metre of increasing depth.

Treatment of mask squeeze is non-specific. Aescin and heparinoid gel assist to relieve swelling, but care must be taken to avoid the eyes. Diving must stop until all bruising clears.

Skin barotrauma

This occurs most commonly when dry suits or baggy wet suits are worn. Pockets of air are trapped between folds in the suit, and descent causes these spaces to contract. The skin is sucked into the folds and welts or bruising can occur. No treatment is required and the diver is invariably pain-free.

Head and body barotrauma of descent (diver's squeeze)

This is the greatest potential fault of freeflow systems using a copper or hard helmet. With freeflow systems, air or a breathing mix is supplied through a hose from the surface to the diver. A constant excess of gas is delivered to flush out exhaled carbon dioxide and prevent accumulation of the gas. If a Standard Diver's hoses break, or if he descends too fast, the surrounding water pressure increases more rapidly than can be maintained by his air supply. In the worst case, his whole body and suit will be squeezed up into his copper helmet. A non-return valve on the helmet prevents this in the event of hose rupture, and careful control of descent is mandatory.

Suit barotrauma of ascent ('blow up')

This occurs classically with a Standard Diving Suit, but can result from accidental underwater inflation of any buoyancy accessory – dry suits, buoyancy compensators and counterlungs in closed-circuit rebreathing units. 'Blow up' in scuba divers most commonly occurs as a result of neglecting to dump air used for buoyancy control at depth once the ascent has begun. Failure to vent expanding air causes the suit or BC bladder to inflate like a balloon (Boyle's Law), and the diver then rockets to the surface (Archimedes' Principle).

This can cause pulmonary barotrauma of ascent, arterial gas embolism, acute decompression illness, diver entrapment in a tightly inflated suit, and diver injury, for example a forceful collision with the bottom of the dive boat.

Pulmonary Barotrauma

Pressure-volume damage inside the fixed space of the chest is *the most dangerous* of all pressure injuries. The two most vital life-support organs in the body — the lungs and the heart — are directly affected, and significant derangement then affects brain function.

As with all barotraumas, a fixed gas space (air in the lungs) is involved, with obstruction of the passage (the bronchial tree) to atmosphere. The problem may be descent or ascent.

Pulmonary barotrauma of descent (chest squeeze or lung squeeze)

Chest squeeze cannot occur while breathing normally on scuba. Regulated air pressure maintains lung pressure at ambient. Among sport divers the condition is limited to breathhold divers who descend beyond their depth limit, which depends on two things:
— the diver's residual volume,
— the distensibility of blood vessels.
As residual volume is the fixed volume of the bronchi and bronchioles in both lungs, it follows that at residual volume depth all the air in all the alveoli is now in the bronchial tree. All the alveoli are completely flattened, the rib cage is tremendously compressed, the diaphragm is sucked up high into the chest, and the lungs are a solid mass of tissue penetrated by more rigid tubules pressurised to the particular depth.

Further descent cannot be compensated for by a decrease in alveolar volume. The large veins in the chest begin to dilate with blood to accommodate continued air volume decrease as maximum breathhold depth is reached. Then rupture of veins, haemorrhage and death occur. Further descent results in crushing and collapse of the ribs and chest.

Causes
1. Breathhold diving, especially attempts at depth records.
2. Excessive speed of descent with Standard Diving Equipment, also leading to diver's squeeze into the helmet.
3. Losing surface pressure with Standard Diving Equipment and the absence of a non-return valve on the helmet.

Treatment
1. Treat for shock (see pp 175, 219).
2. 100% oxygen.
3. Summon emergency medical help.

Pulmonary barotrauma of ascent (burst lung)

This is precisely the reverse of lung squeeze. The diver begins with normal lung volumes safely balanced at depth pressure and then develops overpressurisation and bursting of lung tissue on returning to the surface. It is usually the alveoli that distend and burst because they are the thinnest-walled (one cell thick). Inadequate exhalation of expanding gas distorts their normal grape-like configuration and they distend like blown-up rubber gloves, with their capillary network tautly stretched around them. With total lung involvement, the ribs are forced out tightly and the diaphragm is driven down into the abdomen. The ultimate release of pressurised gas is not a gentle process. When the elastic limit of the lungs is reached, shredding of lung tissue occurs with rapid liberation of pressurised gas.

Causes of pulmonary barotrauma of ascent. The following are the usual causes and, except for the lung disorders, all are related to inadequate underwater techniques:
1. PANIC, with an attempt at an emergency ascent.
2. Free ascents, especially uncontrolled free ascents, and submarine escape training.
3. Skip breathing, with a diver attempting to conserve air by breath-holding and being unaware that he or she is ascending.
4. Buddy breathing at depth becoming uncoordinated and leading to panic.
5. Inability to gain comfortable and relaxed control of the regulator during ditch and recovery training, resulting in the abandonment of the exercise in favour of a hurried return to the surface.
6. Apparatus difficulties, such as a high regulator resistance to inhalation because of an almost empty air cylinder.
7. Water inhalation, causing choking, panic and laryngospasm, with frantic attempts to reach the surface.
8. Lung disorders, such as asthma and chest infections with a high resistance to outflow or mucous plugs blocking bronchioles.

All cause internal air trapping and inadequate exhalation. The degree of damage and the effects on the diver depend on the speed of ascent, the size of the pressure differential, whether the injury is localised to a small area or generalised, and the presence of any underlying lung disorder in the diver, such as asthma or a respiratory infection. Pressurised gas, bubbling or gushing out of torn alveolar units, can cause any combination of the following four presentations:

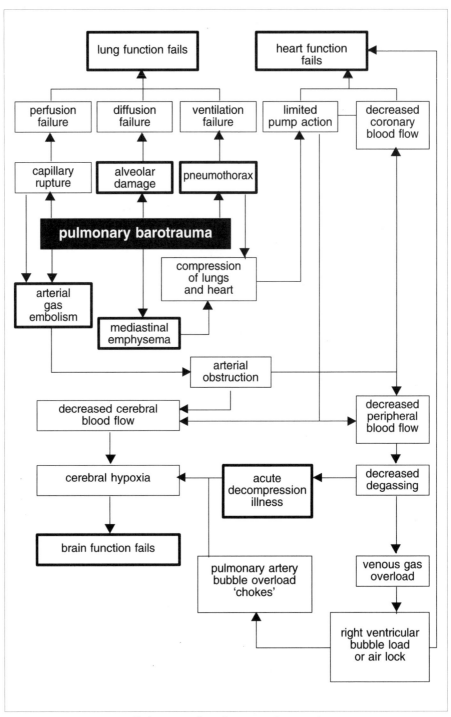

Pulmonary barotrauma of ascent

1. **Lung tissue damage.** Alveolar and surrounding connective tissue damage results in a reduction in the number of functional alveolar units. If extensive, this decreases ventilation ability. Rampant membrane disruption causes diffusion failure and the inevitable accompanying damage to the capillary supply causes perfusion insufficiency, failure of gas exchange, and respiratory failure.

Presentation. At the surface, pressurised gas gushes through the trachea and larynx and whistles out of the mouth as a high-pitched cry. The diver is breathless, has chest tightness or pain, and coughing produces blood-stained sputum. If damage is extensive, death will occur.

2. **Mediastinal emphysema.** Alveolar rupture may be followed by gas tracking along the slack tissue layer around bronchi and blood vessels to reach the root of the lung, the major bronchi and blood vessels, and the heart — all in the mediastinum — the very centre of the chest. The trapping of gas here is called *mediastinal emphysema*. Further tracking can occur — under the pericardium, the fibrous sac lining the heart, to cause a pneumopericardium with free gas around the heart; down through the diaphragm and into the peritoneal cavity, to cause a pneumoperitoneum with free gas around the intestines and swelling of the abdomen; or up into the neck as far as the jaw. Here it can be felt as a 'crackling' under the skin. This is called *subcutaneous* or *surgical emphysema*.

In scuba diving the commonest cause of mediastinal emphysema is ascent with a near-empty air cylinder. The high resistance to inhalation results in long slow inspirations with air expanding in the lungs all the while as the diver ascends to enable the regulator to deliver the last vestiges of air. It is imperative that divers do not delay ascent until their cylinders are virtually empty. At a cylinder pressure of 50 ATA the ascent must begin.

Presentation. As free gas may be present in connective tissue planes anywhere from inside the abdomen to the jaw, the effects on the diver may be variable. With extensive gas tracking, the onset is instantaneous. In milder instances the presentation may be delayed for hours. In most cases the effects of air in the neck and mediastinum are felt, and the onset is delayed. The neck feels 'full', the voice is hoarse or brassy, and chest discomfort and breathlessness are present. Coughing may worsen matters by driving more gas into the mediastinum. The effects of compression become felt. Shortness of breath increases and the diver becomes blue *(cyanosis)*. Pressure on the foodpipe causes difficulty in swallowing; compression of the great veins and heart results in a fast thready pulse with a drop in blood pressure, going on to a decreased blood supply to the brain, unconsciousness and shock.

It must also be remembered that the free gas in the tissues is not stable air. It is postdive gas and the surrounding tissues may have a substantial dissolved nitrogen load. At the surface the free gas obeys Boyle's Law and expands until its pressure is ambient. Degassing of tissues is also occurring and nitrogen will be delivered to adjacent free gas which will increase in volume. Delayed worsening must therefore be anticipated.

3. **Arterial gas embolism.** Simultaneous alveolar and capillary rupture can result in a direct hook-up between the respiratory and cardiovascular systems. Gas in the lungs can be vented directly into the blood to reach the general body circulation. This is *Arterial Gas Embolism (AGE)*.

It does not occur while the lungs are tightly inflated during the ascent from depth because the low-pressure capillaries surrounding the alveoli are stretched and compressed flat by the tightly distended alveoli. It follows the first exhalation after lung-tearing. Blood flow through capillaries then resumes and alveolar air is sucked into them with each inspiration. Once inside the blood, gas bubbles form and pass via the pulmonary vein to the left atrium and ventricle. Within the heart, the powerful pumping of the left ventricle may churn larger bubbles into myriads of tiny bubbles which in turn are sprayed into the aorta and reach the coronary or cerebral arteries, or the arteries of any organ or tissue in the body. Bubbles do not have to be large to be lethal, nor is a large volume of gas required. Bubbles as small as 0.03 mm in the coronary or cerebral arteries can cause grave trouble, and when AGE is accompanied by mediastinal emphysema or lung tissue damage the diver is in very dire straits.

But, once again, the diver may have significant coexisting decompression commitments and AGE with obstruction of the blood supply to an organ or tissue will prevent effective degassing and removal of nitrogen from the area affected. Under these conditions even a minor tissue gas load, not normally requiring any in-water decompression stops, can cause acute decompression illness. Carbon dioxide build-up in oxygen-starved tissues will also drive excess dissolved nitrogen out of solution in those tissues. Computer and table predictions regarding safe decompression no longer apply. They are based on a normal blood supply to tissues. It must not be assumed that a diver who develops AGE after a short non-repetitive shallow dive cannot develop acute decompression illness – he or she can, and precisely in the area already damaged by AGE.

Presentation. Any diver who develops any untoward neurological symptoms immediately after a dive must be presumed to have AGE and this is a diving medical emergency. Do not wait to see what develops! Begin first-aid treatment! Summon trained medical help urgently!

Cerebral Arterial Gas Embolism (CAGE) is the commonest manifestation, probably because the diver ascends and suffers lung-bursting in the vertical position which encourages bubble flow to the head. Placing the diver in the now-prohibited head-down Trendelenburg position would encourage bubble entry into the coronary arteries with resulting additional heart damage.

(a) Brain damage presents in three ways:
 – impairment of the higher faculties, such as confusion, disorientation, unconsciousness and convulsions;
 – impairment of motor function, such as weakness, abnormal gait,

incoordination and paralysis;
— impairment of sensory function, such as blurred vision, blindness, loss of balance, vertigo and numbness.
(b) Heart damage presents with tightness in the chest or constricting chest pain, sweating, extreme paleness, faintness, a rapid, weak pulse with an irregular rhythm, and breathlessness.
Both types of damage may progress to death.

4. **Pneumothorax.** Compressed gas ruptures through the pleural lining of the lung, enters the pleural space and the lung collapses. The effects are identical to those of a tension pneumothorax (see pp 40-41).

Presentation. A pneumothorax is usually a sudden event and presents during the ascent or soon after the dive. The usual features are sudden pain on the involved side — worse on breathing in; the need for rapid shallow breaths with inability to breathe deeply; a feeling of tightness in the chest; and the development of shock.

Examples of pulmonary barotrauma of ascent
• Konrad was a scuba diving instructor, aged 32. He had a cold but had no one else to take his Openwater I class on their first sea dive. After diving for 40 minutes at 12 msw, he surfaced, feeling well. About two hours later, he felt weak, had difficulty in getting enough air and had mild chest discomfort. He went to see his doctor when his voice became tinny. The examination revealed subcutaneous emphysema and the X-ray chest showed air in his mediastinum and neck.
  Diagnosis: Pulmonary barotrauma of ascent with mediastinal emphysema.
  Treatment: He recovered speedily on 100% oxygen alone.
• Harry was on holiday on a tropical island. The water was warm so he dived without his wet suit. At 20 msw he accidentally brushed against a reef of fire coral. Startled by sudden intense pain in his leg, he made for the surface. While swimming toward the moored dive boat, he noticed that his chest was painful and his breathing difficult. His dive leader immediately took him to the local doctor who, worried about possible AGE, decided to recompress Harry in a chamber. At a depth of 18 msw and breathing pure oxygen, Harry's discomfort disappeared. During decompression, breathlessness recurred at 10 msw and Harry was recompressed to 18 msw, this time with only little relief. Any attempt to reduce the pressure caused severe breathlessness and pain. Really worried now, the doctor called his partner who examined Harry in the chamber and diagnosed a pneumothorax. A one-way needle valve was used to drain the free air in Harry's pleural cavity and decompression was safely accomplished while Harry breathed pure oxygen.
• Stan was an inexperienced diver doing his first night dive. On ascent, he became panicky at 12 msw and inflated his BC. He rocketed to the surface, gave a high-pitched cry, coughed up blood, and lost conscious-

ness. He was quickly rescued from the water. He had stopped breathing. Cardiopulmonary resuscitation was commenced and an emergency rescue service was summoned. All attempts at resuscitation were futile and Stan was pronounced dead by the doctor of the emergency team.

Diagnosis: Pulmonary barotrauma of ascent with cerebral arterial gas embolism.

Management of pulmonary barotrauma of ascent
Action
1. Have someone notify the nearest recompression facility to prepare the chamber and summon a diving physician.
2. Administer continuous 100% oxygen via a face mask. This is to ensure that any further bubbles will be oxygen, not nitrogen, and to increase the available oxygen to the brain and tissues.
3. Some authorities recommend the 'knee-elbow' position immediately and up to 10 minutes after surfacing. Beyond this time, it *should not* be used. The diver is placed on his or her knees and elbows with the left shoulder lower than the right. The objective is to gravitate bubbles away from the brain. The position should be maintained for 10 minutes, then the diver should be laid flat.
4. Keep the diver quiet and as relaxed as possible. Further movement or coughing may increase lung damage or cause more air to be vented into the blood.
5. Keep the diver flat. Do not use the Trendelenburg position (head down with body and legs elevated about 30 degrees). If unconscious, the diver should be placed in a 15 degrees left lateral position with the head to the side to avoid inhalation should vomiting occur.
6. Cardiopulmonary resuscitation may be needed. (AIDS awareness!)
7. Set up a Ringer's lactate intravenous lifeline if a trained person is at hand, and urgently transport the diver to a hyperbaric centre by road, helicopter, or low-flying aeroplane, whichever is the fastest.
8. Recompression to 50 m on Table 63 (Royal Navy) or 6A (US Navy) is *only* indicated for neurological AGE. *Do not recompress a pure pneumothorax* − it will convert to a life-threatening tension pneumothorax. With no neurological AGE, chest drainage and *oxygen at surface pressure* are required. If both neurological AGE and a pneumothorax are present, then both chest drainage and recompression are needed.

Gastrointestinal Barotrauma

Gas in the stomach and intestines expands on ascent, and if air is swallowed during the dive, painful and occasionally dangerous distension may occur.

Causes
1. Air swallowing to equalise, especially in the head-down position, when air will enter the stomach.
2. Drinking carbonated beverages under hyperbaric conditions. This occurs occasionally during chamber pressurisations but more commonly among sport divers drinking champagne under water while coordinating a thumb over the opening of the bottle to prove their diving expertise!

Management of gastrointestinal barotrauma
The condition is usually self-limiting, being relieved by belching or passing flatus. The discomfort may also be eased by removing any constricting belts, straps, wet suits, etc.

Decompression

Decompression is a time-dependent process whereby excess inert gas absorbed by the tissues during an increase in environmental pressure is liberated by the lungs on reduction of ambient pressure. In simpler terms, excess nitrogen absorbed by the body during a dive is exhaled during ascent and after surfacing.

Tissue Uptake of Inert Gas during Compression

When a diver breathing air is exposed to increased pressure under water, each contraction of the right ventricle sends a surge of venous blood to the lungs for oxygen renewal and carbon dioxide extraction. It also results in nitrogen loading of blood in divers. The prodigious size of the alveolar-capillary area in the lungs ensures virtually instant saturation of lung capillary blood with nitrogen at the new higher nitrogen partial pressure (Henry's Law and Dalton's Law).

This nitrogen load is carried in the arterial system to the body tissues where capillary-tissue gas transfer occurs. With time and repeated recirculation of the blood volume to the lungs, the tissues will eventually have the same nitrogen partial pressure as the alveoli. The tissues are then in equilibrium with the alveoli and are said to be *saturated* at that partial pressure of nitrogen. No further uptake of nitrogen will occur. This occurs on land too. A person living at Lake Titicaca at an altitude of 3 600 metres above sea level will have a nitrogen partial pressure of about 0.51 ATA in his or her tissues. On arrival at the coast for a diving holiday, tissue nitrogen will equilibrate over 24 hours to the higher coastal air nitrogen partial pressure of 0.79 ATA.

Tissue uptake of a gas depends on:
1. Solubility of the gas in a tissue.
2. Blood supply to the tissue.
3. Time.
4. Depth.
5. Gas gradient.

1. Solubility

Different tissues have different solubilities for the same gas. For example, nitrogen is about five times more soluble in fat than in water. This means that fatty tissues can dissolve about five times more nitrogen than blood can. It also means that fatty tissues take a long time to saturate, and blood, with its lower solubility for nitrogen, rapidly saturates.

2. Blood supply

Although the total capillary-tissue exchange area in the body is incredibly colossal, being around ten thousand square metres in an average individual, blood volume is not (about six litres), so only a limited amount of inert gas can be carried in the blood at any one time. It is also only the arterial portion of the blood that is transporting the higher partial pressure of inert gas from lungs to tissues.

In addition, some tissues have a rich blood supply, such as muscle, the brain and the spinal cord, and saturate quickly. Others, such as fat, have a much poorer blood supply. In the case of fat, it has a high solubility for nitrogen and a poor blood supply and therefore saturates more slowly than any other tissue. But, once saturated, a large nitrogen load is present, which then desaturates very slowly.

3. Time

As tissue saturation depends on blood circulation, time becomes an important factor because blood circulation requires time. Each minute, an average heart circulates about four to six litres of blood through the systemic circulation, and an identical amount through the lung vessels. Long exposures to pressure therefore cause greater nitrogen uptake than short periods.

4. Depth

At depth, partial pressures of inhaled gases increase (Dalton's Law) and the amount of inert gas diffusing from alveoli into blood increases proportionally (Henry's Law). The deeper the dive, the greater the gradient from alveoli to blood to tissues.

5. Gas gradient

At the seaside, a diver is exposed to nitrogen at 0.79 ATA. Body tissues saturate with nitrogen at 0.75 ATA because in the alveoli, inspired air is mixed with outgoing carbon dioxide and water vapour which dilute air nitrogen a little. Should a diver dive to 50 msw, the nitrogen partial pressure in his air supply increases six times to 4.74 ATA. So, at the beginning of his 6 ATA exposure, the gradient between alveoli and tissues increases by 4.74 minus 0.75 ATA or 3.99 ATA.

It is important to appreciate what this really means — a pressure of nearly 4 ATA is not just a number. It is a huge pressure differential. It will burst a motor car tyre! The diver can only survive because the total gas pressure inside his lungs and the water pressure around the body are exactly balanced and equal. But the absolute amounts of nitrogen — in the air supply and in solution in the tissues — are now very different. A pressure head of nearly four atmospheres of nitrogen gas in alveoli is separated from the blood in lung capillaries by only two membranes of extreme delicacy — each one cell thick. Nitrogen gas speedily diffuses through this insignificant and almost ridiculous barrier, passes into solution in blood, and is carried to the tissues and loaded there.

With time, the concentration of nitrogen in muscle, say, increases to 2.74 ATA. The gradient is then 4.74 minus 2.74 ATA or 2 ATA, so nitrogen absorption into muscle slows. The uptake is *exponential* and a progressive slowing of uptake occurs as the gradient falls. Initial uptake is very vigorous and speedy; later uptake progressively slows, then stops when the gradient disappears at saturation.

Inert Gas Loss by the Tissues — Decompression

The biggest difference between the loading and unloading of tissues with inert gas, is that tissue gas loading is *passively receptive* whereas decompression is *actively driven* by tissue gas pressures and can be explosive. While a tissue may be remarkably tolerant to a horrific gas gradient during uptake, Henry's Law can either gently drive a gas from a tissue and along a small gradient to the lungs for exhalation, or send the gas bubbling and boiling out of solution inside a tissue if the gradient is too high. As soon as free gas is present, Boyle's Law operates and expands the free gas volume to ambient surface pressure. This is the picture of acute decompression illness. The complete process is equivalent to preparing soda water — the water passively absorbs carbon dioxide from the gas cartridge during pressurisation, but sudden release of pressure by rapidly opening the bottle causes instant bubbling. The whole idea of using decompression tables is the establishment of gentle gas gradients which avoid bubbling.

Decompression theory

John Scott Haldane, an English doctor, physiologist and President of the Institute of Mining Engineers, did much of the basic work on decompression in the early 1900s. He proposed two hypotheses:

First hypothesis. Both nitrogen uptake and release from the tissues follow an exponential gas gradient, and all the tissues in the body can be represented by five theoretical model tissues having half times of 5, 10, 20, 40 and 75 minutes.

Blood is the fastest tissue with a half time of 5 minutes. This means that during a dive, saturation of blood with nitrogen can be considered in blocks of 5 minutes. In the first 5 minutes blood will absorb half of the maximum volume of gas it can dissolve at that depth. It is half-saturated in 5 minutes. During the next 5 minutes blood will absorb half as much again, i.e. one quarter. It will be three-quarters saturated. After another 5 minutes, half of a quarter or one-eighth will be absorbed and blood will be seven-eighths saturated, then fifteen-sixteenths, and so on. The same applies to the slower tissues, except that they half-saturate in blocks of 10 minutes to 75 minutes. After 6 half times a tissue is saturated.

Release of gas during decompression follows a reverse exponential gradient. Blood would lose half of its excess dissolved nitrogen in the first 5 minutes; half of the remainder in the next 5 minutes; etc. After 6 half times a tissue is desaturated. Blood desaturates in 30 minutes.

Second hypothesis. Divers can tolerate a doubling of the nitrogen partial pressure in their tissues on returning to the surface after a dive and still not suffer from acute decompression illness. Haldane called this *super-saturation.*

He believed that ambient pressure could be halved, so causing the tissue tensions to be twice environmental pressure without bubble formation. That is, decompression could be done from:

2 ATA to 1 ATA (10 msw to the surface),

4 ATA to 2 ATA (30 msw to 10 msw),

5 ATA to 2.5 ATA (40 msw to 15 msw),

etc., in safety. This 2:1 ratio, or *critical ratio* hypothesis, is the basis of many current stage decompression tables. Haldane recommended its use to 50 msw. For deeper dives, the system is inadequate as such.

Combining the two hypotheses into practical terms means that different tissues control safe ascent at different times. Ascent rates, and depth and time of decompression stops must ensure that at no time is any tissue loaded with inert gas by more than 2:1. At the beginning of ascent the 5 minute tissue will dictate safe ascent. When it is desaturated to below 2:1, the 10 minute tissue will begin to set the safe ascent limits, and so on. A decompression stop with any tissue saturated to more than double the water pressure will cause bubbling in that tissue.

Haldane was actively opposed by Leonard Hill, who believed that decompression should be continuous and uniform. Hill's technique is now used in decompression from saturation, i.e. a *linear* decompression, not *staged,* as with Haldane. For very long deep dives, the five model tissue half times are insufficient and many others have been added by different scientists, some using half times of up to 12 hours! The 2:1 ratio was also found to be too simple, because some model tissues have different critical ratios at different depths. The concept of *M values* was introduced by Workman in America. This stipulates the maximum ratio of super-saturation for each model tissue at varying depths.

Behnke's oxygen window. The big question with Haldane's work was, 'Why can tissues retain gas at double ambient pressure without bubbling in the first place?' Work by Behnke showed that one reason is oxygen use by tissues. As oxygen is used by a tissue, its partial pressure falls in the tissue. This means that the total gas pressure in the tissue drops. A 'space' is formed which nitrogen can fill — the so-called *oxygen window*.

Hill's unsupersaturation. Okinawan divers, diving for pearls off Australia, perform 90 msw dives on air for 60 minutes, twice a day, six days a week, without any theoretical tables. Using only the weight of experience, they have developed their own tables. These are about 30 per cent shorter than the US Navy tables, use deeper in-water stops and no stops shallower than about 9 msw. Hill studied these and, in 1966, proposed the concept of *unsupersaturation*. Venous blood and tissues have a total gas pressure which is less than ambient air at the surface — nearly 0.1 ATA less, due mainly to low oxygen. They are technically gas vacuums. So if a diver ascends one metre, nitrogen can take up the 0.1 ATA to saturate the tissue. A nitrogen gradient to alveoli is then established, and more nitrogen is vented. This restores another 0.1 ATA of unsaturation for nitrogen occupation.

The two concepts, oxygen window and unsaturation, permit the tables that enable a diver to ascend safely with nitrogen supersaturation but little or no bubble formation. The *oxygen window* can be increased enormously by breathing pure oxygen (0% nitrogen) during decompression. If no nitrogen is inhaled, a very high gradient for elimination of nitrogen is set up. The gradient becomes the difference between tissue nitrogen content and zero in the inhaled gas — maximum possible gradient at the surface. If a recompression chamber is now used, breathing pure oxygen at pressure further increases the gradient and actively drives oxygen into, and nitrogen from, tissue cells. In addition, the extra chamber pressure effectively keeps all potential bubbles in solution. This is the basis of all oxygen decompression tables and oxygen therapeutic tables for arterial gas embolism and acute decompression illness.

Bubble behaviour

Consider a bubble inside a tissue. Inside the bubble is gas under pressure. Call the pressure in the bubble Pb. If the pressure around the bubble is less than Pb, the bubble will grow. If the surrounding pressure is greater than Pb, the bubble will shrink. The pressure around the bubble consists of:

Ambient environmental pressure (Pressure ambient) — Pa.

Tissue pressure on the bubble (Pressure of tissues) — Pt.

Surface tension of the bubble (Pressure of tension) — Pτ.

The total pressure on the bubble is Pa + Pt + Pτ.

If Pb is greater than Pa + Pt + Pτ, the bubble will enlarge.

If Pb is smaller than Pa + Pt + Pτ, the bubble will shrink.

If Pb equals Pa + Pt + Pτ, the bubble is stable.

If Pb is much smaller than Pa + Pt + Pτ, the bubble will redissolve. It is apparent that to treat or eliminate a bubble (bend), one must increase Pa or Pt or Pτ or all three. To date, there is no way of increasing the surface tension (Pτ). Increasing Pa (ambient pressure) is done, that is, recompression in a chamber. Substances having high molecular weights such as dextran are also available for increasing the osmotic pressure in the blood in an attempt to increase tissue pressure in blood (Pt).

Where do bubbles appear? Bubbles can originate anywhere, but most are found in the venous system because the venous system drains and transports inert gas from all tissues to the lungs during the degassing process. In addition, the veins are very low pressure systems, so venous Pt is low. The arterial system, in contrast, has the highest Pt because of left ventricular pump pressurisation and the lowest inert gas load because arterial blood has been subjected to lung degassing of nitrogen.

Venous bubbles pass through the right side of the heart and into the pulmonary arteries, arterioles and capillaries. Direct transfer of gas from bubbles to alveoli can then occur. Although there is always some venous bubble transport after any dive, under normal conditions most of the inert gas load is transferred in solution to the lungs for exhalation.

If the number of venous bubbles reaching the right ventricle is excessive, or if they coalesce to form big bubbles, an air-lock in the right ventricle may occur, leading to death. Or the pulmonary arteries may become overloaded with bubbles, causing right heart failure and shock — the 'chokes'. Shunts between the right and left sides of the heart can shift bubbles en route to the lungs back into the arterial circulation as nitrogen emboli. (See pp 20-22.)

Bubbles do not have to reach the chest to cause trouble. They can be problematic anywhere. Obstruction in spinal veins can cause paralysis. Bubbles can form directly in brain tissue causing acute cerebral decompression illness; in joints, causing limb bends; in the fluid-filled labyrinth of the inner ear, giving rise to deafness or vertigo. If they form in arteries, they can embolise, for example to the brain, exactly like arterial gas embolism after pulmonary barotrauma.

Acute Decompression Illness

Acute decompression illness is a disease associated with the development of free gas or bubbles in blood or tissues due to a decrease in ambient pressure. Until recently, this disease was called *Decompression Sickness* or *DCS*. This term and its classification into Type I and Type II DCS have been permanently dropped in favour of a new descriptive term — acute decompression illness.

Acute decompression illness is caused by:
— inert gas bubble formation after a dive;
— pulmonary barotrauma of ascent.

Both result in tissue damage or obstruction to blood flow which then interferes with the oxygen supply to the area involved.

Factors Predisposing to Bubble Formation in Sport Diving

1. *Missed decompression or incomplete decompression.* These result in an excessive tissue inert gas load on return to the surface.
2. *Repetitive dives.* If the required surface interval time is reduced or the residual nitrogen time is not included in the next total dive time, nitrogen overload may occur.
3. *Exposure to heat — heat promotes tissue degassing.* Gases are more soluble in cold than warm solutions. A hot shower after diving can cause bubble formation, even if a correct ascent schedule was used.
4. *Exposure to cold — cold promotes tissue upgassing.* A diver inadequately protected by a suit and developing some degree of hypothermia will absorb more inert gas during the dive. Circulation also slows down, causing a later, slower return of nitrogen to the lungs for degassing.
5. *Excessive movement.* Exercise after diving may dislodge bubbles which are harmlessly lodged and are degassing, causing them to embolise. Exercise also increases tissue temperature, causing an increase in bubble size (Charles's Law), or actual bubble development.
6. *Rapid ascents.* Even when decompression stops are not required, rapid ascents may cause too steep a nitrogen gradient for nitrogen solubility in venous blood. That is, more nitrogen is released from tissues than

venous blood can hold in solution to the lungs. Haldane suggested 18 m/min (60 ft/min) as a safe ascent rate. Recent work measuring bubble formation using sonic Doppler methods suggests that 10 m/min (33 ft/min) is safer.

7. *Increased age.* Possibly due to decreased efficiency of tissue blood supply in degassing.

8. *Obesity.* A greater mass of tissue is available to absorb inert gas.

9. *Dehydration.* A drop in the total volume of body fluids results in less available fluid for inert gas dilution and more rapid saturation of the remaining fluid. This can arise from excessive sweating, restricted fluids, vomiting, diarrhoea, etc.

10. *Increased carbon dioxide.* Inadequate ventilation due to skip breathing, deep air dives, dense nitrox mixes, contamination of an air supply, a faulty regulator, or underwater exercise can lead to a high tissue carbon dioxide level. This then 'closes' the oxygen window and reduces nitrogen tolerance.

11. *Alcohol excess.* Alcohol is a diuretic and overindulgence causes an increased urine output, with loss of body water and dehydration. It also predisposes to vomiting, with similar results. Flushing of the skin predisposes to heat loss and hypothermia with increased nitrogen absorption at depth.

12. *Physical injury.* Injury, to an arm or leg for example, causes tissue swelling and distortion of capillary-tissue function. Degassing of the tissue is slowed and bubble formation can occur.

13. *Altitude.* Flying after diving, with the further drop in atmospheric pressure, will increase the size of existing bubbles (Boyle's Law) or trigger new ones. If flying is essential to transport a diver for any medical emergency, the aircraft should be low-flying or pressurised.

14. *Females.* Some workers report a higher incidence of acute decompression illness in women than in men. The usual explanation given is the greater amount of subcutaneous fat, but many studies have not shown a significant difference in divers using conservative modern tables.

15. *Limb flexion.* Sitting with the legs crossed or flexed after diving may cause problems by kinking of veins in the knees and groins. This may occur, for example, by driving a long distance to get home at the end of an active diving weekend.

16. *Previous decompression illness.* If bubbles recur in a diver, they frequently do so at a site of previous injury or bubble formation, such as a shoulder, elbow or knee. This may be due to distortion or damage to tissue-capillary function resulting in inadequate inert gas elimination.

In most cases, a combination of factors is responsible. Standing in the sun in a wet suit after a repetitive dive; going for a jog on the beach, or on a hike a few hours after a dive; diving with a sports injury to a knee or shoulder − all these are common examples of relatively innocent behaviour resulting in bubble development after a technically correct dive.

Diver disbelief

With the exception of severe pulmonary or neurological cases of acute decompression illness, the greatest problem a diving physician has to contend with is diver disbelief. The average diver simply does not believe it possible that he or she has bent. Any number of reasons are given why symptoms such as joint pain, headache, numbness, weakness or excessive fatigue are due to a late night, falling off a horse, or a bump on the dive boat. The presence of acute decompression sickness is disregarded because the dive profiles were impeccable in their performance. The fact that the diver enthusiastically gambolled with a buxom young thing in a tanga is forgotten. So is the game of volley ball and the squatting around the camp fire telling jokes while a few beers numbed a painful knee. Only when the reasons run out a few days later does the diver hesitantly apologise for disturbing the doctor, but...

If unexplained symptoms develop, even if seemingly minor, do not wait. Contact a dive doctor and explain the position. Let a professional handle the dilemma. A few words of advice may be all that is needed, and if chamber therapy is required it can be arranged in good time before things really deteriorate.

Factors predisposing to pulmonary barotrauma of ascent

Lung damage during ascent results from overdistension of lung tissue due to expansion of contained gas. Factors causing inadequate exhalation or obstruction to airways are responsible. These are listed on p 117.

Time of occurrence of acute decompression illness

Acute decompression illness occurs during ascent or soon after the dive.

   Most present within 30 minutes − about 60%
   By 6 hours − about 90%
   By 12 hours − about 99%

The very odd one is delayed up to or over 24 hours. The majority, about 60 per cent, involve joints and skin. Of the remaining 40 per cent, the vast majority affect the brain and spinal cord. But as the bubbles can appear anywhere, any presentation is possible, such as irritability, confusion, weakness, paralysis, headache, coma, blindness, deafness, numbness, memory loss, chest pain, abdominal pain, etc.

Type of diving

The type of diving is important:
1. Sport divers more commonly perform deep air dives with rapid ascents. They beat their blood-alveolar degassing time and develop fast tissue bubbles. As blood is the fastest tissue, and veins are the transport network to the lungs, bubbles develop in venous blood and may then become widespread with lung, brain or spinal cord involvement. Spinal

cord involvement frequently follows acute lung bubble overload (the 'chokes'). Massive bubble formation can lead to blood clotting throughout the entire vascular system (disseminated intravascular coagulation). This is invariably fatal.

2. Saturation divers and medium depth long dives with slow ascents usually develop slow tissue bubbles, e.g. joints and tendons.

   Fast tissue bubbles are unpredictable and dangerous. Slow tissue bubbles are usually predictable.

3. Very deep heliox divers on excursion dives, or at the beginning of their decompression, or on changing breathing mixes, have inner ear bubbles more frequently.

Presentation of Acute Decompression Illness

As the condition is due to the presence of bubbles or trapped gas anywhere in the body, the presentation will depend on the tissue or organ involved. Bubble formation in a joint will present with joint pain after a dive. Features relating to loss of higher function, or motor or sensory function, will follow bubble formation in the brain or cerebral arterial gas embolism after pulmonary barotrauma of ascent. Arterial gas embolism to the coronary arteries will present with chest pain, etc.

The disease is a dynamic one because bubbles may remain constant in size, grow, shrink or move to a different area. Additional bubbles may develop in different tissues, or more gas may be vented into capillaries and be circulated throughout the body after lung damage.

Because the presentation is so variable, systematic recording of any untoward symptom after diving is very important. It will enable a diving doctor to make a clearer assessment of the case and provide proper definitive treatment.

The following must be carefully noted:

1. Evolution

Evolution refers to the disease development from onset to the present moment. It is a description of the dynamic quality of the disease before any recompression in a chamber.

Evolution may be:

(a) *Static*. No change is occurring. Any complaint remains constant – joint pain neither worsens nor improves; headache, dizziness or blurred vision persist, etc.

(b) *Progressive*. The diver's condition is worsening – pain is increasing; confusion develops, etc.

(c) *Spontaneously improving*. The diver is getting better and any symptoms are lessening.

(d) *Relapsing*. After an initial improvement, symptoms recur.

2. **Manifestations**

This describes the details of the complaint. It could be:
— *musculoskeletal* (e.g. limb pain or aching);
— *neurological* (e.g. headache, unconsciousness, ringing in the ears, or vertigo). Neurological assessments must be recorded as detailed on p 254;
— *cutaneous* (e.g. skin rashes or itching);
— *lymphatic* ('orange peel' appearance of the skin);
— *pulmonary* (e.g. breathlessness, coughing, husky voice, chest pain, 'chokes', etc.);
— *constitutional* (e.g. loss of appetite, fatigue, nausea);
— *other* (any other manifestation).

3. **Time to onset**

For each manifestation, the time that has elapsed between surfacing from the dive and the onset of the manifestation must be recorded. If a manifestation occurs during ascent it must be recorded as such.

4. **Gas burden**

This is an estimate of the residual nitrogen overload present after a dive. It gives some indication of the degree of exposure. It could be described simply as minimal, moderate or substantial; or a no-decompression-stop dive, correctly completed decompression-stop dive, missed decompression-stop dive, and an emergency or uncontrolled ascent with missed decompression-stop dive. Accurate dive profiles of all dives performed before the event, including surface intervals, should be provided to the doctor consulted, as well as details of all surface activities — exercise, exposure to heat, or any of the predisposing causes as described on pp 130-131.

5. **Evidence of barotrauma**

Be alert for possible pulmonary barotrauma (e.g. coughing up blood, tight chest, breathlessness, sudden unconsciousness).

6. **Response to treatment**

Any treatment given (e.g. oxygen, pain-killers) must be fully described as well as the results achieved.

If the above points are noted and documented, the attending doctor will be presented with a clear and concise record of the event, without any assumptions, and an ideal matrix for database applications which will facilitate exchange of information between hyperbaric centres. A model report form follows.

ACUTE DECOMPRESSION ILLNESS REPORT

EVOLUTION		NAME:		
STATIC		AGE:	SEX:	DATE:
PROGRESSIVE		ADDRESS:		
IMPROVING				
RELAPSING		TEL. WORK:		HOME:

MANIFESTATIONS
MUSCULOSKELETAL:
NEUROLOGICAL:
CUTANEOUS:
LYMPHATIC:
PULMONARY:
CONSTITUTIONAL:
OTHER:

TIME TO ONSET		GAS BURDEN	
DURING ASCENT		NO DECO STOPS NEEDED	
ON SURFACING		COMPLETED DECO STOPS	
AFTER SURFACING	MINS	MISSED DECO STOPS	
EVIDENCE OF BAROTRAUMA		EMERGENCY ASCENT	
		UNCONTROLLED ASCENT	

RESPONSE TO TREATMENT

Management of Acute Decompression Illness

It is essential to have some knowledge of management as diving physicians or expert help are not always to hand and divers are often dependent on each other's knowledge and expertise. (Although operating a therapeutic recompression chamber is beyond the scope of sport diving, the relevant tables are mentioned for completeness.)

Prevention

Avoidance of acute decompression illness is the basic objective of a diving course. People can already swim and are reasonably drown-proof when they attend a diving school. They are then taught how not to bend or burst. The other dangers of the sea come next in importance.

1. Prevention requires strict avoidance of the factors that predispose to bubble formation and lung overdistension as enumerated on pp 130-131 and p 117.
2. Proper hydration in extremely important. It is fluid that keeps nitrogen in solution and good hydration can ensure gas solubility even when a little latitude is taken with the predisposing factors for bubble formation. Drink 330 ml of water or fruit juice 30 minutes before diving. With the exception of alcohol, drinking and diving is good!

Treatment

Primary aid

1. Send someone to contact a dive physician.
2. Keep the diver relaxed, lying flat, calm and quiet.
3. Administer continuous 100% oxygen with a face mask.
4. Encourage oral fluid intake − 500 ml initially, then 150 ml per hour. Do not try and give oral fluids to an unconscious diver!
5. Keep the diver flat during transport to the recompression facility. The Trendelenburg position is not permitted. If the diver is unconscious, he or she must be placed on the left side and propped about 15 degrees to the horizontal.
6. If breathing or heartbeat fail, administer rescue breathing or CPR. This should be done with the helper taking a breath of pure oxygen before each mouth-to-mouth exhalation. (AIDS awareness!)

Secondary aid

1. Set up a Ringer's lactate intravenous lifeline.
2. Maintain continuous 100% oxygen.
3. Maintain CPR if required. (AIDS awareness!)
4. It is necessary to reduce or eliminate any bubbles and then return the diver to 1 ATA in safety. Bubble elimination involves recompression. It must be decided what depth is needed and at what rate return to surface pressure is required. Victims should be lying down during their decompressions. Gas bubbles tend to rise (i.e. to the head) and gravity

tends to pool the blood in the veins of the legs when sitting or standing, thereby slowing return of blood for nitrogen elimination to the lungs. On reaching the chamber (a doctor must be present):

    If limb-only or skin-related problem — Table 5 USN; 61 RN.

    More severe but no pulmonary symptoms — Table 6 USN; 62 RN.

    If no relief with Table 6 — Table 4 USN (oxygen version).

    If arterial gas embolism or unsure — Table 6A USN; 63 RN. *Do not recompress a pneumothorax with neurological manifestations until a non-return chest drain has been inserted!*

5. If the situation with recompression is out of hand, compress to depth of pain relief *on air* and hold there until additional emergency specialist medical help can be found.
7. Vitamin C — 1000 mg orally.
6. Valium 5 mg by mouth if the victim is very agitated.

Transport of divers with acute decompression illness
1. The principles mentioned in the management must be followed.
2. If the diver is in a remote place, there are two possibilities:
  (a) Transport the victim using 100% oxygen via a face mask. If it is essential to use an aircraft, it must fly as low as possible or be able to be pressurised to 1 ATA.
  (b) Bring a portable recompression chamber to the diver. Use Table 5 or 6 USN (or 61 or 62 RN). Do not place an unconscious victim in a one-man chamber. You will have no control over any of the parameters of CPR, and if vomiting with inhalation occurs, the situation will become desperate. The chamber should be able to couple under pressure to the multiplace chamber at the recompression facility. If it cannot, the diver must be returned from 18 msw in the chamber to surface pressure over two minutes, transferred with an assistant to the therapeutic chamber, and repressurised while breathing pure oxygen. (See pp 251-253.)
  (c) In both (a) and (b), the recompression hospital must be notified in advance and the case discussed.

Management after decompression

Once the diver has emerged from the chamber, feeling well and symptom free, management is not over. Most cases recur to a lesser degree within a few hours. Some require further recompression therapy. Ample liquids plus the use of surface 100% oxygen by mask for 55 minutes, followed by air for 5 minutes, repeated for 6 hours, will help to prevent a recurrence. This may be regarded as too much fuss or too time-consuming, but the results warrant the effort.

Underwater Management of Acute Decompression Illness

Divers have grown enormously in numbers over the past two decades and, throughout the world, wherever there is water, a diver will enter it. Sometimes, the diver is hundreds or even thousands of kilometres away from the nearest telephone or radio. He is faced with the problem of acute decompression illness. Underwater management is his only alternative.

It must be stressed that:

— This is an emergency first-aid procedure for divers in remote areas only.
— It is not intended as a replacement for chamber therapy.
— It must be used for acute pain-only, limb, joint or skin decompression illness.
— It is not intended for severe decompression illness or arterial gas embolism. Placing an unconscious diver on a demand valve and returning him to the water *can never be acceptable or condoned.*

There are two possibilities:

— underwater air recompression,
— underwater oxygen recompression.

Underwater Air Recompression Therapy

This can only and must only be done by very experienced and highly trained divers. It involves taking the diver plus an attendant back into the water to a depth of 30 msw and ascending using Table 1A USN (over 6 hours) or Table 81 RN (nearly 5 hours). A vertical, calibrated shot line must be used, and the ascent timed by surface tenders, using a signal line.

Advantages
None.

Disadvantages (plenty)
1. The diver must be taken to a depth of 30 msw. This usually means the open sea with swells, currents, wind, rain, and perhaps night.
2. An air supply for *two,* adequate for 6 hours, must be available.
3. At 30 msw, wet suits are thin (Boyle's Law), and prolonged exposure

causes hypothermia in the diver and the attendant.
4. Boat difficulties, weather, seasickness, fatigue, inadequate air, hypothermia and narcosis may force the therapeutic dive to be cancelled prematurely. Now the diver will get worse from the increased nitrogen exposure and the attendant will bend too.

This technique is dangerous, and can only be considered when acute limb or skin decompression illness occurs very soon after diving and worsening of the diver with life-threatening acute decompression illness is anticipated.

This anticipation requires knowledge, training and experience and must only be considered when any other help is impossible.

Underwater Oxygen Recompression Therapy

This technique was developed in Australia by the Royal Australian Navy School of Underwater Medicine as a result of acute decompression illness occurring in areas very remote from a proper recompression facility.

It involves returning the diver to the water with an attendant to a depth of 9 msw, followed by an ascent programme.

Advantages
1. The shallow depth allows selection of a protected area, avoiding a return to the open seas, seasickness, narcosis and boat problems.
2. Less compression of wet suits occurs with less likelihood of hypothermia.
3. There is no requirement for extended air supplies.
4. There is no risk of the attendant bending.
5. Terminating the treatment will not worsen the diver.

The principles used are the same as those used in chamber oxygen recompression therapy tables:
— compressing any bubbles and reducing their size;
— avoiding any further nitrogen uptake;
— creating a large gradient for nitrogen from tissues to alveoli;
— increasing oxygen availability to tissues;
— shortening decompression time.

Disadvantages
1. Oxygen must be supplied from the surface.
2. It should be supplied to a full face mask (e.g. Kirby Morgan or AGA), via a non-return valve on the mask. A full face mask reduces the risk of inhalation of water, allows direct communication between the diver and the surface, and permits breathing should consciousness become clouded or vomiting occur in a dizzy or seasick diver.
3. Cerebral oxygen toxicity, although unlikely, must be remembered. The fire risk must also be noted and oil-contaminated fittings and hoses avoided.

4. This is an emergency regime and is not intended to replace chamber therapy. It is a remote-area option.

Method
1. *The preparation*
   (a) A large oxygen cylinder as used in hospitals is needed.
   (b) This is fitted to a two-stage regulator, the first-stage gauge indicating cylinder pressure and the second-stage delivery pressure. This should be set to 550 kPa.
   (c) A 12-metre length of clean hosing is attached to the second stage outlet.
   (d) The other end of the hose is attached to a non-return valve on the diver's mask inlet.
   (e) The diver must be *fully dressed* and negatively weighted, so that there is no difficulty in maintaining depth under water. A tendency to drift upward is contraindicated.
   (f) The attendant will breathe *air* using conventional scuba. Adequate full spare cylinders plus attached demand valves must be available *on* the shot line.
   (g) A shot line clearly marked in metres and adequately weighted is suspended from a buoy large enough to support two divers easily.
   (h) If the recompression cannot be done in a sheltered, quiet area, the buoy must be tethered close to the boat.
   (i) Hand and foot loops, and a seating system must be fitted to the shot line to assist the diver and the attendant.
2. *The recompression*
   (a) The diver and the attendant descend to 9 metres.
   (b) A timed stay of 30 minutes is done in mild cases, 60 minutes in worse cases, and 90 minutes if improvement does not occur.
   (c) Ascent is then commenced at *12 minutes per metre*. Ascent time between stops is included in each 12 minutes.

9 MSW BOTTOM TIME	ASCENT AT 12 MINUTES/METRE	TOTAL TIME
30 MINUTES	96 MINUTES	126 MINS: 2 HR 6 MINS
60 MINUTES	96 MINUTES	156 MINS: 2 HR 36 MINS
90 MINUTES	96 MINUTES	186 MINS: 3 HR 6 MINS

If necessary, this recompression may be repeated twice daily.

Problems Associated with Dissolved Gases

In the waterworld of Fizz, Robert Boyle is king. He reigns over the physical properties of free gases — what happens when they expand and contract when out of solution. The results are dramatic, with burst lungs, squeezes and bends.

There is another world where Dalton and Henry reign. It is a quiet, painless, soporific place but no less dangerous and with much more insidious difficulties awaiting a diver. All the gases in any breathing mixture can cause trouble or kill while dissolved and in solution in the diver's body fluids. They all cause trouble due to high partial pressures in solution. Only oxygen can kill due to low partial pressures in solution.

The gases involved are:

Oxygen

Symbol O. It exists as two atoms linked together — O_2. Its molecular weight is 32. It comprises about 21% of clean, dry air. Oxygen is the *only* essential requirement in any breathing mixture, but the amount in the mix is very important. If its concentration is too low, oxygen deficiency occurs. This is called hypoxia. If its concentration is too high, oxygen toxicity occurs.

Nitrogen

Symbol N. It exists as two atoms linked together — N_2. Its molecular weight is 28. It comprises about 79% of clean, dry air. For easy calculation, air is often taken to comprise 20% oxygen and 80% nitrogen. Under normal surface conditions, nitrogen is inert as far as most living organisms are concerned. For the diver, however, it can cause problems. At high partial pressures, nitrogen in solution exhibits the properties of an anaesthetic. This is called nitrogen narcosis.

Carbon dioxide

Symbol CO_2. It exists as a single atom of carbon bound to two atoms of oxygen. It is the end-product of oxygen-carbohydrate metabolism by the body, and accumulation is toxic. High partial pressures cause carbon dioxide narcosis.

Carbon monoxide

Symbol CO. It exists as one atom of carbon bound to one atom of oxygen. It is highly poisonous and is found as a contaminant of breathing mixtures as a result of petrol or diesel exhaust fumes being drawn into the intake of the supply compressor. High partial pressures cause carbon monoxide poisoning.

Helium

Symbol He. It exists as a single atom – He. Its atomic weight is 4. It is totally inert, as no other chemical element can react with helium under any conditions. It is obtained from natural gas wells, such as those in Mexico and Russia. Helium is used to dilute oxygen at depths below 50 msw, where air or nitrogen cannot be used alone. This presents both advantages and disadvantages.

Advantages
1. It does not cause narcosis.
2. It is very light, making it easy to breathe.
3. Helium-oxygen (heliox) mixtures allow a shorter decompression time to an equivalent air-saturation dive, because helium diffuses very rapidly.

Disadvantages
1. It is expensive.
2. Speech at depth is unintelligible – a descrambler is needed.
3. Helium has a very high thermal conductivity, rapidly transferring heat from or to a diver. This makes the diver very susceptible to hypothermia and hyperthermia.
4. At depths below 100 metres, helium can cause the HPNS (high pressure neurological syndrome).
5. As with nitrogen, acute decompression illness can occur.

Hydrogen

Symbol H. It exists as two atoms linked together – H_2. Its molecular weight is 2, making it the lightest substance of all. A great deal of fascinating research is currently being done in the field of hydrogen-oxygen (hydrox) breathing as an alternative to heliox.

Advantages
1. It is cheap.
2. It is the lightest gas and the easiest to breathe.
3. The HPNS is less likely to occur.

Disadvantages

1. A hydrox mix is potentially violently explosive (e.g. the wreck of the dirigible *Hindenberg*). This can be avoided by keeping the oxygen percentage in the mix below four per cent. Such a mix will not explode, but it can then only be used for dives deeper than 30 metres (ppO_2 = 4% of 4 ATA = 0.16 ATA).
2. Speech requires a descrambler.
3. It has a high thermal conductivity.
4. Acute decompression illness can occur.

Neon, argon, krypton and xenon

These gases, like helium, are all totally inert. Their use is limited to experimental diving and research. They are all expensive, denser than nitrogen, more narcotic than nitrogen, and require longer decompression schedules.

Attempting to memorise the various presentations of different dissolved gas problems is confusing and difficult. Many of the signs overlap. It is vital, though, to have a working approach to a diver who presents with confusion, convulsions or unconsciousness during or immediately after a dive. An attempt has been made to give a practical overview of the situation which requires only understanding and minimal memory effort.

The key to all these gas problems is *hypoxia*. Features either due to or similar to hypoxia are found with all these gases. The other signs which may be present depend on the specific gas.

The details of the dive are extremely important. An unconscious diver who dived to 14 msw on air could hardly be expected to have nitrogen narcosis or oxygen toxicity. In the case of a diver on a pure oxygen rebreather at 14 msw, oxygen toxicity would be your first bet. Similarly, a diver using scuba and not skip breathing* is unlikely to develop carbon dioxide toxicity, because all his exhaled air is being vented into the water. A Standard Diver on an open circuit-freeflow system is in a different position, because if his ventilation flow rate is insufficient, carbon dioxide will build up. The presentation of high gas partial pressures (or low oxygen) may be complicated by acute decompression illness, but even in these cases the ultimate derangement is hypoxia. Inadequate oxygen is being absorbed or is reaching the affected site. As hypoxia is central to the story, it is dealt with first.

---

* Skip breathing is a form of insanity affecting divers in love and newcomers to the sport. They need to impress and show their worth. For some peculiar reason, this means that they must prove that they have low metabolic requirements and breathe less than other mortals, so they hold each breath and exhale slowly while carbon dioxide steadily accumulates in their tissues. On returning to the surface, they proudly announce that their air cylinder is still half-full and swallow a tablet for their splitting headache.

Hypoxia

Hypo = too little; *oxia* = oxygen. Hypoxia is a condition associated with a deficient supply of oxygen to the tissues.

Recall the petrol engine. Hypoxia is equivalent to decreasing the air supply to the engine. This drastically reduces engine efficiency and may stall the engine. The tissue cells (our engines) suffer similarly from oxygen deprivation. Energy output is drastically reduced.

Hypoxia is often wrongly referred to as anoxia. Anoxia refers to no oxygen (*an* = without; *oxia* = oxygen), and is rapidly fatal. This would occur, for example, with strangulation, drowning, or a tankful of pure helium or nitrogen. The closest a diver normally gets to anoxia is breathhold diving.

Causes:

Look again at the route followed by oxygen from gas supply to tissues. A breakdown anywhere will cause hypoxia.

FAILURE OF OXYGEN SUPPLY TO TISSUES

SITE OF BREAKDOWN	CAUSES
Gas supply	1. Breathhold diving. 2. Exhaustion of air supply. 3. Wrong mix e.g. 2% oxygen instead of 20%. 4. Equipment failure e.g. faulty regulator. 5. Too low flow rate in a rebreather.
Airway (mouth, larynx, trachea, bronchi, bronchioles)	1. Inhaled dentures. 2. Laryngospasm. 3. Inhaled foreign material e.g. vomiting under water.
Alveoli	1. Water in alveoli: drowning. 2. Collapsed alveoli e.g. pneumothorax.
Lung capillaries	1. Obstruction with bubbles: 'chokes'. 2. Compressed capillaries due to pulmonary barotrauma.
Arterial blood	1. Failure of circulation of blood e.g. AGE, shock, heart failure, hypothermia. 2. Failure of oxygen carriage e.g. carbon monoxide. 3. Failure of enough blood e.g. haemorrhage.
Tissue capillaries	1. Failure of capillary circulation e.g. inert gas bubbles or AGE in vessels.
Tissues	1. Poisoning of oxygen uptake e.g. carbon monoxide.

This table is not a complete list of possibilities. It is intended to show that understanding, not memory, is the key.

Presentation of hypoxia

The brain has a rich blood supply and is very sensitive to hypoxia. Not surprisingly, then, it is the brain that first suffers when hypoxia occurs. The degree of presentation depends on the degree of hypoxia.

If severe hypoxia: sudden unconsciousness, e.g. ascent after breathhold diving.

With lesser hypoxia: *any* feature of a drop in brain oxygen, e.g. confusion, headache, fatigue, apathy, overconfidence, blurred vision, slurred speech, vertigo, stupor, etc.

So, with any change in:
- *higher cerebral function,*
- *the senses* (hearing, vision, touch, taste, smell),
- *motor ability,*

straight after diving, think of hypoxia, then consider the possible causes in the ladder from gas supply to tissues.

Failure between gas supply and the lungs causes inadequate oxygenation of blood. The bright red arterial blood becomes darker and the diver becomes blue. This is called *cyanosis.*

A cyanosed diver with blue lips and tongue *must* be considered to have hypoxia.

A blue diver is hypoxic.

Management of hypoxia

The causes involve gas supply, airways and circulation. So does the management.

1. *A, B, C, + Oxygen* (AIDS awareness!)

   A = Airways. Ensure that these are clear by clearing the mouth of foreign material such as vomit, water, blood, etc. Do not forget to do this before beginning resuscitation.

   B = Breathing. Check that the diver is breathing. If not, begin mouth-to-mouth rescue breathing (see p 178).

   C = Circulation. Is the heart beating? Listening with an ear on the left chest or feeling for the carotid artery will determine effective heartbeat. If not, begin CPR (see p 175). Is the diver bleeding? Haemorrhage must be stopped.

   Oxygen. When A, B and C have been attained, give 100% oxygen by face mask or Ambubag.

2. *Summon medical assistance.*

Example
- Mike and Jimmy decided to dive on the wreck of *De Kelders*, which sank with a cargo of snooker balls. Mike, as usual, was meticulous in his

preparation, but Jimmy wanted to try an old twin-hose, two-stage set he had stolen, complete with a full, old rusty cylinder. (What he did not know was that the cylinder and set were three years old.) During the descent, Jimmy began breathing and swimming erratically and rushed back to the surface, where he gasped and spluttered and choked. The rusting in the cylinder had reduced his air to 4 per cent oxygen, causing hypoxia.

Oxygen Toxicity (Hyperoxia)

Oxygen toxicity is a condition caused by a high partial pressure of oxygen in the inspired gas supply.

This relates to Dalton's Law:

Oxygen partial pressure = Percentage oxygen x Ambient pressure
- Increasing the percentage can cause toxicity.
- Increasing the pressure can cause toxicity.
- Increasing both percentage and pressure can cause toxicity.
- All cause an increase in oxygen partial pressure.

Causes

1. Pure oxygen rebreathers.
2. High percentage oxygen mixes. Among sport divers, nitrox breathing has resulted in a number of deaths.
3. Pure oxygen in decompression schedules.
4. Pure oxygen in therapeutic tables.
5. Prolonged exposure under pressure e.g. saturation diving.

Time is required for oxygen toxicity to develop. It is this time that permits the use of oxygen under pressure. Consider what is happening. On exposure to pressure, oxygen is used to replace or reduce inhaled inert gas uptake and reduce or eliminate decompression time. A level of just under poisonous concentrations is set (i.e. 2 ATA when under water and 2.8 ATA in a chamber). When used in decompression, oxygen creates a large gradient from tissues to alveoli for inert gas.

Time is used to remove the inert gas before poisoning a diver with oxygen. The length of time depends on the oxygen pressure used and on the diver. Some divers are sensitive to a high oxygen pressure and present with toxicity early. This is used as a selection test for divers in some navies.

Features of oxygen toxicity

As far as a diver is concerned, two tissues are primarily involved:
- brain,
- lungs.

Brain (cerebral) oxygen toxicity. The brain can tolerate an oxygen partial pressure of 2 ATA continuously in a chamber for about 2 hours, before toxicity becomes obvious. At this point, reducing the oxygen pressure, for example by breathing chamber air, rapidly reduces the toxicity. In water, tolerance to oxygen is much less. The USN oxygen in-water depth-time limits (expressed in msw) are:

NORMAL OPERATIONS		EXCEPTIONAL OPERATIONS	
DEPTH (msw)	TIME (mins)	DEPTH (msw)	TIME (mins)
3	240	9	45
4.6	150	10.7	25
6	110	12	10
7.6	75		

In a chamber at 10 msw, 120 minutes is considered safe. In water at 9 msw, 45 minutes is considered safe under exceptional operations. Why should there be a difference? If ducks are ducks, and apples are apples, oxygen at 2 ATA should be oxygen at 2 ATA. There are two reasons. The first is that in a chamber, divers are resting, whereas under water they are swimming, working, fighting currents, and controlling their depth in a swell. Work reduces the time for the onset of oxygen toxicity and rest increases it, allowing an oxygen pressure of 2.8 ATA in chambers. The second reason is that submerged divers are committed to their gas supply (oxygen), whereas men in chambers are not. They can remove their oxygen masks and take air breaks at regular intervals. This reduces the toxic effect of oxygen.

The effects of oxygen toxicity on the brain are very complex and incompletely understood. A number of metabolic processes are interfered with, including oxygen utilisation by the tissues. Famine in the midst of plenty occurs, and features *similar to hypoxia* appear (see p 156):
— changes in higher cerebral function;
— changes in the senses;
— changes in motor ability.
In addition:
— *twitching,* especially of the face, is common;
— *pallor:* pure oxygen causes intense constriction of blood vessels causing the skin to become very pale (if you observe a diver emerging from a chamber after an oxygen decompression schedule or an oxygen therapeutic table, he or she is always very pale);
— vertigo and nausea are common (as with hypoxia);
— convulsions can occur (as with hypoxia).

Remember:
An unconscious *blue* diver is hypoxic.
An unconscious *white* diver could be oxygen toxic, depending on the gas supply being used. (Shock and hypothermia also cause *white* divers.)

Management of cerebral oxygen toxicity
The objective is the reduction of oxygen partial pressure in the inhaled gas.

Prevention of cerebral oxygen toxicity
1. *Avoid very deep air dives.*
   Among sport divers cerebral oxygen toxicity is rare. It can occur during chamber oxygen therapy for acute decompression illness, but is also possible with very deep dives on air. Despite the risk of severe nitrogen narcosis, dives have been done to 90 msw at which depth the oxygen partial pressure is 2.1 ATA. At shallower depths or with strenuous underwater exercise, individual sensitivity to oxygen and carbon dioxide build-up may result in cerebral oxygen toxicity.
2. *Don't muck about with Dalton's Law.*
   The use of nitrox mixes in sport diving is to be condemned. Although the objective (the reduction of decompression time and nitrogen narcosis by diluting nitrogen in the breathing mix with oxygen) is very understandable, the effect can be lethal. If one considers a scale of concentrations with pure nitrogen and narcosis at one end and pure oxygen and toxicity at the other, clean and dry air lies close to the 79% nitrogen-21% oxygen point. It is biased towards narcosis and deficient in toxicity. Adding oxygen to the mix slides danger along the scale towards oxygen toxicity. So air or nitrox breathing becomes a choice of potential dangers. Narcosis limits air diving and oxygen toxicity determines safe nitrox depth. With oxygen toxicity, the first sign may be a convulsion under water. The diver can do absolutely nothing to save his or her life, and the emergency rescue of a convulsing diver by a buddy can easily cause added pulmonary barotrauma of ascent.
   Sport diving is precisely that – sport diving. Air tables allow an advanced diver to descend to 50 msw without worrying about sudden unconsciousness under water. Nitrox is insidious stuff and has no place in sport diving. If a diver wants to breathe nitrox, then he or she must do a scientific or commercial diving course and have the back-up of an expert surface supervisor, diving helmets, underwater speech communication, an unlimited and variable breathing gas supply, and diving bells and deck decompression chambers immediately available should anything go wrong. Anything else is a dangerous game played by amateurs with nothing to gain: they are simply risking their lives to prove that what is already well known is possible. Professional divers have safely exceeded 600 msw. Using sport diving equipment to breathe mixes is quite simply mucking about with Dalton's Law.

Treatment of cerebral oxygen toxicity
1. *In a recompression chamber:*
   (a) Remove the diver's oxygen mask and allow the diver to breathe chamber air.
   (b) Encourage hyperventilation of chamber air for about 30 seconds.
   (c) If convulsions occur, immediately notify the chamber operator of

the situation. It is essential to maintain the pressure constant in the chamber until the convulsions stop.

(d) Gently but firmly restrain a convulsing diver from injury due to forceful collision with surrounding hard objects. Try to keep the diver's head extended back. This ensures an airway when breathing recommences and prevents the tongue from flopping back into the throat. Tongue depressors, although often recommended, are difficult to insert into a convulsing person's clenched mouth, and can break teeth or cause mouth bleeding with subsequent respiratory difficulty.

2. *Under water*

From a scuba-diving point of view, this refers almost entirely to sport divers who decide to use an oxygen-enriched breathing supply. A *deep diver rescue* must be performed.

(a) *Do not* bring a convulsing diver to the surface. The diver is not breathing, the jaws are clenched, and the risk of pulmonary barotrauma of ascent is very high. This requires extremely good nerves from a buddy, as natural instinct will prompt an immediate rescue ascent.

(b) Ditch the diver's weight belt. Wait until the convulsion stops (it always will).

(c) Turn the diver's head to one side and remove any foreign material by sweeping your forefinger around the mouth from cheek to cheek.

(d) Ascend steadily, holding the diver upright with the jaw well up and the mouth open. Keeping the diver's neck extended will allow expanding lung air to vent freely from the mouth during the ascent. Water will not enter the airway under these conditions. If air does not vent and the airway is clear, laryngospasm is present. *Wait for it to pass* before continuing the ascent − air will then bubble freely from the mouth.

(e) Do not attempt buddy breathing with a semi-conscious diver. Perform a controlled emergency ascent. Breathe normally on your rig, and ensure free exhalation by the diver. Be careful that the ascent does not become an uncontrolled buoyant ascent.

(f) On reaching the surface, inflate the diver's BC and signal for help. Check for diver breathing. If no breathing is evident, begin mouth-to-snorkel rescue breathing. This is easier to do than mouth-to-mouth rescue breathing in a choppy sea. Position yourself behind the diver. Ensure that the diver's snorkel is drained of water and that his or her mask is properly fitted on the face. With one hand, hold the snorkel mouthpiece in the diver's mouth, lift the jaw up and, using the thumb and forefinger, pinch off the diver's nostrils through the mask nosepiece. Tilt the diver's forehead back with your other hand. Blow slowly and deeply into the snorkel, then allow the diver to exhale passively. Repeat this 10 times.

(g) Rescue the diver from the water, with frequent stops for rescue breathing.

(h) On land or on the boat, lay the diver flat and face-down. Straddle the diver's hips. Lift the pelvis to drain any water from the airway.

(i) If the diver is breathing, place him or her in the unconscious left lateral rescue position.

(j) If no breathing is evident, roll the diver on to his or her back and begin mouth-to-mouth rescue breathing or CPR (see pp 175-182).

(k) Do not forget about any missed decompression stops!

Pulmonary oxygen toxicity. The brain is rapidly sensitive to a partial pressure of oxygen exceeding 2 ATA. The lungs develop slow toxicity changes at oxygen partial pressures above 0.5 ATA for continuous long periods.

Pulmonary oxygen toxicity is not seen in usual short-duration oxygen dives. It requires long exposures:

— repetitive oxygen therapeutic tables;
— saturation diving.

The exact mechanism, as with cerebral oxygen toxicity, is incompletely understood. The alveolar-capillary system is affected, with collapse of alveoli, filling of alveoli with secretions, and capillary breakdown. Eventually, extensive lung scarring may occur.

Presentation of pulmonary oxygen toxicity
1. 'Tickling' or 'scratching' feeling in the throat.
2. Coughing which becomes uncontrollable.
3. Burning chest pain.
4. Breathlessness, becoming worse and worse.

Management of pulmonary oxygen toxicity
Reduce the oxygen partial pressure of inspired gas to between 0.2 and 0.5 ATA. If treated early, the pulmonary effects revert to normal.

Nitrogen Narcosis (Rapture of the Deep)

Nitrogen narcosis is a condition associated with a decrease in intellectual and physical ability due to a high partial pressure of nitrogen in the inhaled mix. It is equivalent to being stone drunk under water, and limits sport diving to 50 msw.

Narcosis also occurs, and even more readily, with the heavier inert gases — neon, argon and krypton. Xenon narcoses even at the surface. In addition, the condition is caused by anaesthetic gases, for example nitrous oxide, the 'laughing gas' used by dentists. Helium has not been shown to cause narcosis.

Note: Narcosis is a 'nitrogen on descent' effect. The nitrogen is in solution in tissues. Acute decompression illness is a 'nitrogen on ascent' effect. The nitrogen is out of solution as bubbles.

Causes of nitrogen narcosis

Nitrogen at high partial pressures has an effect similar to that of an anaesthetic gas. The exact mechanism, as with oxygen toxicity, is not clear. It is believed that nitrogen is rapidly absorbed into brain cells which:

— have a rich blood supply; and
— have a high fat content in membranes.

The increased amount of dissolved gas may cause osmotic swelling of brain cells, interfering with membrane function and the delicate interrelationships between brain cells. No metabolism of nitrogen or any inert gas occurs. It appears to be a purely physical osmotic effect.

Presentation of nitrogen narcosis

As with hypoxia and cerebral oxygen toxicity, there are:

— changes in higher cerebral function,
— changes in the senses, and
— changes in motor ability.

Changes in higher cerebral function. This is usually the first presentation. Between 30 to 50 msw there is a feeling of well-being and overconfidence, similar to the effects of alcohol. Learning, attention, memory and concentration are impaired (the diver may forget what was done or noted at depth). At greater depths mental function gets worse, and hallucinations, sleepiness, stupor, coma and death can occur.

Changes in the senses. Vision is most commonly affected, sight becoming blurred or tunnel vision developing — the visual field becomes narrowed, rather like looking through a tube or tunnel.

Changes in motor ability. Movements become awkward and automatic, then incoordinated and ineffectual.

Nitrogen narcosis occurs suddenly on reaching depth, but does not get worse with time. It occurs more intensely with very rapid descents (a very high gradient for the absorption of nitrogen is suddenly set up). The depth of occurrence is variable. Some divers become narcosed at relatively shallow depths, while others are affected only beyond 50 msw. With regular diving, tolerance develops and the diver becomes less prone to narcosis. It is aggravated by cold, alcohol, drugs, fatigue and anxiety. Nitrogen narcosis disappears rapidly during the ascent.

The danger of nitrogen narcosis is usually not so much the narcosis itself, but the likelihood of injury or a fatal mistake under water, equivalent to driving a motor vehicle when drunk.

Management of nitrogen narcosis

Narcosis disappears with ascent. It can be prevented by the addition of helium to the gas supply (trimix). This dilutes and reduces the partial pressure of nitrogen as well as the risk of oxygen toxicity.

Naturally this has led to groups of trimix sport divers who confidently mix their own gases and gas switch-over depths, working purely on Dalton's Law of partial pressures to avoid narcosis and oxygen toxicity, and Haldane's exponential assumptions for upgassing and degassing. Factors such as variable compressibility of gases, gas mixing and analysis equipment, variable tissue solubilities, diffusion and counterdiffusion rates, differing half times at different depths, and emergency back-up support are ignored. They dive deeply, frequently bend, and invariably knew someone who died.

Carbon Dioxide Toxicity

Carbon dioxide is a gaseous toxic waste product produced by metabolism and unless a diver promptly removes it by effective exhalation, poisoning will occur.

1. Carbon dioxide is produced by the tissues in amounts proportional to oxygen used and work done. Production increases with exercise, including the work of breathing a dense mix at depth.
2. Carbon dioxide production is *independent* of depth alone.
3. Carbon dioxide is the *prime* stimulus for breathing. A rise in circulating blood carbon dioxide stimulates breathing.
4. In a freeflow system, e.g. inside a decompression chamber, or when using a hard helmet, the maximum carbon dioxide partial pressure permitted in inspired gas is 0.02 ATA. This is:
    - 2% at the surface (1 ATA);
    - 0.2% at 90 msw (10 ATA);
    - 0.07% at 290 msw (30 ATA).

With increasing depth, carbon dioxide control becomes more and more exact and demanding. An increase in the amount of carbon dioxide in the body is called *hypercapnia* and leads to carbon dioxide toxicity, then carbon dioxide narcosis.

Causes of carbon dioxide toxicity

As with hypoxia, the causes are found from gas supply to tissues.

1. *Gas supply*
    (a) Contamination of the gas supply with carbon dioxide.
    (b) Failure of absorbent in scrubbers.
    (c) Poor ventilation flow in helmets and decompression chambers.
2. *Airways and lungs*
    (a) Breathhold diving.
    (b) Inhaled dentures.
    (c) Laryngospasm.

(d) Inhaled foreign material, e.g. vomiting under water; near-drowning.
(e) Inadequate ventilation of alveoli. Breathing a dense mix at depth can be hard work in itself and becomes dangerous with any resistance to breathing due to tight suits, harnesses or flotation jackets. Not only does the diver have to work harder to breathe, but this increased work produces more carbon dioxide and demands more oxygen.
3. *Failure of carbon dioxide transport from tissues to lungs*
    (a) Failure of circulation due to shock, hypothermia or heart failure.
    (b) Failure of enough blood, e.g. haemorrhage.
4. *Excess tissue production of carbon dioxide.* Under normal circumstances, the blood and lungs easily handle carbon dioxide production. Under conditions of heavy work, if any of the foregoing causes are even moderately present, carbon dioxide will accumulate.

Note: In most cases carbon dioxide toxicity and hypoxia develop concurrently. Using nitrox mixes, carbon dioxide toxicity and oxygen toxicity can occur simultaneously. A convulsion is almost inevitable.

Presentation of carbon dioxide toxicity

1. Once again features similar to those of hypoxia occur (see p 156):
    — changes in higher cerebral function,
    — changes in the senses, and
    — changes in motor activity.
2. Carbon dioxide is the most powerful respiratory stimulus of all. It activates the inspiratory centre in the brain stem, and the diver starts breathing rapidly and deeply.
3. Carbon dioxide causes *dilation* of blood vessels, so the diver becomes flushed and sweaty.
4. The blood vessels in the head also dilate, causing a throbbing headache.
5. If the carbon dioxide level rises too high, it no longer stimulates breathing, but *depresses* it. Unconsciousness or convulsions can occur
    — carbon dioxide narcosis.

The flushing and sweating will not be noticed under water. The diver may think that his increased depth and rate of breathing are due to the exertions of diving. He may then convulse, stop breathing or lose consciousness under water *without any further warning.*

Management of carbon dioxide toxicity

Prevention. This is, as always, the most important part of management and involves:
1. Meticulous attention to scrubbers.
2. Constant care to ensure adequate freeflow volume.
3. Monitoring carbon dioxide levels in chambers, bells and habitats.
4. Ensuring no contamination of the air mix with carbon dioxide.

5. Avoiding restraining equipment and dense mixes.
6. A diver must be aware of the problem. This can be difficult as the first obvious signal may be sudden unconsciousness.

Treatment
1. If carbon dioxide toxicity under water is suspected, stop swimming and relax (less carbon dioxide production and oxygen use).
2. Signal to the buddy that something is wrong (unconsciousness may occur at any moment).
3. Begin the ascent.
4. At the surface hyperventilate atmospheric air.
5. If a diver sees an unconscious buddy, perform a deep diver rescue as described on p 149.

Example
• Pete Muckitt decided to make a mix to go diving for abalone and crayfish at 8 msw in a protected natural reserve. Creeping into his neighbour's garage at night, he quietly filled his cylinder to 80 ATA from a light Brunswick green bottle (containing carbon dioxide) which looked black (oxygen bottle) in the dark. Happily sneaking home, he topped up his cylinder to 200 ATA with air. Next day, he dived to 5 msw on his mix, promptly lost consciousness and convulsed. The local inspector, who had been watching from his boat, retrieved Pete from the water, resuscitated him and arrested him.

The High Pressure Nervous Syndrome (High Pressure Neurological Syndrome; HPNS)

The HPNS is a condition caused by rapid compression using helium or hydrogen to depths greater than 150 metres. It presents with fine tremors progressing to dizziness, impaired consciousness and stupor below 300 metres. HPNS is today the limiting factor to the depth that man can dive.

High pressure increases electrical activity and excitability in the brain. In animals, it progresses from tremor to drowsiness to convulsions to coma and finally death. Pressures well in excess of 200 ATA (over 2 000 metres) have been used experimentally in animals.

The onset of the HPNS is delayed by:
1. Narcosis-inducing gases, sedatives and anaesthetics.
2. Slow compression rates.

1. Narcotic gases

Narcotic gases such as nitrogen, as well as anaesthetics and sedatives such as barbiturates, can delay or reverse HPNS. The opposite also occurs — very high partial pressures of helium reverse anaesthesia.

The concept of a sedated, anaesthetised diver working alertly and efficiently at very great depths arises for the future. Nitrogen is commonly used for its narcotic effect. The mechanism is still unclear, but it appears that high-pressure helium tends to compress brain cell membranes. Nitrogen is believed to cause brain cell swelling. Possibly the effects are mutually counteractive, but much research is still being done to clarify the situation.

So nitrogen the narcoser, the scourge of shallow diving, has a happier side in very deep diving:

(a) It is cheap and reduces the cost of the mix.
(b) It reduces the heat loss by the diver in pure heliox atmospheres.
(c) It helps to reduce the garbled speech of helium.
(d) It prevents or delays the onset of HPNS.

2. Slow compression rates

With deeper and deeper dives, slower and slower compression rates are necessary to avoid HPNS. For example, a diver can be taken to a depth of 100 msw at a rate of 30 metres per minute without causing HPNS. To reach 200 metres, a rate of 15 metres per minute will cause the syndrome and to reach 300 msw, the compression must be below 1 metre per minute. It has been computed that if a compression rate of 10 metres per hour is used, the limit before HPNS convulsions occur in man would be about 84 ATA (855 metres). If sedatives, narcotic gases and anaesthetics are used, this limit will probably be exceeded. (See Saturation diving p 210.)

TABLE OF DIVING DISORDERS

	EFFECTS OF DESCENT		ASCENT
0 m			
O₂	OXYGEN TOXICITY *Cerebral:* Convulsions, pallor, twitching + *FSH** *Pulmonary:* Scratchy throat, cough, burning chest, breathlessness	SQUEEZE Lung, ear, sinus, mask, suit, diver.	ACUTE DECOMPRESSION ILLNESS; OSTEONECROSIS BAROTRAUMA OF ASCENT
10 m	OXYGEN TOXIC **FSH*	**FEATURES OF HYPOXIA** 1. **Higher cerebral function**	Arterial gas embolism;
AIR		Irritability, anger, fear,	Pneumothorax; Mediastinal
	NITROX TOXIC NITROGEN NARCOSIS **FSH*	laughter, irresponsibility, hysteria, hallucinations, apathy, sullenness, stupor, uneasiness, illusions,	emphysema; Lung tissue damage; Sinus barotrauma
50 m	SEVERE NARCOSIS	confusion, automatism, amnesia, unconsciousness.	of ascent; Ear barotrauma of ascent;
AIR	Dense air → more work to breathe → CO₂ TOXICITY flushing, headache, breathlessness + **FSH*	2. **Changes in the senses** *Visual:* blurring, double vision, tunnel vision, blindness, dazzle. *Hearing:* deafness, ringing in the ears	Gut barotrauma of ascent; Suit blow-up.
90 m	Absolute limit to air dive − ppO₂ = 2 ATA CEREBRAL OXYGEN TOXICITY	(tinnitus), loss of balance with nausea, vertigo, vomiting. *Touch:* Numbness, itching, pins and needles, burning. *Taste:* Loss of taste, or abnormal taste awareness.	
100 m	DIFFICULT TEMP REGULATION	*Smell:* Loss of smell or abnormal smell awareness.	
He + O₂ mix	Hypothermia Hyperthermia Garbled speech Strict ppO₂ + ppCO₂ + gas purity control	3. **Changes in motor activity** Weakness, loss of balance, incoordination, tremor, abnormal gait, twitching, slurred speech, paralysis.	
150 m	HPNS Tremors + **FSH* Deep saturation diving	**FSH:* Features similar to those of hypoxia.	
600 m **? limit**	Liquid breathing???		

Inhaled Gas Contamination

Contamination of a diver's air supply is an insidious but potentially lethal hazard. It invariably occurs only when compressors are used for air diving. Only rarely will commercially obtained gases such as oxygen, nitrox, trimix or heliox be contaminated.

The contamination comes from:
— the air,
— the compressor,
— the storage tank.

Contamination from the Air

Jimmy wants to dive in Emmarentia dam in Johannesburg. It is winter, and the glorious air in Johannesburg contains the following:
1. Carbon monoxide from hundreds of home fires belching smoke, and from thousands of motor cars.
2. Oxides of nitrogen and nitric acid from chemical factories.
3. Oxides of sulphur and sulphuric acid from the same factories.
4. Dashes of chlorine, bromine, lead, mine dust, pollen and other exotica.

All these gases must be filtered out during compression. The presence of abrasive dusts guarantees that the compressor will have a happy but short working life.

Contamination from the Compressor

Compressors have two possible points for contamination:
— from the engine driving the compressor,
— from the oil used to lubricate the compressor.

From the compressor engine

By far the commonest method of driving a compressor is a petrol motor. If one visits a dive resort on a weekend, one can witness dozens of divers happily sucking their own and other people's exhaust fumes into their breathing mix, together with a little barbecue smoke for flavour. Using an electric motor to drive the compressor eliminates one's own petrol exhaust fumes, but not those of one's neighbours, nor the exhaust fumes from the diesel engine on the ship supplying the generated electricity. The air-inlet hose to a compressor must always be *upwind* of any contamination source.

From the compressor oil

All compressors used for air-breathing supply should be in perfect running order, and use a vegetable oil as lubricant. These oils should also have a high resistance to breakdown on heating, and any oil which may enter the receiver or cylinder is less toxic than mineral oil.

Unfortunately, compressors are expensive and divers are poor, so a 'make-do' is often the result, with a grossly overheating compressor labouring to fill a neglected and out-of-date cylinder. The overheating is the main reason for contamination.

Causes of overheating
1. Restriction of the air-inlet by a filthy filter or a kinked narrow-bore inlet hose.
2. Damaged cylinders, rings, pistons and valves causing excessive friction.
3. Leaky valves, gaskets and fittings, causing a higher-than-designed final compression ratio to reach the required pressure.
4. Failure to cool the compressor.

Oil is not the most stable substance in the world. With high temperatures and pressures it can:
— vaporise, producing oil gas which reaches the receiver;
— 'crack', or break down into smaller, more volatile hydrocarbons;
— 'flash', or burn like diesel fuel, releasing carbon monoxide.
For all these reasons, *filters and traps* are used. A filter is needed on the outer end of the air inlet hose (which should be wide bore to reduce resistance). This eliminates leaves, dust, bits of sausage and other large particles.

Between stages (there are commonly three stages on a high pressure compressor), are finned cooling coils, which cool the air before it is further compressed by the next stage. This cooling causes moisture from the air to condense (rather like breathing on a cold mirror). Water traps are therefore used after each set of cooling coils between stages and they should be regularly vented.

After the third stage, the air is:
— at high pressure (say 200 ATA),
— fairly dry,
— contaminated with oil,
— contaminated with hydrocarbons and other gases,
— generally unbreathable.
Filters are now used. There are a variety of filters available. Very strict standards of air purity are set by the controlling authorities in most

countries. These should be strictly adhered to. They dictate the maximum amount of water, carbon monoxide, carbon dioxide, oxides of nitrogen, oil, odour and taste acceptable in an air mix.

Common filters in use are
1. Silica gel or activated alumina gel to remove water.
2. Activated charcoal to remove oil vapour and hydrocarbons.
3. Molecular ceramic sieves to remove oil and hydrocarbons.
4. Sodalime and baralyme to remove carbon dioxide.
5. Centrifugal filters to remove water and oil.
6. Cryogenic filters to freeze out carbon dioxide and water.
7. Oil-free compressors are available, but they are very expensive and rarely used by sport divers.

Testing for purity. Ideally, the air from a compressor should be checked after filtration. A number of simple test kits are available (e.g. the Draeger Multi-Gas Detector). This involves a simple gauging device which draws a sample of air through a small tube containing chemicals and indicator dyes specific for the gas being tested. Colour changes and tube markings indicate the degree of contamination for carbon monoxide, carbon dioxide, oxides of nitrogen, oil, hydrocarbons, chlorine, etc.

Contamination from the Receiver or Cylinder

The diver's air cylinder could contain:
— oil from previous faulty fillings;
— rust from water, either from the compressor or from a water cooling bath allowing water to enter an empty cylinder through an open valve.

Effects of Air Contamination on the Diver

Divers are believers. They believe that they will be safe under water and they believe that the air in their scuba cylinders is pure and breathable. Several problems relating to inspired air contamination await:

Oxygen (permissible range in air 20-22 per cent)
   (a) Low oxygen content could occur with a long-forgotten filling followed by cylinder rusting causing a reduction in the partial pressure of contained oxygen.
   (b) High oxygen concentrations follow the addition of oxygen to air, and can cause oxygen toxicity or a fire hazard in a chamber.

Carbon dioxide (maximum permissible 0.05 per cent or 500 ppm).

The presence of carbon dioxide and the effects of increasing its partial pressure have been discussed on p 153.

Carbon monoxide (maximum permissible 0.001 per cent or 10 ppm).

Carbon monoxide is an extremely dangerous contaminant. It has three actions:
— it competes with oxygen for haemoglobin;
— it delays or prevents the release of oxygen from haemoglobin to tissues;
— it poisons tissue utilisation of oxygen.

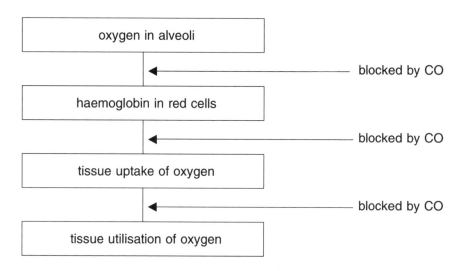

Effects of carbon monoxide on the oxygen pathway

Carbon monoxide has an affinity for haemoglobin (the carrier pigment for oxygen in red blood cells) which is 200 times that of oxygen. The presence of carbon monoxide causes gross hypoxia in the presence of normal amounts of oxygen. If the carbon monoxide partial pressure is 1/200th that of oxygen, half of the haemoglobin will be bound to carbon monoxide, and half to oxygen. As the oxygen partial pressure in air is 0.21 ATA (21%), a carbon monoxide concentration of 1/200 x 0.2 or 0.001 ATA (0.1%) is enough to halve the available oxygen.

In addition, the presence of carbon monoxide interferes with the release of oxygen from the remaining oxygen-haemoglobin complex (oxyhaemoglobin) to tissues, further aggravating the hypoxia. Finally, carbon monoxide poisons the metabolism of oxygen once within the tissues.

The maximum carbon monoxide permissible is 0.001 per cent (10 ppm), which would reduce oxygen carriage by 0.5 per cent.

Divers on air are protected to some degree by increased pressure, because as the partial pressure of oxygen rises with depth (Dalton's Law), more oxygen can be carried in free solution in plasma. This oxygen is not bound to haemoglobin and is more readily available to the tissues, but tissue utilisation will also be hampered by carbon monoxide which obeys Dalton's Law too.

The problem really becomes critical in saturation diving, where the partial pressure of oxygen is kept between 0.2 and 0.5 ATA, to avoid pulmonary oxygen toxicity. With a saturation dive of 90 msw using mixed gas and an oxygen pressure of 0.21 ATA (the same as in air at sea-level), if the amount of carbon monoxide was only one-hundredth of one per cent of the chamber atmosphere, half of the divers' available haemoglobin would be bound to carbon monoxide and they would die.

Causes of carbon monoxide poisoning
1. Carbon monoxide in the air.
2. Carbon monoxide formed in the compressor by flashing of oil.

Presentation of carbon monoxide poisoning
1. The features of hypoxia are evident (see p 156):
   — changes in higher cerebral function,
   — changes in the senses, and
   — changes in motor ability.
2. In addition, carbon monoxide forms a bright red stable complex with haemoglobin. The poisoned diver may therefore have cherry red lips and 'healthy' red cheeks. This is not a reliable sign, however, and its absence need not mean the absence of carbon monoxide poisoning.
   Carbon monoxide poisoning can cause irreversible brain damage which persists after resuscitation and treatment.

Management of carbon monoxide poisoning
Prevention. Poisoning a sport diver with carbon monoxide can only mean sloppy technique.
1. Ensure that the compressor air intake is upwind of petrol and diesel exhausts. Keep an eye on the direction of the wind. If it changes, move the intake hose.
2. If you have your own compressor, keep it serviceable. Have it maintained by someone who is knowledgeable and reliable.
3. Test the purity of the compressed air being pumped into your cylinder. It only takes a moment to draw a sample into a hand-held tester.

Treatment. The principle involved is to induce a high oxygen gradient into the tissues and a high carbon monoxide gradient from the tissues via the blood to the lungs for exhalation. This is identical to the management of acute decompression illness. Pure oxygen is therefore used, either at surface pressure or preferably a short therapeutic oxygen table (Table 5 USN).

Example
• Jimmy was diving at 25 msw. During the dive he began to feel dizzy, felt his vision fading and became very breathless. He decided to ascend and, halfway to the surface, became blind and had to fight to retain consciousness while hauling himself hand over hand up the shot line.

Back on the dive boat he was flushed, confused and disorientated. As a chamber was not to hand, he was given oxygen by mask, and over the next two hours gradually improved. Examination of the air compressor showed that the wind had changed direction, and the diesel fumes from the boat's generator exhaust were blowing directly into the compressor's inlet filter. Jimmy had suffered carbon monoxide poisoning and resultant hypoxia.

Oxides of nitrogen (maximum permissible less than 1 ppm)

Nitrogen reacts with oxygen to produce a variety of oxides:
— nitrous oxide — used in anaesthesia,
— nitric oxide — a pungent colourless gas,
— nitrogen dioxide — a pungent brown gas.
Other oxides exist, but they are unstable and break down to nitric oxide and nitrogen dioxide. These are intensely irritating and very poisonous. They affect chiefly the eyes, nose, throat and lungs, producing coughing, wheezing and difficulty in breathing, and in severe cases, death.

Oil and hydrocarbons (maximum permissible 1 mg/m^3)

Contamination causes a characteristic oily taste. A chemical pneumonia may follow, especially if mineral oils are used. Oil and hydrocarbons are inflammable, and the risk of fire becomes great when hydrocarbon vapours are mixed with air under pressure. The air cylinder on a diver's back becomes a potential bomb, equivalent to the inside of a petrol engine during the compression stroke. All it needs is one bright spark.

Altitude Diving

Diving at altitude causes diver confusion. All the standard decompression tables are based on the fact that a dive begins at sea-level (1 ATA; 760 mm Hg; 101 kPa; etc.) and ends at sea-level. What is the position in Johannesburg at an altitude of about 6 000 feet or 1 830 metres above sea-level? Here, besides air pollution and mugging, special traps lurk for our gentle coastal aquanaut. These traps are not immediately obvious, and make altitude diving a constant grey area in the average sport diver's knowledge.

The first thing a diver needs to know is the local atmospheric pressure at the area.

Determination of the Local Atmospheric Pressure

The air we breathe is not simply an even envelope of gas surrounding the Earth. The higher one goes, the lower the air pressure. Fortunately for diving calculations, the drop in pressure from sea-level to 3 600 metres (Lake Titicaca in South America — the highest lake in the world) is just about linear. For every metre one rises, the atmospheric pressure drops about 10 pascals or 0.01 kPa; or for every thousand metres one rises, the pressure drops about 10 kPa or 0.1 ATA.

Sea-level atmospheric pressure drops 10 per cent for every 1 000 metre rise.

As a formula:

$$\text{Local atmospheric pressure (kPa)} = 100 - \frac{\text{altitude (metres)}}{100}$$

or

$$\text{Local ambient pressure (ATA)} = 1 - \frac{\text{altitude (metres)}}{10\,000}$$

In Johannesburg:
    Altitude = 1 830 metres
    Local atmospheric pressure = 100 − 18.3 = 81.7 kPa
    Local atmospheric pressure = 1 − 0.183 = 0.817 ATA

So what? Jimmy dives to 50 msw at the coast, where the pressure is 6 ATA. What's 0.183 ATA compared to 6 ATA? Now we have reached the trap. It is essential to realise that absolute pressures are not important. Ratios are, and it is the ratio of change that will bend you.

Example
• Pete Muckitt is hiding from the police for catching crayfish in berry. Taking refuge in Mafikeng he decides to dive at Wondergat nearby at an altitude of 1 430 metres. He has heard the rumour that a packet of diamonds was once thrown into the water there so, setting up a surface-supply system, he spends five hours looking for the fabled loot at 10 metres of fresh water (mfw). (He thinks that he can spend an unlimited bottom time at 10 mfw and then surface without in-water decompression stops.) Finally, cold and hungry, he surfaces in disgust and returns to Mafikeng to lose some money at the casino. While standing at the one-armed bandits, Pete suddenly develops a terrible headache and blurred vision and, calling a doctor, is rushed to Pretoria for a therapeutic recompression under the beady eye of the police. What happened?

It's back to John Haldane. Many of the decompression tables are based on the fact that the majority of divers can tolerate a doubling of their tissue nitrogen without developing obvious bends. A coastal diver can ascend from a long dive at 30 msw (4 ATA) to 10 msw (2 ATA) for decompression; or from a long dive at 10 msw (2 ATA) to the surface (1 ATA) for decompression. A 2:1 ratio is usually tolerated due to the 'oxygen window'. (See p 128.)

   Look at Pete Muckitt's dive. The surface of Wondergat is at an altitude of 1 430 metres.

$$\text{The local ambient surface pressure} = 1 - \frac{1\ 430}{10\ 000}$$

$$= 1 - 0.143 \text{ ATA}$$

$$= 0.857 \text{ ATA}$$

Wondergat contains fresh water:
   33 feet or 10 metres of sea water $\equiv$ 1 ATA
   34 feet or 10.3 metres of fresh water $\equiv$ 1 ATA
   10 metres of fresh water $\equiv$ 0.97 ATA

At 10 mfw: pressure is 0.857 (atmospheric) + 0.97 (water) = 1.827 ATA

The ratio therefore is 1.827 : 0.857 = 2.132, so Pete bent.

It is obvious that a correction must be made for altitude diving. There are two ways to do this:
1. *Easy way.* Use a specially prepared altitude table. This clearly defines depth, dive times and decompression stages. The following tables were compiled by Professor A.A. Buehlmann of the University Hospital of Zurich, and were kindly made available for this section.

NO-DECOMPRESSION LIMITS — AIR DIVING DECOMPRESSION TABLE

Altitude 0–700 m above sea level

Safety stop: 1 min at 3 m • Ascent rate: 10 m/min

Depth m	BT min	Stop 6	Stop 3	RG
12	125		1	G
15	75		1	G
15	90		7	G
18	51		1	F
18	70		11	G
21	35		1	E
21	50		8	F
21	60		16	G
24	25		1	E
24	35		4	E
24	40		8	F
24	50		17	G
24	60	4	24	G
27	20		1	E
27	30		5	F
27	35		10	F
27	40	2	13	G
27	45	3	18	G
27	50	6	22	G
30	17		1	D
30	25		5	E
30	30	2	7	E
30	35	3	14	F
30	40	5	17	G
30	45	9	23	G

m	min	9	6	3	RG
33	14			1	D
33	20			4	D
33	25		2	7	E
33	30		4	11	F
33	35		6	17	G
33	40	2	8	23	G
36	12			1	D
36	20		2	5	D
36	25		4	9	E
36	30	2	5	15	F
36	35	2	8	23	G
39	10			1	D
39	15			4	E
39	20		3	7	E
39	25	2	4	12	F
39	30	3	7	18	G
39	35	5	9	28	G
42	9			1	D
42	12			4	D
42	15		1	5	E
42	18		4	6	F
42	21	2	4	10	F
42	24	3	6	16	G
42	27	4	7	19	G

m	min	12	9	6	3	RG
45	12				5	E
45	15		3		5	E
45	18		2	4	9	F
45	21		3	5	13	F
45	24		4	6	18	G
48	9				3	E
48	12			2	5	E
48	15		3	4	6	F
48	18		3	4	10	F
48	21		4	6	16	G
51	9				4	E
51	12			3	6	E
51	15		2	4	8	F
51	18		4	5	13	F
51	21	3	4	7	18	G
54	9				5	E
54	12		1	4	6	E
54	15		3	4	10	F
54	18	1	3	6	17	G
57	9			2	5	E
57	12		2	4	8	E
57	15	1	4	5	11	F
57	18	3	4	7	18	G

Altitude 701 m – 2 500 m above sea level

Safety stop: 1 min at 2 m • Ascent rate: 10 m/min

Depth m	BT min	Stop 6	Stop 4	Stop 2	RG
9	238			1	G
12	99			1	G
12	110			4	G
15	62			1	F
15	70			4	G
18	44			1	F
18	50			4	F
18	60			11	G
21	30			1	E
21	35			2	F
21	40			5	F
21	45			9	G
21	50	1		13	G
21	55	3		17	G
24	22			1	F
24	30			3	F
24	35			7	F
24	40		2	11	G
24	45		4	16	G
27	18			1	D
27	20			2	E
27	25			4	E
27	30		2	7	F
27	35		4	11	G
27	40	1	6	16	G

m	min	9	6	4	2	RG
30	15				1	D
30	20				3	E
30	25			2	6	F
30	30		1	4	11	G
30	35		2	7	15	G
30	40	1	5	10	20	G
33	12				1	D
33	15				2	E
33	20			2	4	E
33	25		2	3	9	F
33	30	1	3	6	14	G
33	35	2	4	9	20	G
36	10				1	D
36	15			1	3	D
36	20			3	6	E
36	25	1	3	5	12	G
36	30	3	3	8	19	G
39	9				1	D
39	12				3	D
39	15			2	4	E
39	18		2	3	7	E
39	21		3	4	10	F
39	24	2	3	6	15	G
39	27	4	4	8	18	G

m	min	9	6	4	2	RG
42	8				1	D
42	12			1	4	E
42	15		1	3	5	E
42	18		3	4	8	F
42	21	3	3	4	13	G
42	24	3	4	7	18	G
45	9				3	D
45	12			3	3	D
45	15		3	3	6	E
45	18	2	3	4	11	F
45	21	2	4	7	16	G
48	9				4	E
48	12		1	3	4	E
48	15	2	2	5	9	G
48	18	4	2	5	14	G
51	6				2	E
51	9			1	3	E
51	12	1	2	3	5	F
51	15	3	3	4	11	G
54	6				2	D
54	9		1	3	3	E
54	12	2	3	3	7	F
54	15	2	4	6	13	G

REPETITIVE DIVE TIME-TABLE 0 — 2 500 m above sea level

Surface Interval Times

								A	2	2
RG at start of						B	20	2	2	
surface interval					C	10	25	3	3	
				D	10	15	30	3	3	
			E	10	15	25	45	4	3	
		F	20	30	45	75	90	8	4	
	G	25	45	60	75	100	130	12	5	
	G	F	E	D	C	B	A	hrs	hrs	
RG at end of surface interval										

"0" ➤ Example:
Previous dive: 24 m, 35 min =
Repetitive Group **(RG) = F**
— after 45 min at surface: **RG = C**
— after 90 min at surface: **RG = A**
  (intermediate time: use next
  shorter interval time)
— after 4 hrs: flying is permitted
— after 8 hrs: **RG = "0"**, no more
  Residual Nitrogen Time **(RNT)**

RG for No-Decompression Dives and RNT for Repetitive Dives
Repetitive dive depth m (intermediate depths: use next **shallower** depth)

RG	9	12	15	18	21	24	27	30	33	36	39	42	45	48	51	54	57
A	25	19	16	14	12	11	10	9	8	7	7	6	6	6	5	5	5
B	37	25	20	17	15	13	12	11	10	9	8	7	7	6	5	5	5
C	55	37	29	25	22	20	18	16	14	12	11	10	9	8	7	7	6
D	81	57	41	33	28	24	21	19	17	15	14	13	11	10	9	9	8
E	105	82	59	44	37	30	26	23	21	19	17	16	14	13	12	11	10
F	130	111	88	68	53	42	35	30	27	24	21	19	17	16	15	14	13

Example: RG = C at end of surface interval. Planned depth of repetitive dive = 27 m. **RNT = 18 min**, to be added to Bottom Time (BT) of repetitive dive.

(side text: BUEHLMANN TABLE; © A.A. Buehlmann, University of Zurich/Switzerland 1986)

2. *Hard way.* Calculate the correction required for a particular altitude using standard tables. This is necessary if altitude tables are not available, if the bottom times exceed the altitude tables, or if special decompression techniques are used e.g. surface recompression and decompression using oxygen.

The calculation is actually very simple. The idea is to think in *local atmospheres.*

At the sea the local atmosphere is at 100 kPa or 1 ATA. At 10 msw the pressure doubles, at 20 msw it triples, etc. At Wondergat, the local atmosphere is 0.86 ATA or 86 kPa. Therefore at 8.6 msw (if it contained sea water) the pressure doubles, at 17.2 msw it triples, at 25.8 msw it quadruples, etc.

Note: As fresh water is less dense than sea water, allowance must be made for the difference. (The calculated depth must be multiplied by a factor of 1.03). This means that at 8.9 mfw the pressure doubles, at 17.7 mfw it triples, at 26.6 mfw it quadruples, etc.

To put it another way, at Wondergat, an 8.9-metre dive is equivalent to a 10-metre sea dive; a 17.7-metre dive is equivalent to a 20-metre sea dive; and a 26.6-metre dive is equivalent to a 30-metre sea dive.

Example
• Martin Martin decides to dive to 36 metres at Lake Titicaca on a second

honeymoon with his wife Dulcinea. The altitude is 3 600 metres. The local atmospheric pressure is:

$$100 - \frac{3\ 600}{100} = 100 - 36 = 64 \text{ kPa}$$

or

$$1 - \frac{3\ 600}{10\ 000} = 1 - 0.36 = 0.64 \text{ ATA}$$

Every 6.4 x 1.03 metres of fresh water depth is equivalent to 10 metres of sea water.

So 36 metres of actual fresh water depth at an altitude of 3 600 metres is equivalent to:

$$\frac{36 \times 10}{6.4 \times 1.03} = 54.6 \text{ msw}$$

Using Royal Navy Tables, Martin Martin must plan his dive on a 57-metre schedule. If no decompression in water is needed, there is no further problem.

But, on a 57-msw apparent dive there are decompression stops. Martin Martin decides to dive for 20 minutes at 36 metres at Lake Titicaca.

He calculates that his apparent depth is 57 metres, and looking at the table sees that he must spend:

5 minutes at 9 msw
10 minutes at 6 msw
20 minutes at 3 msw

Trap number two opens.

At an altitude of 3 600 metres water depths of 3, 6 and 9 metres are not the same as at sea-level. The total pressure (ambient atmospheric + water pressure) is less.

The water stop depths must be *reduced* in depth. Just as the actual depth was 36 metres although a 57 metre table was used, so the decompression stops are equivalently shallower.

In this case:

$$\text{The 9-metre stop is done at } \frac{6.4 \times 1.03 \times 9}{10} = 5.9 \text{ metres}$$

$$\text{The 6-metre stop is done at } \frac{6.4 \times 1.03 \times 6}{10} = 4 \text{ metres}$$

$$\text{The 3-metre stop is done at } \frac{6.4 \times 1.03 \times 3}{10} = 2 \text{ metres}$$

These reduced stops give the same ratio of pressure change as the tabled 9-, 6- and 3-metre stops at sea-level. Times spent at the bottom and on decompression stops remain the same.

To summarise:

Apparent depth (metres) $= \dfrac{\text{Actual depth x 1 ATA}}{\text{Local ATA}}$

or even more simply $= \dfrac{\text{Actual depth}}{\text{Local ATA}}$

Using kPa: apparent depth $= \dfrac{\text{Actual depth x 100 kPa}}{\text{Local pressure in kPa}}$

The depth of decompression stops is exactly the same calculation, but with sea-level and local pressures transposed.

Decompression stop (metres) = Tabled stop x Local ATA

$= \dfrac{\text{Tabled stop x Local kPa}}{100}$

Finally, when diving at altitude:
1. Remember that fresh water is involved and an actual chosen *fresh water* depth must be divided by 1.03 to convert it into sea water density equivalence.
2. A chosen table sea water depth must be multiplied by 1.03 to obtain fresh water equivalence.
3. Remember to think in terms of local atmospheric pressures.
4. Remember that all depth corrections are only ratios of sea-level tables.

Flying after Diving

The question of flying home after diving is one which often worries sport divers. Altitude after depth can precipitate acute decompression illness due to both reduced ambient pressure and a reduced partial pressure of oxygen (which then decreases tissue tolerance to a nitrogen load). There are two very important variables:
— the inert gas load of the diver;
— the imposed physical conditions in an aircraft.

The inert gas load of the diver

The higher the inert gas load a scuba diver has dissolved in his or her tissues before a flight, the higher the risk of acute decompression illness. It takes any saturated tissue six half times to degas (see p 127). Blood, with a 5-minute half time takes 30 minutes to degas. To degas the 120-minute tissues requires 12 hours. For safety, this is the minimum time permitted between surfacing after short exposures and flying in an aircraft. Longer exposure to diving requires more surface time.

Daily exposure to diving	Accumulated bottom time	Any deco stops in last 48 hrs	Minimum time before flying
48 hours or less	Under 2 hrs	No	12 hrs
48 hours or less	Under 2 hrs	Yes	24 hrs
48 hours or less	Over 2 hrs	No	24 hrs
Multi-day	Unlimited	No	24 hrs
Multi-day	Unlimited	Yes	24-48 hrs

The imposed physical conditions in an aircraft

If a diver has an inert gas load, it is the venous system that transports this load from the tissues to the lungs for degassing. Platelet clumping, leading to blood sludging and clotting, occurs much more readily in nitrogen-loaded venous blood. Flying aggravates sludging in the venous system by inducing dehydration and by limiting movement:

— The cabin humidity in a commercial aircraft is only eight per cent. Breathing dry air rapidly depletes tissue fluids, including blood.

— Alcohol and caffeine (tea or coffee) stimulate urine production without adequately replacing the resultant fluid loss.

— Eating large fatty meals causes shunting of peripheral blood to the gut. Peripheral venous blood flow becomes sluggish and slow.

— Sitting for extended periods in an aircraft seat drastically reduces venous blood flow in the lower limbs. This is especially dangerous in divers. Acute decompression illness may occur with numbness or pain in the legs. In addition, swelling of the feet and pooling of blood in the calf veins leading to deep vein thrombosis is not uncommon.

Flying also exposes one to infection. Forty to sixty per cent of the air in an aircraft is recirculated. This means enforced sampling of a pot-pourri of perspiration, human body odours, assorted brands of cigarette smoke, and a polyculture of bacteria and viruses. Behind the plasticised decor and piped background music lurks an air-borne bacterial colony nearly thirty times greater than that found in an average sleazy bar. Upper respiratory infections, presenting two to three days after a flight, are very common.

What should divers do before, during and after a flight?

Before flying home, the last dive of the holiday should preferably be a short, deep dive. If you are planning a deep dive (25-30 msw), save it for last and keep it well within no-decompression time limits. This primarily loads the fast tissues which then have ample time to degas while you wait the required surface interval before flying. Should you ever have any untoward symptoms before a flight, which you think may be related to acute decompression illness, *do not fly*. Reducing altitude could be disastrous. Contact a diving doctor immediately.

During a flight, eat frugally and drink copious amounts of water, fruit juice and non-carbonated beverages. These prevent dehydration and induce the desire to urinate which then means a walk down the aisle and improved circulation in the legs — so move about regularly.

After a long international flight to a diving destination, drink lots of fluids, spend the first day of the diving holiday swimming and snorkelling, and go to bed early. Don't dive on day one — let your body recover from the insults of cramped, polluted aviation.

Drowning and Near-drowning

Drowning is death due to inhalation of fluid.

If a person survives immersion, drowning did not occur. The victim *nearly* drowned, so survival after fluid inhalation is called *near-drowning.*

There are three basic causes:
— accidental,
— suicidal,
— homicidal.

Only accidental drowning is relevant to divers. Obviously, anyone could drown anywhere, but there is a pattern:
— swimming pools: mostly babies and very young children;
— rivers, dams, and the seaside: mostly teenagers and young adults;
— boatsmen and fishermen at sea: mostly adults;
— bathtubs: mostly babies and the aged.

Predisposing Factors

Most accidents are preventable and drowning is usually very preventable.

Lack of supervision of children

Strict parental care is critical — leaving an unattended baby by a pool or in its bath while chatting on the phone or answering the doorbell is potentially tragic negligence. Pool fencing, 'drown-proofing' lessons, and learning to swim come next as safety measures.

Alcohol and drug abuse

About 80 per cent of adults who drown took alcohol before entering the water. Alcohol, drugs and swimming *never* mix. Look at the. reasons. Alcohol causes:
— overconfidence — risks are taken beyond training, fitness and ability;
— inability to react adequately to the situation resulting in panic;
— hypothermia due to skin flushing and rapid heat loss;
— increased likelihood of vomiting, with inhalation of vomit and water;

— possible suicidal tendencies.

General state of health

Underlying illnesses such as heart disease, high blood pressure, diabetes and epilepsy can place the victim in a drowning situation. Injuries from sharks and boat-propellers can do the same.

Diving

Divers do it in water so the spectre of drowning always lurks. What are the causes of drowning in divers?
— Panic
— Gas problems
  — hypoxia
  — oxygen toxicity
  — carbon dioxide toxicity
  — carbon monoxide poisoning
  — nitrogen narcosis
  — HPNS (theoretically)
— Pulmonary barotrauma (ascent and descent)
— Hypothermia
— Seasickness, vomiting and inhalation
— Marine animal stings and attacks
— Underwater injuries or entrapment
— Underwater explosions
— Underlying medical problems — known and unknown

Mechanism of Drowning

Much of the early research on drowning was done on experimental animals, by introducing sea water or fresh water into the lungs of the anaesthetised animals. Large quantities of water were poured into their lungs — up to 20 ml/kg body weight.

Two types of drowning were then described:
— freshwater drowning,
— salt-water drowning.
The following applies to experimental drowning of animals only. It does not happen in human drowning.

1. Freshwater drowning

Blood contains a great assortment of salts, proteins, glucose, hormones, and other chemicals. These *concentrate* the blood, making it more dense than water.

The presence of fresh water in the alveoli results in the water moving from an area of low concentration (alveoli) to an area of high concentration (blood in the lung capillaries). This dilutes the blood and increases blood volume. In addition, the red blood cells within the blood absorb water from the diluted blood and swell and then burst, releasing free haemoglobin into the blood. The increased blood volume causes heart overload and the rupture of red blood cells means reduced oxygen-carrying capacity and hypoxia. Heart failure then causes lung congestion and more hypoxia. Death results from cardiac arrest or ventricular fibrillation.

2. Salt-water drowning

Sea water contains many dissolved salts which make it even more concentrated than blood. So salt water in the alveoli causes water movement in the opposite direction to fresh water. Water moves from the blood in the lung capillaries to the alveoli. This causes marked lung congestion with water and decreases blood volume. The red cells lose water to the concentrated plasma and shrink.

Note: In both sea-water and freshwater drowning, lung congestion occurs. In freshwater drowning, because of heart overload with damming back of blood in the lungs due to pump failure, and in sea-water drowning through movement of water from the blood into the alveoli. Both cause boggy, fluid-filled lungs. Movement of oxygen through the flooded alveoli is impeded and there is interference with circulation through the lungs – both factors cause more hypoxia.

What happens in human beings?

The deliberate drowning of anaesthetised people by pouring 20 ml/kg of fresh water or sea water into the lungs will cause the police to raise their eyebrows. In a 70 kg man this would amount to the introduction of 20 x 70 ml or 1.4 litres of water. In human drowning, only about 2 ml/kg is usually inhaled. This is too little to cause the clear picture of experimental drowning.

Therefore:
- there is very little change in blood volume;
- rupture or shrinkage of red cells is very uncommon;
- dilution or concentration of blood is rare;
- ventricular fibrillation does not occur.

Why are human beings different from experiments?

1. *Diving reflex.* Immersion of the face in water causes reflex breath-holding and slowing of the heart, especially in babies.
2. *Laryngospasm.* Inhalation of water causes immediate spasmodic closure of the vocal cords, shutting off the larynx so water (or air) cannot enter. Only when death by hypoxia is imminent will the spasm relax. The victim is no longer attempting to breathe so water will not enter unless the person is head-up and face-up in the water. Most drowned victims are face-down.

3. *Hypothermia*. Cooling of the victim in cold water protects the brain and heart by reducing oxygen requirements. Babies have a relatively large surface area compared to adults and hypothermia occurs rapidly in infants.

These three factors:
— diving reflex,
— laryngospasm, and
— hypothermia
decrease water inhalation and prolong possible survival time under water. With vigorous resuscitation, survival with no apparent damage has been reported in people submerged for up to 40 minutes in cold water.

Presentation

The following is the sequence of events in drowning:
1. The victim submerges.
2. The diving reflex operates — breathholding occurs. How long the breath can be held depends on fitness, fatigue and fear.
3. Meanwhile, oxygen is being used and carbon dioxide produced in the body. The rising carbon dioxide eventually forces the victim to inhale.
4. Water is inhaled and laryngospasm occurs, keeping the victim's lungs more or less dry.
5. Oxygen is still being used and hypoxia worsens. Consciousness is lost. The heart begins to fail, causing lung congestion.
6. Still more hypoxia occurs. Breathing attempts stop and the laryngospasm relaxes. Passive flooding of the lungs may now occur if the victim is head-up and face-up in the water.
7. Death occurs.

Depending on the water temperature, how fat the victim is, and how much clothing is being worn (insulation), hypothermia will protect the victim to some degree. Theoretically, a skinny, naked victim should do better than a fat, dressed victim.

Rescue before death reveals the following:
1. The victim is unconscious and limp.
2. The skin is pale.
3. The skin is cold.
4. No breathing is evident.
5. There is no pulse or heartbeat.
6. The pupils do not react to light.
7. Copious frothy blood-stained foam may be flowing from the mouth due to lung congestion — secondary to heart (pump) failure from hypoxia.

Management of Near-drowning

Most people die after immersion because resuscitation was started too late or stopped too soon. If breathing is absent it should be assisted in the water, while bringing the victim to shore or to the boat. Supporting the head in the water and giving mouth-to-mouth or mouth-to-snorkel resuscitation may make all the difference. *Resuscitation should be continued until a doctor calls off the attempt because of definite death.* The method used is aimed at restoring breathing and circulation – Cardiopulmonary Resuscitation or CPR.

Note: The disease AIDS had made CPR a potentially dangerous procedure for the rescuer. It has become essential that rescuers protect themselves if any bleeding is present by using a non-return airway, gloves, goggles and a plastic apron, unless the victim is known to be HIV-negative.

Cardiopulmonary resuscitation (CPR)

Do not rush blindly into administering CPR. A 20-second initial assessment of the victim is vital. Six essential questions must first be answered.

Assessment

1.	Are the victim and the rescuer in a safe place?	H	HAZARDS?
2.	Is the victim rousable?	H	HELLO?
3.	Is anyone on hand to help?	H	HELP?
4.	Is the airway clear?	A	AIRWAY?
5.	Is the victim breathing?	B	BREATHING?
6.	Can a pulse be felt?	C	CIRCULATION?

1. *Are the victim and the rescuer in a safe place?* Both must be in a safe place – out of the water and on the beach beyond the tidal action of the sea, on the deck of the dive boat or, if inland, out of the way of oncoming traffic or chemical, electrical, thermal or physical hazards.

2. *Is the victim rousable?* Assess whether the victim is rousable by gently shaking his shoulder and yelling 'Are you OK?' Use your shouting voice, and not forceful shaking, to gain attention. Violent shaking may aggravate spinal or internal injuries.
(a) *The victim responds:* check for injuries, render assistance, summon help if required, then wait with the victim until trained aid comes.
(b) *The victim does not respond:* yell for help and immediately clear the victim's airways.

3. *Is anyone on hand to help?* If available, you need two kinds of help:
    – someone to summon emergency trained assistance (see p 248),
    – someone to assist with resuscitation of the victim.

4. *Is the airway clear?* Quickly partially unzip the victim's wet suit or slacken any tight neckwear.
(a) *Perform the 'head tilt-chin lift' manoeuvre:*
    – Place one hand on the victim's forehead and *tilt* the victim's head well back. This straightens the windpipe and provides a good

Basic life support

It's as simple as the ABC of CPR (Cardio Pulmonary Resuscitation)

Assess

Assess Alertness/Responsiveness

- Hazards?
  - Ensure safety of scene and rescuer
  - Beware of electrocution, noxious gases, oncoming traffic, etc.
- Hello?
  - Try to arouse victim by gently tapping the shoulder
  - Shout: 'Are you okay?'
- Help?
  - Call for assistance

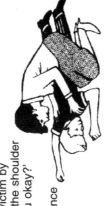

If Responsive →

Check for Injuries

- Look for injuries and treat as necessary
- Get help if needed
- Reassess victim
- Keep victim comfortable until help arrives

Not Responsive →

Breathing

Assess Breathing

- With the fingers of one hand, lift the bony part of the chin forwards while tilting the head back with the other hand.
- Remove obvious obstructions from mouth
- Place ear next to victim's mouth and nose
  - Look for movement of chest
  - Listen for breath sounds
  - Feel for breath on your cheek
- Take five seconds to determine if breathing

Adequate Breathing →

Place in Recovery Position

- Support head with one hand, and turn victim as a unit onto his side, ensuring that no twisting of the head or neck occurs
- Get help
- Keep checking breathing and pulse
- Stay with victim until help arrives

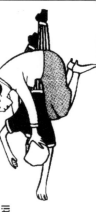

Circulation

- Keep head tilted back
- Slide two fingers into the groove between the 'Adam's Apple' and the muscles of the neck.
- Press gently
- Feel for a pulse for five seconds

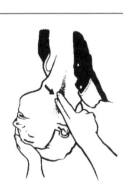

Pulse Present →

- Pinch nose closed with thumb and index finger of hand on victim's forehead
- Place mouth over victim's mouth, forming a tight seal, while lifting bony part of chin up with fingers of other hand
- Give 10 slow, full breaths, ensuring that the chest rises and falls with each breath
- Get help then reassess and continue rescue breathing if pulse present
- Reassess pulse after every 10 rescue breaths

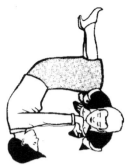

No Pulse →

Don't Delay

Get Help and Start CPR

- Call the emergency services immediately
- Commence CPR:
  A – Airway: Lift chin up and tilt head back
  B – Breathing: Give two slow full breaths
  C – Circulation: Place heel of one hand on lower half of breastbone, two finger-breadths above lower end of ribcage in the midline
- Place measuring hand on top of first hand and start chest compressions

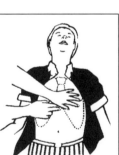

Do CPR →

Start Chest Compressions

- Compress breastbone to a depth of 4-5 cm, at a rate of 80 compressions per minute
- Count: 1-and, 2-and, 3-and, etc with each compression
- Lift chin, and give 2 full, slow breaths after every 15 compressions
- Continue until professional help arrives, or pulse and breathing returns.

Calling the emergency services:
1. Dial 10177 (otherwise 1022 or ....)
2. Indicate emergency (CPR in progress)
3. Give exact location (street name and number/cross-street/landmark/etc.)
4. Replace receiver last (answer all questions)
5. Return to the victim

Compiled by Dr WGJ Kloeck (Jan 93)

airway. (This is essential. Try it yourself — it is impossible to breathe properly with the head flexed forward on the neck.)
- Use the fingers of your other hand to *lift* up the front of the victim's jaw — this pulls the tongue forward and prevents it from flopping backwards and blocking the airway.

(b) Look inside the mouth. Quickly remove any foreign material. Clear away any vomit, blood or water by wiping the mouth from cheek to cheek with a forefinger wrapped in a piece of cloth.

(c) *Dentures, unless very loose or ill-fitting, must be left in place* — they will support a proper lip seal with mouth-to-mouth resuscitation.

(d) *In near-drowning there is often copious pink froth welling up from the lungs.* This must continuously be wiped away.

5. *Is the victim breathing?* While maintaining the head tilt-chin lift position, use the next 5 seconds:
- to listen for breathing next to victim's mouth and nose,
- to feel for any movement of breath with your cheek,
- to watch the victim's chest for movement.

(a) *The victim is unconscious and breathing:* turn the victim as a unit (head and body together to avoid worsening possible neck trauma) into the left lateral recovery position:
- victim lying on the left side with the left leg extended,
- head resting on the left arm extended in line with the body,
- right knee flexed and resting on the ground in front of the victim,
- right elbow flexed and resting on the ground in front of the victim.
This position ensures that the tongue cannot obstruct the airway and allows drainage of vomit, blood and water. Summon emergency help, then wait with the victim until professional aid comes, constantly monitoring satisfactory pulse and breathing.

(b) *The victim is not breathing:* feel for a *carotid* pulse.

6. *Can a pulse be felt?* The carotid arteries are the large arteries in the neck supplying blood to the head. They are easily found by placing the fingertips on the larynx and then moving them round to either side *into the hollow* next to the neck muscles and gently pressing back. A pulse is normally easily felt. It is essential to spend 5 to 10 seconds in finding a pulse. A very slow or weak pulse will not be found with a too rapid or cursory feel. Do not:
- try to find a wrist pulse — it is invariably impalpable,
- use a thumb to find a carotid pulse — you will feel your own pulse,
- press too hard — you will not feel a weakly pulsating artery.

(a) *The victim is not breathing but a pulse can be felt.* Perform mouth-to-mouth rescue breathing immediately.

Mouth-to-mouth rescue breathing:
- Ensure that the victim is on a firm, flat place.
- Roll the victim as a unit on to his or her back.

- Ensure the head tilt-chin lift position.
- If available, and especially if the victim is a stranger, place a disposable non-return airway between the victim's lips, with the thin plastic skirt of the airway covering the victim's face.
- Pinch off the nostrils, using the thumb and forefinger of the head-tilt hand. (Do not forget to pinch off the nose. It is pointless to commence blowing through the victim's mouth and venting through his nostrils.)
- Inhale deeply, then place your mouth firmly over the victim's mouth or the non-return airway. Blow slowly and fully into the victim's mouth or the airway. *Take a full 2 seconds to do this.* Allow the victim to exhale passively while you take another deep breath. Repeat this ventilation *10 times.* There should be very little resistance. Watch the victim's chest. It should rise when you blow. Be sure that it is not the victim's stomach that is rising. If this happens you are filling the stomach with air which will predispose to vomiting. *If the victim's chest does not move, it means obstruction or leakage.* Then:
  - ensure that the head is tilted well back,
  - ensure that the jaw is well lifted,
  - ensure that the nostrils are pinched closed,
  - ensure that the victim's mouth is partially open,
  - ensure a good mouth-to-mouth or mouth-to-airway seal.
- If the chest still does not rise when you blow slowly and fully, there is foreign material in the airway. Then:
  With the victim flat on the back, straddle the victim's upper legs. Place the palm of one hand on the back of the other and link your fingers. Place the heel of the lower hand on the victim's abdomen just above the navel and well below the breastbone. Push sharply upwards and inwards. Repeat this thrust up to 5 times. This will force inhaled foreign material from the airway. Clear this away by sweeping your forefinger around the inside of the cheek and behind the material. Listen, feel and watch for breathing. If no breathing is evident, recommence rescue breathing.
- When the victim is being ventilated properly, there will be passive exhalations between breaths. Mouth-to-mouth ventilation must be done at a rate of 10 to 12 breaths per minute in an adult, checking the carotid pulse after each cycle of 10 breaths.

(b) *The victim is not breathing and no pulse can be felt.* Summon emergency assistance — CPR and defibrillation are required.

Cardiopulmonary resuscitation
- Send someone to make the emergency call. If you are alone, make the call yourself before starting CPR. It is essential to ensure that advanced life support is rushing to help you. Quickly telephone your private rescue service or dial 1022 anywhere in South Africa.
- Tell the rescue service that CPR is about to be performed or is being done. Do not waste time explaining the case. *Say 'CPR'.*

- Be calm and relay all asked-for information clearly (see p 248).
- Go back to the victim immediately after the rescue service hangs up.

Remember:
- ventricular fibrillation is uncommon in true human drowning,
- ventricular fibrillation is commonly caused by cold water stress in adults and death is then due to cardiac arrest, not drowning.

Commence CPR and continue until professional help arrives.

One-rescuer CPR

In order to maintain proper sequence in extremely emotional and confusing circumstances, it is essential to call out each step.

A = AIRWAY. Call A and perform the head tilt-chin lift manoeuvre.

B = BREATHING. Call B and deliver two slow deep breaths to the victim. Watch that chest movement occurs.

C = CIRCULATION. Call C and place the heel of one hand on the centre of the chest two fingerbreadths above the lower end of the breastbone.

Now place the other hand on top of the first with your fingers off the chest and facing away from you.

- *Keep your elbows straight.*
- *Keep your shoulders directly above the victim's breastbone.*
- *Keep your fingers off the victim's chest.* You must press on the breastbone, not on the ribs.

Press *smoothly* downward, using the weight of your upper body to push the breastbone down 4 to 5 centimetres. Do not jerk downwards – you will break ribs and damage internal organs. Release the pressure, allowing the chest wall to spring back, but without losing your hand position on the breastbone.

This process compresses the heart between the front of the chest and the spine, forcing blood from the ventricles. On releasing pressure, the ventricles refill from the venous system. If done properly, a pulse will be felt in the neck with each compression.

Repeat this compression 15 times, while loudly reciting, 'One and, two and, three and, four and...' Compress with each number and release with each 'and'. You will achieve a rate of 80 to 100 compressions per minute.

You have completed one cycle of ABC. This must be repeated in cycles of 2 breaths then 15 compressions (2:15) until help arrives, or the victim breathes or moves. If you are alone do not waste time trying to find a carotid pulse again – it will break your rhythm and timing.

Call A and return to the airway.

Call B and give 2 slow, deep, mouth-to-mouth breaths.

Call C and commence 'One and, two and...'

It is hard and desperate work, but persistence is vital. If spontaneous breathing recurs, place the victim in the left lateral position, give 100% oxygen by mask if it is available, and stop CPR.

Two-rescuer CPR

If you have someone to assist you, perform the initial six-question assessment:

1. Are the victim and the rescuers in a safe place? H HAZARDS?
2. Is the victim rousable? H HELLO?
3. Is anyone on hand to help? H HELP?
4. Is the airway clear? A AIRWAY?
5. Is the victim breathing? B BREATHING?
6. Can a pulse be felt? C CIRCULATION?

Then proceed as described above and determine whether the victim still needs any rescue breathing or CPR. If either is required, one rescuer begins immediately while the other summons emergency help and then returns.

The first rescuer kneels on one side of the victim's head − he will be in charge of *airway and breathing*. He ensures the airway is clear, then ventilates the victim with *one* deep, slow exhalation.

The second rescuer kneels on the opposite side next to the victim's chest (the two rescuers can then see each other and coordinate their actions) − he will be in charge of *circulation*. He places his hands correctly over the victim's breastbone, *waits for the victim's chest to inflate,* then performs 5 smooth compressions at a rate of 80 to 100 compressions per minute while calling, 'One and, two and...'

This cycle of one breath to 5 compressions (1:5) is repeated continuously until a spontaneous pulse and breathing return, or emergency help arrives and takes over.

Note

The rescuer in charge of circulation must wait for two seconds after each fifth compression, while the first rescuer administers one rescue breath. If the chest is compressed during the rescue breath, most of the delivered air will not enter the victim's lungs − it will be blown back into the first rescuer's mouth or diverted into the victim's stomach and predispose to vomiting and aspiration.

The two rescuers must monitor each other:
− the rescuer in charge of airway and breathing must feel for a pulse in the carotid artery with each chest compression;
− the rescuer in charge of circulation must watch that the chest expands with each rescue breath.

Every few minutes stop CPR for 5 seconds while a carotid artery is checked by the airway rescuer for the reappearance of a spontaneous pulse. The rescuers can take advantage of this time to change places if the circulation rescuer is tiring. The airway rescuer always restarts CPR by giving a rescue breath − it is pointless to compress the chest 5 times without an initial charge of new lung air. If a pulse is felt, test for spontaneous breathing too.

If a third person is present and oxygen is available, he or she should hold the oxygen mask against the airway rescuer's face while he waits for the 5 chest compressions to be performed. The airway rescuer will then deliver a much higher oxygen partial pressure to the victim with each mouth-to-mouth exhalation.

Emergency equipment
An Ambubag is a very valuable piece of emergency equipment. It consists of a rubber bag which forces air into a face mask through a one-way valve when the bag is squeezed. On releasing pressure on the bag it refills through another one-way valve. Oxygen can be piped into the patient inlet so that
- unpleasant and potentially dangerous mouth-to-mouth contact is avoided,
- oxygen can be administered during ventilation.
A plastic airway is another useful tool. It has a curved plastic tube, flattened to fit the mouth, and ensures that the tongue is kept from rolling back. The airway should not be too long nor too short. It should extend from the lips to the angle of the jaw. Together with an Ambubag, superior control of breathing is at hand.

Always bear in mind that a near-drowned diver may also have substantial decompression requirements, arterial gas embolism, or both. In this case, administer CPR until expert help takes over and then transports the victim to a recompression facility. Always remember to notify the facility so that qualified help is waiting and the chamber can be prepared in advance.

Signs of improvement
CPR is a dire measure for someone who performs it for the first time. Any sign that it is working will give courage and strength to aching arms and back:
- The victim's lips become pinker.
- The pupils start to react to light. They become smaller when a torch or other light is shone into them.
- Spontaneous heartbeat starts. Stop chest compressions.
- Spontaneous breathing begins. Stop rescue breathing and give oxygen by mask.
Even when full recovery of a near-drowned person appears to have occurred, in that he or she is breathing, the heart is beating and consciousness has returned, medical help must be obtained and the patient admitted to hospital for observation. The secondary effects of near-drowning and hypoxia can kill the recovered victim hours later (see secondary drowning).

Vertigo Under Water

Vertigo is a subjective illusion of directional movement — to the left or right, upwards, downwards, or round and round like a merry-go-round. The diver may feel either that he or she is spinning or falling in a particular direction, or that he or she is quite still but that the environment is suddenly moving or turning topsy-turvy.

Vertigo is extremely disorientating, is frequently accompanied by intense nausea and vomiting and, when it occurs under water, can be a rapidly life-threatening condition. It must be clearly understood that vertigo is not dizziness, faintness, light-headedness or giddiness. There is always a profound hallucination of movement which can render a diver totally incapable of any safe, or even life-saving, reaction.

In the scuba diving mode, vertigo is invariably caused by:
— sensory deprivation,
— disorders of the ear, or
— inhaled gas toxicity, including hypoxia and hypocapnia.

Sensory Deprivation

Under conditions of poor visibility due to turbid water or night diving, disorientation is very common. In inexperienced divers disorientation may proceed to true vertigo, due to any combination of hyperventilation, loss of gravity, sound and visual reference or anxiety which then reduces the inner ear threshold for the onset of vertigo.

Disorders of the Ear

External ear

Vertigo as a result of a disorder of the external ear can occur if one external canal is obstructed.

Caloric vertigo. The external ear can induce vertigo if the temperature of the water entering the external ears varies. The temperature of the water in each external ear affects its respective inner ear. If one external ear canal is blocked by wax, a foreign body such as an ear plug, bony thickening (exostoses), or obstruction by swelling due to swimmer's ear, then cold water cannot easily enter that canal and the information relayed to its semicircular canal in the inner ear will differ from the much colder news delivered to the other side. It is the horizontal semicircular canals that are especially relevant.

In the upright position on land, the horizontal semicircular canals relay information about sideways movements of the head to the brain. If a diver is descending head-down with the angle of the head at 30 degrees to the horizontal, the horizontal semicircular canals become vertical. Under these conditions, any partial obstruction to an external ear can induce profound temperature-induced or *caloric* vertigo. Vertical information from one ear is interpreted by the brain as horizontal and intense disorientation results.

The solution is simple: if the diver assumes a vertical position under water the vertigo disappears.

External ear barotrauma of descent. Total obstruction of one external ear canal by wax, a foreign body or inflammation prevents water from filling the canal during descent (see p 107). The air space trapped between the obstruction and the ear drum contracts and the ear drum bulges outwards, pulling the bony chain of the middle ear with it. Pulling on the stirrup reduces the pressure of the footplate in the oval window on the affected side. A difference in pressure in the inner ears results and vertigo can occur.

In this case, the diver is often in a vertical position under water and changing position does not relieve the vertigo. Ascent is required.

Middle ear

Middle ear barotrauma of descent (ear squeeze). If a diver fails to equalise but persists with descent, the shrinking air volume in the middle ear sucks the ear drum inwards (see pp 107-110). Haemorrhage into the middle ear may occur to equalise pressure, and vertigo can result.

Ear drum perforation. If haemorrhage into the middle ear to compensate failed equalisation during continued descent does not occur, the ear drum bursts inwards. The diver hears a sudden noise, then experiences intense vertigo as cold water gushes into the middle ear. This is the second cause of *caloric* vertigo (see above). Rapid warming of the cold water to body temperature occurs and the vertigo passes. On returning to the surface, the diver notices deafness in the ear, often accompanied by bloody fluid leaking from the affected ear.

Middle ear barotrauma of ascent (alternobaric vertigo). During ascent, air in the middle ear expands with reducing ambient pressure. If release of the excess volume through the Eustachian tubes is unequal, the resulting pressure variation in the two middle ears can cause unequal inner ear stimulation and vertigo. This is called *alternobaric vertigo* (literally, 'vertigo due to two kinds of pressure').

If one Eustachian tube is blocked by blood or mucus from a previous middle ear squeeze, nasal allergy or infection, the ear drum may rupture outwards during ascent (see p 110). In this case the diver clearly hears gas bubbling out of the ear as he ascends; water does not enter the middle ear because of the vigorous passage of expanding gas through the external ear; and vertigo may not occur.

Inner ear

Inner ear barotrauma. Trauma to the inner ear, including round window rupture, can follow a very forceful equalising attempt (see pp 110-112). Vertigo may be immediate or, if the leak of inner ear fluid is slight, delayed for days.

Seasickness. With unequal or aberrant stimulation of the vestibular apparatus, intense seasickness with vertigo can occur above and below water (see pp 73-76).

Acute inner ear decompression illness. Acute decompression illness involving only the inner ear is very rare in sport divers. Invariably any vertigo is only part of more widespread and serious neurological involvement. Pure inner ear decompression illness is far more common with deep heliox saturation diving.

Caloric stimulation. Some divers have different caloric responses to the same cold temperature from the vestibular apparatus in each ear. This third type of cold-induced vertigo occurs without any equalising difficulty, external ear obstruction or ear drum injury. The diver equalises easily, reaches bottom depth effortlessly and then develops disabling vertigo about five to ten minutes after starting the dive.

This type of caloric vertigo can usually be prevented by wearing a hood.

Gas Toxicity

A diver depends for his life on the purity and safety of his breathing mix. Several gas-induced disorders can present with vertigo. It is essential that a diver recognises vertigo for what it is, signals his buddy for help, and then commences an assisted ascent.

Nitrogen narcosis

At depths below about 40 msw nitrogen narcosis can present with giddiness. True vertigo is uncommon but if a feeling of rotation begins it will always be relieved on ascent.

Oxygen toxicity

Breathing pure oxygen or nitrox mixtures rapidly induces toxicity when the oxygen partial pressure exceeds 2 ATA. The onset of vertigo is indicative of an incipient convulsion under water.

Hypoxia

In the sport diving situation, hypoxia occurs most commonly with breathhold diving. The other causes are considered on p 144. Vertigo is one of the usual presenting features.

Carbon dioxide toxicity

Skip breathing, breathing dense nitrox mixtures, air supply contamination, or the use of faulty rebreathers can result in vertigo due to inner ear and cerebral carbon dioxide build-up.

Hypocapnia

Hyperventilation at the surface by breathhold divers, or under water by anxious scuba divers, causes the alveolar and arterial carbon dioxide levels to drop. An increase in the alkalinity of the blood occurs and vertigo is frequent.

Carbon monoxide poisoning

Air supply contamination by exhaust fumes leading to carbon monoxide inhalation under water regularly presents with vertigo.

Management of Underwater Vertigo

Vertigo under water is a life-threatening event. It is impossible for an affected diver to react rationally to a sudden and spinning loss of orientation, and total reliance on a vigilant buddy is all that can be done. The onset of nausea and vomiting, disorientation, inhalation of water, panic and frantic attempts to reach a non-discernible surface make an assisting buddy's task extremely difficult. Firmness is essential. The affected diver must be returned to the surface. It is impossible to perform any required in-water decompression stops under conditions of vertigo. In most cases, beginning the ascent will at least reduce the vertigo. In extreme cases with profound vertigo and uncontrollable disorientation, initiating a controlled buoyant ascent may be necessary. The consequences of missed decompression stops and possible pulmonary barotrauma of ascent must then be considered and acted on, and the buddy must remember that he too has missed decompression stops.

Common Infections in Scuba Divers

It is axiomatic that divers expose themselves to water, so water harbouring bacteria, viruses, fungi, yeasts and parasites can cause problems in divers. Infection can occur whenever contaminated water gains entry into a diver's body:
— through the skin,
— via the mouth,
— into the ears,
— into the lungs,
— into the eyes.
Infection can also occur when an intermediate host harbours a developmental stage of an infecting organism and then directly or indirectly causes diver infection.

All divers should consult their doctors for expert advice before leaving on a diving holiday or expedition.

All divers should maintain their immunity to tetanus by having tetanus toxoid booster injections every three years.

All divers should be immunised against hepatitis B.

Skin Infections

Infections of the skin are common in divers. They usually occur following skin injury, e.g. coral cuts and fin blisters, or by allowing the skin to become excessively soggy, predisposing to yeast and fungal invasion.

Tinea pedis (athlete's foot)

This fungal infection of the skin of the feet follows barefoot exposure to contaminated wet areas such as showers and decks, or sharing rubber diving bootees. The skin, commonly between the toes, becomes very white and soggy. Small blisters appear which later burst and are followed by skin ulcers and peeling. Pain is not usually a feature unless secondary bacterial infection occurs in the broken skin.

Treatment
1. Keep the skin dry. Exposure to sunlight dries out the blisters.
2. Bathe the feet in 0.05% potassium permanganate solution (about ⅓ teaspoon in 5 litres of water) twice a day when the blisters are first noticed. Dry carefully with paper towels.
3. Apply topical antifungals such as ketoconazole, zinc undecanoate with undecanoic acid, tolnaftate, or miconazole for three to four weeks.

Tinea versicolor

This superficial fungal infection of the skin is caused by the fungus *Malassezia furfur*. It presents with many brownish spots over the body, especially the chest and back. It is usually very mild and is only noticed after sunbathing when the skin becomes tanned everywhere except for untanned paler spots affected by the fungus.

Treatment. The application of half-strength Whitfield's ointment, 15% sodium thiosulphate solution, or 5% salicylic acid in alcohol for three to four weeks cures the condition. The conazole group of antifungal creams is also effective.

Coral abrasions and cuts

Inadvertent skin contact with the hard corals frequently results in skin nicks and grazes which are only noticed on return to the surface. Infection is almost invariable if calcific fragments, nematocysts and contaminating bacteria are not thoroughly removed from the wound. Infection becomes apparent after a few days with swelling, redness and heat in the area, then spreads to surrounding normal tissues. Skin wounds sustained by divers do not do well if diving is continued. Repeated wetting removes antiseptic or antibiotic creams, reinfects the wound, and causes bogginess of the skin. Under these conditions healing can be very much delayed.

Treatment. If possible, a doctor must be consulted.
1. Avoid direct contact with coral. This usually occurs due to excessive negative buoyancy in inexpert divers and students.
2. Wash any coral injury thoroughly with antiseptic solution such as cetrimide and chlorhexidine. It is essential to ensure that all foreign debris has been removed.
3. Apply an antiseptic cream, e.g. povidone iodine, or an antibiotic cream such as neomycin, mupirocin or fusidate.
4. If infection spreads as evidenced by increasing pain, swelling and redness, consult a doctor. An oral antibiotic such as broad-spectrum penicillin or tetracycline is necessary.

5. Treat any non-diving related cut or blister with frequent applications of antibiotic or antiseptic cream. Any diving or immersion in water may aggravate these injuries too.

Infections via the Mouth

Swallowing water contaminated by sewage can cause a host of illnesses, including bacterial gastroenteritis, amoebic dysentery, cholera, typhoid and paratyphoid. If the measures described on pp 97-98 are ineffectual in controlling any episode of diarrhoea and vomiting, expert medical advice becomes essential.

Avoid sewage-contaminated water like the plague − it can cause it!

Ear Infections

External and middle ear infections have been discussed on pp 68 and 71.

Lung Infections

Inadvertent inhalation of water or a near-drowning episode may be followed by secondary lower respiratory infection such as pneumonia or abscesses in the lungs. This is one of the reasons for seeking urgent medical attention after a near-drowning experience. In addition, a delayed chemical pneumonia due to irritation of the lungs by only small volumes of sea water can place the victim in dire straits hours after apparent full recovery from near-drowning. Hospitalisation, oxygen therapy and antibiotics become essential.

Contamination of regulators is another source of respiratory infection. Failure to clean regulators after diving is the cause. The condition has been labelled *scuba disease*. Bacteria, commonly *Pseudomonas* and *Moraxella,* as well as other marine bacteria, survive inside the regulator and are inhaled with the next dive. Thorough cleansing and drying of regulators and cylinder HP outlets are an essential part of safe diving practice.

Eye Infections

Exposure of the eyes to chlorinated water or sea water may result in chemical irritation or infective conjunctivitis. Chemical or allergic irritation presents with red, burning or itchy eyes and is rapidly relieved by the use of 0.9% saline eye baths followed by antihistaminic drops containing antazoline, oxymetazoline or phenylephrine. Bacterial conjunctivitis (pink eye) requires antibiotic therapy. A doctor should be consulted before these are used. Numerous preparations are available, containing antibiotics such as neomycin, chloromycetin, fusidic acid, gentamycin, polymixin and sulphacetamide. Eye preparations containing cortisone derivatives should never be used without medical opinion, as corneal ulceration and scarring can occur with viral eye infections.

Infections via an Intermediate Host

Aside from direct infection with contaminating organisms in water, divers are often exposed to diseases which possess a more complex infective pattern. These are carried in intermediate hosts — other creatures that harbour the disease and pass it on to man. The route of infection may be oral, e.g. paralytic shellfish poisoning (PSP) following the eating of contaminated molluscs, or by penetration of the skin by the organism or the intermediate host.

Tick-bite fever

Divers camping in African and Mediterranean countries may be bitten by ticks harbouring *Rickettsia conori*, the causative organism of tick-bite fever. After a few days, a black sore develops at the site of the tick bite, followed by painful enlargement of nearby lymph glands. Fever, severe headache and a spotted rash appear. The disease is self-limiting, even without treatment, and is rarely fatal.

Treatment
1. Adequate precautions must be taken to avoid being bitten, including the use of insect repellents.
2. Any ticks found on the skin must be removed. Do not pull off the tick. It usually breaks in two, leaving the head embedded in the diver's skin. Apply a drop of petrol, paraffin or diesel on to the tick. This will induce it to let go. It can then be removed using tweezers.
3. Not all ticks carry tick-bite fever and most tick bites simply heal. Only if the tick itself is harbouring the organism will a black sore develop and the disease occur.
4. Tetracyclines cure tick-bite fever, but should not be given to children under 13 years as staining and damage to unerupted teeth can occur.

Malaria

Malaria is carried by the female *Anopheles* mosquito and infection occurs following a mosquito bite and the injection of the insect's saliva containing the malaria parasite into the wound. The disease occurs in many parts of the world and is caused by a parasite called *Plasmodium*. There are four species of *Plasmodium,* the most dangerous of these being *Plasmodium falciparum.*

The parasite multiplies in red blood cells, which swell and then burst to release more parasites. These then attack other red cells and multiply. In severe cases the urine becomes blood stained with excretion of clumps of released haemoglobin from billions of destroyed red cells. Obstruction to microscopic kidney tubules disrupts their filtering capacity and can lead to kidney failure. This is the picture in the serious complication of malaria called blackwater fever.

Presentation. Malaria usually presents initially with flu-like symptoms — headache, muscle and joint aches, and fever. Severe shivering attacks (rigors) and high fever then occur, and recur in a cyclical pattern every third or fourth day. *P. falciparum* can cause massive invasion and destruction of red cells and obstruction of capillaries anywhere in the body. Involvement of brain capillaries leads to cerebral malaria. Paralysis, convulsions, coma and death may result.

Prevention. No drug provides 100 per cent cover against malarial infection. Prophylaxis must involve both mosquito avoidance and antimalarial drugs.

Mosquito avoidance involves:
— meticulous application of insect repellent to exposed skin *and* clothing — the repellent of choice is N,N-diethyltoluamide (e.g. Peaceful Sleep, Mylol and Tabard lotion and stick);
— wearing long-sleeved shirts or blouses, slacks and socks between sunset and sunrise (the feeding time of the *Anopheles* mosquito);
— moving continuously when outdoors at night (mosquitoes prefer a static meal);
— mosquito screening on all doors and windows;
— spraying insecticide inside living quarters every day at dusk;
— burning insecticide coils in the sleeping quarters at night;
— sleeping under insecticide-impregnated mosquito nets tucked in under the mattress.

Antimalarial drugs. The drug of choice depends on the area visited, the presence or absence of drug-resistant *P. falciparum* malaria, personal allergies and idiosyncrasies to antimalarial medication, drug interaction with any maintenance medication a diver may be using, pregnancy, age, health, and the availability of the drug. Consult your doctor to determine the best choice of medication and to ensure that no untoward side-effects or contraindications are present.

In South Africa, with the exception of the Ingwavuma and Ubombo districts, all species of malaria are to date chloroquine-sensitive. A combination of pyrimethamine and chloroquine (Daraclor) is usually effective. Preventative treatment should begin 24 hours before entering an endemic area. In adults and children over 12 years, two tablets are taken initially, repeated weekly on the same day while in the area, then weekly for 4 weeks after leaving the area. Children aged 6 to 12 years take one tablet; aged one to 5 years ½ tablet (or 10 ml of syrup); aged 6 weeks to 12 months 5 ml of syrup.

Dapsone and pyrimethamine (Maloprim) is an alternative preventative measure, and should also begin 24 hours before entering a malarial area. Adults take one tablet weekly and continue for 3 to 4 weeks after leaving the area. Children aged 5 to 10 years take ½ tablet.

In areas where drug-resistant *P. falciparum* prevails (South-east Asia including the Philippines, Thailand, Burma and China, Gabon and most of sub-Saharan Africa, and the Ingwavuma and Ubombo districts of South Africa), other antimalarial drugs are required. These are tabulated below.

Drugs recommended in the prevention of resistant *P. falciparum* malaria

Preventative drug	Dose in adults	Dose in children
Mefloquine Trade name: — Lariam	250 mg each week on the same day. Start 24 hours before entering the area and continue for 4 weeks after leaving the area. *It can cause vertigo and divers are advised not to use it if at all possible.*	Do not use in children under 15 kg. 5 mg/kg body mass per week, at the same time intervals as adults. *Contraindicated in pregnancy and breast-feeding.*
Chloroquine Trade names: — Nivaquine — Anoclor — Plasmoquine	400 mg each week on the same day. Start one week before entering the area and continue for 6 weeks after leaving the area. Usually taken in combination with proguanil.	5 mg/kg body mass per week, at the same time intervals as adults. *Safe in pregnancy.*
Proguanil Trade name: — Paludrine	200 mg daily. Start 24 hours before entering the area and continue on a daily basis for 6 weeks after leaving the area. *Must only be taken together with chloroquine.*	Under 1 year: 25 mg/day. 1-4 years: 50 mg/day. 5-8 years: 100 mg/day. 9-14 years: 150 mg/day. *Safe in pregnancy.*
Doxycycline Trade names: — Cyclidox — Doxyclin — Doxylets — Doxymycin — Dumoxin — Thedox — Vibramycin	100 mg daily. Start 48 hours before entering the area and continue on a daily basis for 4 weeks after leaving the area. *Skin sensitisation and severe sunburn may occur.*	*Do not use in children under 8 years.* 8-15 years: 3 mg/kg daily as for adults. *Contraindicated in pregnancy and breast-feeding.*

Self-treatment of malaria. Divers in remote malarial areas and without access to immediate medical treatment may be faced with the problem of unexplained fever, headache, body aching and rigors. If malaria is suspected, use Fansidar (pyrimethamine/sulphadoxine) as a single dose (3 tablets in adults; 2 tablets aged 9-14 years; one tablet aged 4-8 years; ½ tablet under 4 years). This is a temporary measure only – a doctor must be found and consulted.

Bilharzia

Named after the physician Bilharz, the disease occurs in tropical and subtropical areas. It is contracted by swimming near the banks of dams and rivers infested with the *cercarial* larval form of one of the human blood flukes belonging to the *Schistosoma* genus. Their life cycle is amazingly complex. Cercariae in the water digest and burrow through the diver's skin and capillaries and enter the bloodstream to reach the veins of the liver. Here they mature into adult worms and then migrate to the veins in the membranes of the gut or pelvic veins where they live for several years. The female worm begins to produce eggs (over 1 000 per day) which are excreted in the urine or stool, depending on the species involved. The eggs must now reach dam, or sluggishly flowing river water where they hatch within a few minutes into an intermediate larval form *(miracidium)*. To achieve this, urine or stool contamination of water has to occur. Once hatched, the miracidia have less than 24 hours to find and penetrate the skin of a specific species of water snail. If they fail to find a snail, they die. Inside the snail, the miracidium makes its way to the digestive gland and begins to produce thousands of cercariae. A single miracidium can produce over 200 000 cercariae. Burrowing out of the snail, the cercariae are released in puffs into the water to complete the life cycle. They have two to three days to find a swimmer to invade, or die.

Inland divers in bilharzia-infested water are obviously at risk. Their wet suits afford protection, but any exposed skin may be a target site for cercarial penetration.

Presentation. Bilharzia eggs have sharp spines, exude digestive enzymes, and work their way through blood vessels and tissues in the bladder and bowel to reach the inside of the organ involved. Blood in the urine (frequently the last few drops) or stool may be a presenting sign, or difficulty with urination or diarrhoea may occur. Generalised fatigue, and loss of appetite and energy reserves may develop due to anaemia. If untreated, later severe scarring results due to the passage of millions of spiked eggs through involved organs, with ulceration, obstruction, and interference with the function and venous drainage of the abdominal organs. Cancer of the bladder is not uncommon in late cases.

Management of bilharzia
Prevention. Bilharzial areas should be avoided. All divers who do swim in water suspected of harbouring bilharzia should wear full wet suits, hoods, gloves and bootees. They should have their blood tested twice a year to

exclude undiagnosed bilharzia. Unexplained fatigue should also be checked to exclude possible bilharzia.

Treatment. The drug of choice for proven bilharzia is praziquantel (Biltricide). It is a single-dose oral treatment but must only be given with a proven diagnosis of bilharzia. This requires finding schistosome eggs in urine or stool specimens, or in the tissues of the rectum or bladder on biopsy.

Schistosome dermatitis (swimmer's itch)

If non-human schistosome larvae (whose hosts normally are migratory water birds or muskrats) penetrate human skin, an itchy inflammation of the skin at the area can occur. These cercariae invade man by accident and cannot survive in the wrong host. They are destroyed by the human inflammatory response.

Treatment. Soothing creams or lotions, e.g. calamine lotion, or zinc oxide with salicylic acid and ichthammol, are all that is required.

Burns

Aside from fungal or bacterial skin infections, divers are prone to skin damage as a result of sun exposure and burns or scalds at camp fires.

Sunburn

Exposure to excessive ultraviolet radiation causes inflammation of the skin presenting with redness, pain and swelling. In tropical and subtropical areas, 30 minutes of sun exposure is enough to cause sunburn. Symptoms only appear after several hours — excessive morning exposure presents with pain and redness the same night. With extreme exposure, the skin becomes very red and painful, blistering occurs over the next 24 hours, and skin peeling follows.

Depletion of the ozone layer by the world-wide use of chlorofluorocarbons has resulted in much harder and intensely active ultraviolet light reaching the earth's surface. These radiations induce cancerous change in skin and the incidence of malignant melanoma, a highly malignant tumour of the skin, has risen in recent times.

Predisposing factors to sunburn

Retinoids. The diving population is generally a young one and acne, with all of its cosmetic and social implications, is common among divers. Medicine has addressed the problem of acne and several oral and topical medications, based on vitamin-A retinoid precursors, are available which achieve very gratifying results in acne management. The problem is that the use of retinoids such as topical tretinoin and oral isotretinoin sensitises the skin to sunlight and predisposes to severe sunburning and its complications. An additional problem with oral isotretinoin is its effect on the membranes of the nose and throat. Severe drying of nasal membranes is a common side-effect, predisposing to nose bleeds, Eustachian tube dysfunction, and middle ear barotrauma of descent and ascent. Oral isotretinoin is contraindicated with diving.

Antibiotics. Other antibiotics commonly used in acne management are tetracyclines and sulphonamides. These also sensitise the skin to sun damage.

Management of sunburn

Prevention
1. Divers unaccustomed to sun exposure must protect their skin. Many barrier creams are available, offering partial to total protection from ultraviolet light. These must be reapplied after diving, as water exposure will tend to wash off the protective screening layer.
    The use of barrier creams or moisturising preparations can produce mask problems under water. The mask may tend to slip and slide over oiled skin, and wiping the glass surface of the mask with greasy hands can result in blurring of vision under water.
2. Skin-sensitising medications should be avoided.

Treatment
1. Moist bandages offer relief to areas of painful sunburn.
2. The use of half-strength cortisone creams in a moisturising base increases the soothing effect of moist bandages.
3. In severe cases of sunburn with generalised symptoms such as fever, nausea, vomiting and malaise, a doctor must be called. Oral cortisone may be indicated.
4. Antihistamines, by mouth or in cream form, do not help sunburn.
5. Oral pain-killers will afford some relief.

Burns and Scalds

Burns are skin damage caused by fire or hot solids. Scalds are damage caused by hot liquids or steam. Both are common injuries in a camping environment. The depth and extent of injury are very important in determining management. First degree burns cause skin reddening and swelling only, and peeling occurs after a few days. This is very similar to moderate sunburn. Second degree burns result in blistering under the epidermis of the skin, often with bleeding into the blisters. Third degree burns cause full-depth destruction of the skin and permanent scarring is inevitable.

If second degree burns involve more than nine per cent of the skin (equivalent to a whole arm, half a leg, or half of the back or front of the torso) hospitalisation and intensive local and intravenous treatment are essential. The same applies to third degree burns affecting more than two per cent of the skin area.

Treatment
1. Move the victim to a safe area.
2. Drench the burnt area immediately with copious cold water and continue water cooling for 30 minutes. Speed is essential so do not

waste time first removing bits of burnt clothing. Hot skin continues to suffer more damage until the temperature of the skin and underlying tissues cools down.

3. Rinse off loose bits of burnt clothing and dead skin with very dilute antiseptic solution. Do not remove adherent charred skin or clothing.
4. Leave blisters alone — do not deroof or remove blisters.
5. *Do not apply sugar, honey, flour, powder, etc. to a burn!*
6. Medical help must be sought if the burn is more than first degree.
7. If medical help is not available, leave small blisters alone and use a sterile syringe and needle to drain large blisters. Once drained, blisters flatten and form a 'biological bandage' over the area.
8. Apply synthetic dressings such as OpSite Flexigrid, Granuflex or Omniderm if they are available. They maintain a humid environment under the dressing, allow oxygen and carbon dioxide transfer, are effective bacterial barriers and, being transparent, permit visual examination of the burn. These dressings should be changed every 5 to 7 days.
9. If synthetic dressings are unavailable, cover the burnt area with a non-adhesive dressing impregnated with silver sulphadiazine or furacin cream; or apply vaseline/antibiotic-impregnated gauze such as Sofra-tulle or Fucidin tulle.
10. Cover the dressing with layers of gauze, then cotton wool, and bind gently in place with a crepe bandage. Change the dressing daily.
11. Before changing any dressing, thoroughly soak the area with dilute antiseptic solution to loosen any sticking of the dressing to the wound.
12. Oral pain-killers should be given.
13. If the wound becomes septic, broad spectrum antibiotics are needed.
14. In severe cases, and if paramedically trained:
    (a) Set up a Ringer's lactate drip. The volume (in millilitres) required is determined by the formula weight (kg) x % burn x 4. Half must be given in the first 8 hours and the rest in the next 16 hours.
    (b) The victim must be catheterised. Urine output must be 30-50 ml/hour (1 ml/kg/hour in children). Fluid administration should be increased if required.
    (c) Give intravenous morphine 0.1 mg/kg as a single dose, then titrate as required.
    (d) Use mask oxygen if flame or smoke inhalation has occurred.
    (e) Transfer urgently to hospital.

Hypothermia

Hypothermia is the process that occurs when a warm diver gets into cold water. The normal central body temperature or core temperature is 37°C. It is a fine balance between heat production from metabolism and heat loss to the environment. If heat production equals heat loss, a stable temperature exists. If heat production is less than heat loss, the body temperature falls — hypothermia occurs. If heat production exceeds heat loss, the body temperature rises — hyperthermia occurs.

Hypothermia is a drop in core temperature as a result of heat loss being greater than heat production.

The process is comparable to inert gas elimination after a dive where *gas* is exhaled as a result of a gradient between a high tissue concentration and a lower environmental concentration. With hypothermia, *heat* is lost along a gradient from a higher core temperature to a lower environmental temperature.

What is the environmental temperature?

The sea has an extreme range of temperatures from −2°C to 25°C. A diver therefore has a possible heat loss gradient of 39°C to 12°C between core temperature and the water. In addition, water conducts heat about twenty-five times more efficiently than air, causing rapid diver cooling.

How is heat lost?

Several processes occur:
1. *Conduction.* Direct mass transfer of heat occurs along a gradient from a warm diver to cold water. The diver cools down and the water in the immediate vicinity warms up.
2. *Convection.* Water warmed by conduction is less dense and rises, so more cold water moves in to take its place. This puts our poor diver in the unfortunate position of trying to warm up the sea. Convection is increased by movement, especially swimming. Certain areas when measured by thermograms (infra-red photographs of hotter and colder areas) show a high heat loss. These are:
   — the head and neck (up to 50 per cent of heat loss occurs here);

- the axillae (armpits);
- the sides of the body;
- the groins.

These four areas arc thc grcatcst sites of heat loss. The amount of heat lost can be reduced by flexing the head on to the chest, folding the arms across the chest and drawing the knees up to the body. This diminishes the exposure of these key sites to the water. It is a position similar to that of an unborn baby in its mother's womb — the foetal or spheroidal position.

Swimming exposes these areas, increasing conduction, and movement increases convection. Alcohol and marijuana decrease skin arteriolar constriction and promote flushing, so further increasing heat loss.

3. *Breathing.* Every inhaled breath of air is warmed by the respiratory passages and the lungs. Every exhaled breath means heat loss from the body. Helium and hydrogen have a high thermal conductivity, being much more efficient in conducting heat than nitrogen. The use of these gases in the breathing mix will cause much greater respiratory heat loss.

4. *Urine output.* Exposure to cold causes the blood vessels in the skin to constrict. The skin becomes pale. When blood vessels constrict, the blood volume within them decreases. This blood must go somewhere and it is to the warmth of the core that it goes. This increases the core blood volume. As kidneys are in the core, the kidney blood flow increases, which in turn means increased urine production. This now causes heat loss when the warm urine is voided as well as a decrease in the total fluid content of the diver, including his blood volume.

Suppose a warm diver in a swimming costume only, falls into water at 2°C:

1. Sudden cold exposure can cause a *gasping response* with abnormal heart rhythm or even cardiac arrest. So, sudden death can occur.

2. *Diving reflex:* Exposure of the face to cold water causes *breathholding* and *a slowing of the heart rate* in diving animals such as whales and seals. The diving reflex is also associated with intense constriction of arterioles throughout the body, except those of the heart and brain. Virtually the entire blood supply becomes an oxygen store for these two organs alone. Shunting of the blood from the skin also means less heat loss to the water. In man, this reflex is very poorly developed. An acceleration in heart rate may occur, with the development of an irritable and excitable heart muscle. This can result in the development of abnormal heart rhythms and death. (See p 19.)

In infants, the reflex appears to be more efficient, so with facial immersion in cold water:
- breathholding,
- slowing of the heart rate, and
- oxygen conservation due to shunting of blood to the heart and brain occur. This is of immense importance in cold-water drowning.

What happens with hypothermia?

A diver can tolerate a maximum drop of 12°C in body temperature before death occurs, that is, a fall from 37°C to 25°C. Think about what is happening. Heat from the central warm core is being transferred by the bloodstream to the periphery, where it is being lost to the water. The cold peripheral blood is then returned to the core, causing core cooling. With each repeat cycle, further cooling occurs.

Divers experience three phases of cooling as their body temperature falls:
— they react to the cold,
— they become passive, then
— they lose consciousness.
1. At a core temperature of 37°C to 34°C, the diver feels cold, begins shivering and becomes pale. Shivering is an attempt by the body to produce more heat by muscle contraction. In the sea this is obviously a futile exercise. At about 34°C, shivering is replaced by muscle rigidity. Movements become difficult and awkward, power decreases and swimming ability falls.
2. Between 34°C and 30°C, the effects of cold on the brain appear. The blood becomes more viscous or 'thicker'; transfer of oxygen from haemoglobin to tissues decreases; and hypoxia begins. Confusion, disorientation, lack of judgement and amnesia occur. In the absence of some flotation device the diver will now drown. Human heart muscle becomes very irritable with hypothermia and irregular rhythms develop. Breathing becomes shallow and slow.
3. Between 30°C and 25°C, consciousness is lost, going on to deep coma and death by ventricular fibrillation (uncoordinated 'rippling' contractions of the muscles of the ventricles, without any pumping effect — similar to muscle shivering).

Protection against hypothermia

The above effects of hypothermia are very bad for business in the diving industry. An immense amount of research and expense has gone into solving some of the problems.

Heat is lost by:
— conduction,
— convection,
— breathing,
— urination.
One cannot do too much about convection in the ocean, nor can one stop divers from urinating if one wants to maintain their interest in diving. Conduction and breathing have been the object of intense research in diving technology.

Reducing conductive heat loss. Reduction of the amount of heat conducted by a diver to the water means *insulation.* Fat is a good insulator and fat people exposed to very cold water survive longer than thin people. Fatties also have a body shape closer to that of a sphere, giving a maximum volume to minimum surface area for heat loss. Lanky, long divers have small volumes and large surface areas. It is possible to encourage divers to eat more but, aside from the expense, fat divers are more prone to acute decompression illness, flatulence within the confined space of a decompression chamber, and other diseases, so this is not done. Long-distance swimmers, however, do use the insulating properties of fat − they grease themselves before entering the water.

Divers use protective suits. These not only reduce heat loss, but protect against contact with stinging marine life and rough surfaces. There are several types:
− Wet suits
− Dry suits
  − constant volume
  − variable volume
− Heated suits
  − thermochemical
  − electrical
  − hot-water
The choice depends upon the water temperature, the depth, and the duration of the dive.

1. *Wet suits*
   These are composed of closed-cell expanded neoprene varying in thickness from 3 mm to 8 mm or more. The bubbles in the neoprene sponge are poor heat conductors but good insulators.

   Wet suits are effective at shallow depths, but with increasing depth lose their efficiency. This is because the bubbles in the neoprene sponge obey Boyle's Law. As pressure increases, bubble volume decreases, so the suit becomes thinner and thinner while the water becomes colder and colder. This also reduces buoyancy and the diver becomes more negative at depth (Archimedes' Principle).

   Wet suits, as their name implies, allow water in
   − through the neck,
   − through the cuffs, and
   − through the zippers.
   This water soon warms up though, forming a warm layer between the diver's body and the neoprene sponge suit.

2. *Dry suits*
   These suits rely on underwear and a layer of insulating air for warmth. Water must not be allowed access into the suit. There are two types − constant volume and variable volume dry suits.
   (a) *Constant volume dry suits.* Made of incompressible rubber or neoprene-impregnated fabric, no trapped bubbles are present in the material so they do not change thickness with depth. The suit

material has constant volume. Alone they have very little insulating capacity against cold, but they are made large and baggy, allowing very warm polyamide-nylon undergarments to be worn — 'woolly bears'.

These suits, being large and loose, are liable to cause suit squeeze on descent. Adding an inflation device powered by a suit-bottle or the LP stage removes the 'wrinkles' and provides a layer of insulating air; care must then be taken to avoid an uncontrolled ascent — so a dump valve is fitted. Holes or leaks into the suit allow water entry, converting it into a bulky, negatively buoyant, waterlogged and soggy bag containing one miserably cold diver.

(b) *Variable volume dry suits.* These are foam-neoprene suits, usually double-lined with nylon. The presence of the foam neoprene adds insulation and buoyancy. As with the constant volume suits, undergarments are worn and inflation and dump devices are fitted. Inflation of the suit provides a water seal at the cuffs and neck. The variable volume dry suit is superior in insulation to both wet suits and constant volume dry suits. Air is a good insulator and the foam neoprene adds the advantage of further insulation. Warm undergarments then provide a warm, dry and happy diver who looks and feels like a contented teddy bear. Again, a leak guarantees misery.

3. *Heated suits*

Instead of trying to prevent the diver's body warmth from seeping into the sea, heated suits dispense with baggy and bulky insulation and provide external heat to the diver. They are the ultimate in diving suits but require energy input.

(a) *Thermochemical.* The simplest method involves a chemical reaction with water. A wet suit is used and porous bags containing iron filings and magnesium are placed inside the suit. Contact with water starts a heat-evolving reaction providing body warmth to the diver. Placing small bags within the gloves provides hand warmth. Leaving the water stops the reaction.

(b) *Electrical.* Electrical suits have built-in heating elements much like an electric blanket. Their power source may be carried (but this means a bulky power pack as an extra diver burden), or surface- or bell-supplied. Repeated kinking with movement, for example at the elbows and knees, can cause interruption of electrical flow due to wire breakage.

(c) *Hot-water suits.* These are the most efficient heated suits, but also the most expensive to power. Sea water is heated at the surface and then pumped down a hose to the diver. A bypass valve fitted to the suit allows the diver to select whether the water enters the suit or is dumped into the sea. Within the suit are perforated tubes supplying hot water to the neck, arms, hands, body, legs and feet. The water then exits the suit through the cuffs into the sea and is constantly replaced by more hot sea water from the surface.

Temperature is adjusted at the surface to provide optimal diver comfort, but as this is a very subjective means of temperature control, care must be taken to avoid over-heating and hyperthermia. Local 'hot spots' of water entry can cause scalding, and should the hot-water supply fail, a very cold and angry diver soon results.

Reducing breathing heat loss. With each exhaled breath, a diver loses heat. In addition, when gas passes from a high to a low pressure (e.g. from an HP scuba cylinder to an LP regulator), it cools down. The diver therefore inhales gas which is even colder than the sea.

Prewarmers have been devised to warm the inhaled air as well as countercurrent insulating devices to limit exhaled heat loss. The problem really is fitting a bulky warmer to a diver's face, which is already overloaded with high-precision contraptions.

Management of Hypothermia

The most important message in the management of hypothermia is the understanding that a diver in deep hypothermia may appear to be *dead*. Never assume a cold diver to be dead. True stories abound of hypothermic and comatose people regaining consciousness without help in a mortuary. 'Dead' children presumed to have drowned, have recovered spontaneously, being protected by their hypothermia.

Only a warm dead diver is a dead diver.

Management of mild hypothermia

This is rarely a problem.
1. Remove the diver from the cold water.
2. Place the diver flat in a protected place.
3. Cover the diver with a space blanket, normal blankets, sleeping bags, body-to-body contact, etc.
4. Encourage the diver to drink warm fluids.

Management of deep hypothermia

The understanding of the active management of deep hypothermia requires an initial explanation of *afterdrop*. Afterdrop is a phenomenon where core temperature (as measured rectally) continues to drop during active rewarming of a hypothermic victim in a bath of water at 43°C. It has long been presumed that the heat of the bath caused the blood vessels in the arms and legs to dilate, sending a flush of cold peripheral blood returning to the core, causing further central cooling and precipitating ventricular fibrillation and death. For this reason, arms and legs were kept out of the warm bath and were just covered. Afterdrop is a rectal fact only and does not reflect true core temperature, as core mixing of venous blood is poor in a passive, hypothermic diver. Rectal afterdrop is due to continuing mass tissue conduction of heat from a relatively warmer lower body to colder upper legs during the initial minutes of rewarming.

As the diver's heart and brain are of greater concern to us than his rectum, what then does cause the ventricular fibrillation that kills up to twenty per cent of hypothermic divers after rescue and during rewarming? If it is not a surge of cold blood to the heart, what is it?

There are several causes. Let's look at the cardiovascular system of an immersed hypothermic diver. This involves:
— blood,
— the heart,
— blood vessels.

With severe cold exposure, increased urine output decreases the total body water. As tissue cells lose water, their contents becomes more concentrated. Water moves from the blood into tissue cells and into the spaces between tissue cells; the blood becomes more viscous and total blood volume is decreased.

A hypothermic heart contracts slowly. Heart rate is low and each contraction (systole) of the ventricles takes longer, but the filling time of the ventricles as they relax between beats (diastole) is short. The coronary arteries, which supply blood to the heart muscle itself, are the only arteries in the body that depend on ventricular relaxation for filling. As their filling time decreases, the heart muscle is supplied with less blood and oxygen, and that blood is thicker and its flow more sluggish.

When the diver is immersed, the water supports the blood vessels in his limbs. There is no gravity-induced pooling of blood in the limbs. We now rescue the diver from the water. Gravity suddenly causes blood to pool in dangling legs and arms. Heart rate increases to circulate these columns of blood. The coronary artery filling time, already reduced, becomes border-line for adequate heart muscle oxygen supply. As the rescuers rush the diver to safety, they move his or her arms and legs. Further reflex acceleration of the heart rate occurs, blood supply to the heart with its increased work becomes inadequate, and ventricular fibrillation and death occur. In addition, exercise and movement do promote cold venous return from the limbs, and this can cause sudden further cooling of the core. Conscious, intensely cold divers must be discouraged from any unnecessary voluntary movement, and extreme care must be taken to keep the limbs of unconscious hypothermic divers immobile and horizontal.

Remember two things:
1. *The diver may appear to be dead:*
   — there may be no discernible heart beat;
   — there may be no obvious breathing;
   — the pupils may be fixed and unreactive;
   — no blood pressure may be measurable.
2. *Do not move or handle the diver too much.* Grabbing a diver in an emergency situation by the arms and legs, handling the neck roughly, pounding the chest and frantically giving mouth-to-mouth resuscitation can precipitate ventricular fibrillation which will *kill* the diver.

(a) Be gentle. Do not move the limbs unduly.

(b) Check the airways — if obstructed, clear very gently.

(c) Check breathing — if the diver is breathing, even very shallowly and slowly, *leave the diver's chest alone.*

(d) Check the heartbeat — if a heartbeat is present, even if very indistinct or slow, *leave the diver's chest alone.* Do not try to improve circulation by thumping the chest.*

(e) If a low-reading clinical thermometer is available, gently check the diver's rectal temperature. If the temperature is above 34°C, the diver is not in hypothermic coma. Then treat for an unconscious diver (see p 242) plus passive rewarming.

(f) *Rapid rewarming.* Leave the diver in his or her wet suit if one is being worn. This avoids excessive manipulation of the limbs, protects against scalding, and the rubber support retards pooling of blood in the limbs.

Circumstances will dictate the method available. Generally, active rewarming in water is done. If a bath is unavailable, a hole in the ground with a tarpaulin in it will do. The bath water provides hydrostatic support for the limbs, reduces gravity-pooling and decreases the forward load on the heart. If the diver is wearing a hot water suit, reconnect it to a warm water supply and circulate the water through it.

Note: While the bath is being prepared, cover the diver with blankets, warm bottles, sleeping bags or body-to-body contact in a sheltered place out of the wind.

The bath should be as hot as possible without causing scalding — i.e. hot enough for the helpers to tolerate without flinching. This is about 43°C. The diver is placed in the bath for 20-30 minutes. The limbs *should be included* in the bath. Disturb the diver as little as possible. Do not perform CPR in a bath of hot water as you will drown the diver as well. Keep the water hot by adding more as required.

(g) *Monitor the pulse rate continuously* — placing a hypothermic diver in the warm bath *does* cause dilation of arterioles in the periphery and can drop blood pressure. This will then cause the heart rate to accelerate in an attempt to maintain the blood pressure. Note that this does not occur immediately, but over a period of 15-20 minutes after immersion. If the pulse rate starts to accelerate, *quickly cool the water down again until the rate settles.* Then continue with hot water. If the diver is conscious, keep him or her in the bath until sweating starts.

---

* Active cardiac massage and mouth-to-mouth ventilation may cause ventricular fibrillation. If no breathing is discernible using a mirror in front of the mouth to look for condensation, and no carotid pulse is felt or heartbeat heard by an ear on his left chest, then CPR could be given at one chest compression per 2 seconds or 30 beats per minute, and one chest inflation after every fifth compression or 6 breaths per minute). The use of CPR in hypothermic coma is dangerous.

After the bath:
- — the diver must lie flat in a warm place with liberal blankets;
- — encourage warm drinks.

Accidental cold-water exposure

This could occur by falling overboard or with a boat capsizing. *Swimming* is the danger. It exposes the body to increased conduction and convection, with a greatly increased speed of heat loss. In cold water below 10°C an uninsulated man of normal build without a life-jacket will not manage a one-kilometre swim. Stay with the boat. Adopt the foetal position to conserve heat. If several people are in the water, link elbows to form a 'hot-tub' and adopt the foetal position.

Mixed Gas and Sport Diving

In recent years, groups of sport divers in several countries have broken away from traditional air diving and are using nitrox or trimix as their breathing source.

Two nitrox mixes are commonly used:
- nitrox I (oxygen 32 per cent, nitrogen 68 per cent),
- nitrox II (oxygen 36 per cent, nitrogen 64 per cent).

The use of nitrox followed the publishing by NOAA of guidelines for the use of nitrox in commercial saturation diving. The original concept was aimed at *preventing* pulmonary oxygen toxicity at shallow saturation depths. The maximum permissible oxygen partial pressure for prolonged periods is 0.5 ATA. This would allow air saturation at a depth of only 13.8 msw. At deeper depths the amount of oxygen must be *reduced* and nitrogen *increased*. This reduces the depth at which nitrogen narcosis occurs and makes nitrox saturation diving safe only in a very limited and shallow depth range. Air, with a higher oxygen pressure, is then used on shallow downward excursions from saturation depth.

The whole thing has been turned topsy-turvy. Pulmonary oxygen toxicity cannot develop in sport diving. It takes days of continuous high exposure to develop. So instead of avoiding pulmonary oxygen toxicity, nitrox sport divers change the objective and aim at reducing nitrogen uptake by increasing the oxygen in the mix. This then reduces the risk of acute decompression illness and can nearly double maximum bottom time. But it increases the risk of cerebral oxygen toxicity which takes minutes, not days, to develop at depth.

Among sport divers, the maximum safe oxygen partial pressure is set at 1.6 ATA. Air then has a maximum safe oxygen depth of 66 msw. Nitrox I has a maximum safe depth of 40 msw, and nitrox II 34 msw. This would seem to make nitrox the ideal breathing mix for the shallow diving depths of most reefs because nitrogen uptake and the chances of bends would be substantially reduced.

It would be, except that nitrox divers have died. There will always be cowboys and instead of aiming at increased shallow dive durations, the objective changed again. This time, nitrogen narcosis was targeted. If the mix had a lower nitrogen content it stood to reason that nitrogen narcosis would occur at deeper than air-breathing depths. This resulted in deep nitrox dives with no nitrogen narcosis, but sudden cerebral oxygen toxicity, underwater convulsions and drowning.

Requirements for Safe Nitrox Mixing

Accurate mixtures

Making a nitrox mix by using Dalton's Law of partial pressures is dangerous. Oxygen is the problem. It does not quite obey Dalton's Law. Oxygen is physically more compressible than nitrogen and if compressed air is mixed with oxygen until the calculated pressures are reached, the mix will not be the required one. It will contain too much oxygen. This means that oxygen analysers are necessary and these are expensive and require precise calibration with known standard mixes. In commercial use, mixes are made by precise flow (not pressure) mixers with continuous analysis facilities.

Oil-free compressors

Increasing the oxygen content increases the fire and explosion risk. Standard sport diving air compressors are not oil-free and using them to top up a cylinder containing pressurised oxygen is hazardous.

Nitrox and Carbon Dioxide Build-up

Nitrox is denser than air so the work of breathing nitrox causes more carbon dioxide production than air breathing does. The big problem with any carbon dioxide build-up due to exercise, tight gear, skip breathing, etc., is that it dilates brain blood vessels and increases blood supply to the brain. If the blood is also loaded with a high concentration of oxygen in solution, unconsciousness and convulsions can occur without warning.

Should Sport Divers Use Nitrox?

It is true that nitrox at shallow depths is safe. It is also true that it does increase safe permissible dive duration. What nitrox does not do is increase available gas supply. Whether air or nitrox are breathed, the volume-pressure demands of Boyle's Law must still be met to avoid squeeze. This means that the diver must carry a larger, heavier cylinder, or use twin cylinders.

The diver must also be sure that the mix is correct; the correct tables are being used; or the dive computer is calibrated to the nitrox mix. There is no surface back-up in case of trouble.

Major sport diving training centres such as NAUI, PADI, SSI, and YMCA have shunned nitrox for recreational diving. A diver unable to control buoyancy or inadvertently or deliberately going too deep can suddenly die. This has happened on several occasions and, should it continue, it is inevitable that legislation banning the use of nitrox will emerge. Nitrox and other gas mixes are special mixes designed for specialist working applications. They require specialist handling, equipment and back-up, and should not form part of a sport diver's life-support system.

Breathing Mixtures in Saturation Diving

Of all the gas mixes used by saturation divers, only oxygen must be included in any mix. Nitrogen, helium and hydrogen have all been used as diluents for oxygen, the determining factors in mix selection being depth and cost.

Air is the cheapest mix, but nitrogen narcosis limits its usefulness to about 60 msw, that is, relatively shallow dives. It is interesting that divers saturated for two weeks on air at a storage depth of 17 msw during the SCORE programme at Duke University in 1976 were able to dive effectively for up to 60 minutes on deeper excursions to 90 msw without disabling narcosis. Cerebral oxygen toxicity then became the limiting factor (oxygen partial pressure = 2.1 ATA). The nicest way of interpreting this was that the divers had simply adapted to narcosis by acclimatising to the high nitrogen partial pressure. Work by Hamilton and Kizer in 1985 has indicated that there may be some degree of physiological adaptation to nitrogen narcosis, but the effect seems to be largely one of learning to cope.

Nitrox has been widely used in saturation diving, the idea being that increasing the percentage of oxygen in the breathing mix reduces the percentage of nitrogen and so extends the depth limit before narcosis becomes significant. It is a method of providing a deeper equivalent nitrogen partial pressure but is really only a compromise. It is a sliding scale between narcosis on the one hand and cerebral oxygen toxicity on the other, but is useful if the application is right. Expertise in nitrox diving was derived from the US Navy and the National Oceanic and Atmospheric Administration (NOAA). The US Navy undertook the SHAD, Nisat, Surex and Minisat programmes and NOAA began the NOAA OPS programme (NOAA OPerationS) in 1973.

A habitat on the sea-bed allows marine scientists to live close to their working sites. The depth of the habitat is called the storage depth. From there they can make vertical excursions, either deeper or shallower. Tables were developed by NOAA OPS, limiting time-depth-gas profiles. In almost all the experimental series it was found that downward excursions from the storage depth rarely caused problems. Upward excursions to shallower depths were problematic, however, with the development of itches and 'niggles' and even overt joint bends.

When commercial companies received news of the NOAA OPS technology, a commercial adaptation of nitrox habitat diving appeared, with divers living in a surface deck-decompression chamber on a ship and excursing to and from the bottom worksite in a pressurised diving bell. As commercial diving companies need mobility and flexibility of operations, it made good sense for them to use pressurised bells for depth transfer rather than the fixed location of habitat diving. They were also rarely interested in shallower excursions from the surface storage depth except during final decompression from saturation. They needed long hours at one location, whereas scientists wanted to visit many sites around their habitat and usually several times per day. Commercial companies traditionally keep their dive tables top secret. They are in fierce competition and sell their expertise at a very high price. But, following the published reports of Comex, Seaway Diving, Oceaneering, and others, it became apparent that commercial diving companies generally avoid the problem of decompression sickness by saturating at storage depth close enough to the depth of the worksite to perform daily 8-hour downward excursions without any decompression requirements. These reports led to the development of a set of commercial nitrox-excursion tables sponsored by the UK Department of Energy and published by CIRIA, the British Industrial Research Association in 1985.

Everything was not all roses, however. Avoidance of the bends could largely be achieved by juggling depth-time parameters, but cerebral and pulmonary/chronic oxygen toxicity demanded attention. The nitrox techniques did not permit more than one excursion dive each day. The tables also did not allow for emergency ascents, nor for dealing with bends that might occur as a result of the diving operation. The final decompression techniques following each mission also needed more reliable choices.

In 1988 NOAA published their REPEX report, detailing the methods for repetitive excursions, surfacing techniques, and oxygen procedures for habitat diving. Over the past years many computerised mathematical algorithms have been devised, some tables being highly lauded and hugely sophisticated, and others super secret. At the end of the day, however, no table is infallible and the well-trodden path of testing a profile, revising it, and then retesting it always had to be followed. No table is bends-proof. The human body is not so easily predictable. The best that can be achieved is a high probability of successful decompressions. All today's decompression tables are both empirical and computational. They are 'reliable' rather than 'safe'. The REPEX experiments developed precursory tables, which are preliminary stabilising tables used before commencing final decompression on the main table. The divers are recompressed on air to a depth which varies according to the depth of the deepest excursion in the last 36 hours. (The 36-hour period was arbitrarily chosen as conservatively reasonable.) The use of air provides an oxygen window, allowing a preliminary increase in pressure without substantially increasing the nitrogen load. The ascent rate is designated RRate or Reciprocal Rate in min/ft. It describes minutes per depth unit and is used for practical reasons only. It is simple to decompress a chamber by one foot every nine minutes but how does one ascend at 0.11 ft/min?

Oxygen toxicity in saturation diving

Nitrox saturation diving generally uses an oxygen partial pressure of 0.3 to 0.5 ATA at the storage depth to avoid pulmonary oxygen toxicity, and 'air' (20 per cent oxygen) during excursions. If a maximum of 1.5 ATA of oxygen is allowed for deeper excursions, this means a maximum depth of 75 msw on 'air'. The fact that 'air' has a substantially higher oxygen pressure than the storage mix means that the diver also has a very useful downward vertical range without adding to his nitrogen gas loading – an oxygen window of descent.

Exactly the same principles apply to helium/oxygen (heliox), hydrogen/oxygen (hydrox), and helium/nitrogen/oxygen (trimix) saturations – a lower oxygen partial pressure at storage depth with a richer oxygen mix on downward excursions.

It is obvious that oxygen toxicity is inherent in saturation diving.

Central nervous system (CNS) oxygen toxicity (Paul Bert effect) with the development of epileptiform seizures may occur with exposure to high partial pressures of oxygen. The time to onset is very variable, ranging from a few to many minutes in different individuals. Generally, exposures above 1.8 ATA, especially if exercise or carbon dioxide accumulation are also factors, may lead to a convulsion after a variable number of minutes.

Chronic oxygen toxicity presents differently and is generally caused by longer exposures to lower levels of oxygen. Pulmonary oxygen toxicity (Lorrain Smith effect) is a subset of chronic oxygen toxicity, and is usually the presenting symptom in a broader syndrome. The limiting partial pressure is 0.5 ATA. Levels above this for several days may invoke symptoms. The amount of chronic oxygen exposure is monitored by bookkeeping the CPTD (Chronic Pulmonary Toxicity Dose). This is measured in CPTUs (Chronic Pulmonary Toxicity Units), one CPTU being an exposure of one minute to a partial pressure of oxygen of one atmosphere. At a constant oxygen pressure of 0.5 ATA a total dose of 720 CPTUs/day can be maintained indefinitely without symptoms.

Heliox is commonly used at depths below 50 msw. Obviously the avoidance of narcosis is the prime reason for substituting helium as a diluent for oxygen, but the low density also makes breathing easier at depth with far less reduction in the maximal minute volume as compared to nitrogen breathing. There are disadvantages too. Speech distortion makes descrambling necessary. High thermal conductivity makes precise environmental temperature regulation essential to avoid hypo- and hyperthermia. The gas is much less soluble than nitrogen and diffuses more rapidly so that saturation of tissues is fast. Although this means a lower total gas load during saturation and a shorter time for final decompression compared with an equivalent air dive, it also means easier bubble formation with bends on ascending excursions with habitat diving, or with long bottom times before returning to storage depth. HPNS is a further problem, necessitating very slow rates of compression for dives deeper than 100 msw.

Hydrox has the great advantage of being cheap. It has the great disadvantage of being explosive when the mix contains more than 4 per cent oxygen. Generally 2 to 3 per cent oxygen is used, which means that the mix cannot be used at depths shallower than 60-90 msw to maintain a minimum normoxic oxygen partial pressure (0.21 ATA). In other respects it behaves much like heliox, with speech distortion, high thermal conductivity, and rapid diffusibility. HPNS occurs too, but is reputed to occur less readily.

Trimix is a mixture of helium, nitrogen and oxygen. Nitrogen the narcoser delays and even prevents the onset of HPNS by helium the stimulator. This beneficial effect of nitrogen is also shared by barbiturates and ketamine. The converse also applies. High pressure helium reverses anaesthesia. HPNS appears to be the limiting factor to the ultimate depth to which man can dive. It is fascinating to contemplate a future diver working alertly at depths well below 1 000 msw only because he is sedated with barbiturates, nitrogen and anaesthetics!

The future of saturation diving probably lies in trimix diving, with faster and safer compressions, deeper diving, and less expense, heat loss and voice distortion. By 1989 commercial diving had outstripped systematic research. Divers were routinely working at 450 msw, empirically developing their techniques, keeping their tables secret, and without the backing of systematic deep diving research to develop routine operational procedures.

In April 1989, a new international research and development programme was begun at the German Underwater Simulator (GUSI) at Geesthacht near Hamburg, Germany. Scientists from the US, the UK, Norway and Germany are participating in the project. The aim is the development of safety and quality in underwater technology, by making simulated dives to 450 msw. The project is ongoing and eight areas are being researched:
- Underwater work techniques, especially wet and dry welding by divers and mechanised robotic and orbital welding to 1 200 msw.
- Diving techniques and diving equipment.
- Training procedures for divers and operators of diving systems.
- Health protection, both short and long term, including risk assessment and the prevention of diving illnesses.

- Quality assurance methods.
- Computerised underwater handling systems and robotics to support future diverless technology.
- Independent underwater systems for exploitation of oil and gas fields. This is extremely high-tech work and involves the establishment of deep, large multi-chambered habitats actually incorporating the drill wellhead, and with people living in saturation at plus 600 msw at the ocean bed and without surface back-up. The concept poses major challenges in multiphase transport technology and underwater energy supply.
- Structural and fluid mechanics with computerised analyses of highly stressed underwater welds and complete structures.

GUSI is one of the largest and most sophisticated simulated deep diving facilities in the world. Manned diving tests are done to 600 msw and unmanned tests to 2 500 msw. The main chamber has a maximum operating depth of 1 000 msw and permits welding 24 hours a day. Divers can be transferred using a three-man diving bell from their living chamber to the work chamber. Twelve to eighteen divers can be accommodated. A TUP (transfer under pressure) facility is available for hyperbaric evacuation. More than ten other chambers are available for unmanned tests to 2 500 msw.

HPNS is one of the major limitations to very deep diving. A trimix (He-N_2-O_2) breathing mixture is used at GUSI which permits diving to 600 msw without HPNS. It is called Trimix 5 and comprises N_2 5%; O_2 0.5 ATA; He the rest. Very careful and sophisticated monitoring of divers, involving physiological, psychological and neurological assessments, is made predive, during the dive, postdive and annually thereafter. Since 1986 no cases of acute decompression illness have occurred, nor any cases of HPNS except small, temporary and insignificant decrements of short-term memory and visual concentration. No nausea, tremors, undue fatigue, sleep problems or personality changes occurred. (One diver spent five months between 300 and 450 msw.) No significant increase in brain wave activity occurred on EEG. Associative memory and auditory selection tests showed no decrement. A set of compression and decompression profiles have been issued by GUSI for routine use to 600 msw.

Marine Animals That Bite

Sharks

Of all the potential man-eaters in the sea, sharks are invariably the beasts that come to mind first. Virtually fully evolved well over a hundred million years ago, and perfectly designed for their environment, they are the lords of the fishes. Over 250 species have been described, but only 27 have been definitely implicated in attacks on humans. They range in size from 0.4 metres in some dogfish (Squalidae), to over 15 metres in whale sharks *(Rhincodon)*. As with panic, there are three dimensions to a shark attack:
— the shark,
— the victim, and
— the environment.

1. The shark

All sharks, even the smallest or reportedly most docile ones, are potentially dangerous, simply because sharks are so perfectly designed for attack. The ragged-tooth shark *(Carcharius taurus)*, despite its ferocious appearance, is usually docile and relatively indifferent to visiting divers. The mako shark *(Isurus glaucus)*, blue shark *(Prionace glauca)*, hammerheaded sharks (Sphyrnidae) and tiger sharks *(Galeocerdo)* are all man-eaters. Although the most feared shark is the great white shark *(Carcharodon carcharias)*, the most dangerous shark of all, found only in warm open seas, is the long-finned shark *(Carcharhinus longimanus)*. Large, ugly, muddily-mottled, small-eyed and vicious, they have huge rounded fins tipped with white circles. They are aggressive and never scared off by an approaching diver.

Sharks use a number of senses in detecting their prey, and their perfection in integrating these senses is the reason behind the incomparable environmental adaptation of sharks. Their vision is poor in detail and colour but is well equipped to see a moving diver against a bright surface background, even when the shark is twisting or turning. In contrast to humans, who focus by changing the shape of the lens of the eye, sharks have a fixed round lens which is moved in and out like a camera lens to accommodate for distance. To accommodate for dim light, sharks have a tapetum, a carpet of crystalline doubly-refracting silvery plates in the choroid layer behind the retina. These refract light back into the eye, resensitising the retina to the same rays of light. In bright light, dark pigment-containing cells at the base of the silvery plates migrate over the surface of the tapetum, covering it and preventing resensitisation. A shark's sense of smell is very acute in detecting blood and food in the water. The entrance to each nostril is channelled by a Schneiderian fold, forming a canal through which water flows and is tested. The entire skin of the shark is equipped for tasting – sensorial crypts, especially around the head, continuously sample and taste surrounding water for possible prey. Running from around the eyes, and then along the lateral lines on the sides of the shark, are sensorial canals with radar-like sensitivity to vibration and pressure waves, and, at the tip of the nose, pressure-sensitive flasks, the ampullae of Lorenzini, detect minute changes in sound at amazing distances and with savage accuracy. Compare this militant combination of radar and sonar to *Homo scubiens* who, for hearing under water, depends on simple bone conduction in his head, and is hopelessly unable to distinguish sound direction.

Sharks have two feeding patterns. Their normal feeding pattern consists of one or a few sharks seeking food and proceeding with slow, purposeful movements. The frenzied feeding pattern occurs when there is suddenly a large amount of food in the area (e.g. following an aircraft or ship disaster with injured people in the water, or ships throwing garbage into the sea). Sound also appears to play a role in frenzies. Cousteau has reported that a shark biting into soft fish flesh gets little reaction from other sharks in the immediate area. The grating of teeth into bone, however, or the crunching of a fish head, appears to be a clarion call to other sharks. The sharks become erratic, snap savagely and dementedly at anything in sight, and move rapidly and jerkily. Even cannibalism has been reported. During deliberate attacks, however, they tend to select their victim out of a collection of swimmers and concentrate their attention on that person.

A shark's lower jaw is situated well back and below the snout. Just before striking, the jawbone is moved forward and the snout is lifted up and back, almost at a right angle to the axis of the body. At the instant of biting, the shark's jaw is actually forward of the head and not below it. Utilising the mass of his body, the shark savagely jerks and scissors rows of razor-sharp teeth into the victim, instantly ripping off a large chunk of flesh.

2. The victim

Much can be done to avoid becoming *Homme tartare*. Avoid swimming or diving alone, as single divers become the prime target. A buddy diver may also be able to warn you of a shark's presence in time to take avoidance action. During the day, and with good visibility, meeting one or two sharks should present no immediate peril. Should three or more sharks appear, look for some type of underwater back-up shelter. Sharks do not immediately attack submerged divers. They will circle the divers, disappear, and then guardedly return, giving the divers ample time calmly to decide whether to continue the dive or return to the boat. Spear fishermen should avoid baiting themselves by tying their catch to their weight belts, and avoid provoking the shark by spearing it or pulling its tail. If you have been cleaning your fish catch, wash yourself thoroughly with soap and water before diving. Avoid young sharks. Although small, they are audacious and can inflict savage wounds. Sharks naturally and fearlessly attack any floating object. Even outboard motors have been attacked. Do not splash about on the surface. Keep water entries and exits short — these are the times when divers are in most danger. Do not put your trust in chemical, sonic or electrical shark repellents. They are not reliably effective. Avoid turbid waters and night diving in known shark-infested areas. Open wounds and bright shiny suits can attract sharks. Dress conservatively — it is preferable for you to wear black than for your relatives to do so.

3. **The environment**

Most shark attacks occur during the day, in warm weather, during holidays and within 30 metres from the shore. This is probably simply because this is when bathers enter the sea in large numbers. The water is mostly about chest deep. Big man-eaters feed towards evening and at night; favour murky water containing garbage; swim further out from shore in deeper water; and lurk in drop-offs. If bathers adopted these swimming habits the incidence of attacks would no doubt increase. But these are often the habitual areas for divers.

What to do when confronted by one or two sharks while diving

1. Remain submerged, if possible.
2. Use slow, soft, purposeful movements, as panicky and erratic movements will excite the shark. Avoid any sudden positional changes.
3. Do not attempt to swim away. Stay calm — sharks can somehow sense fear. Keep facing the shark and try to get a reef or wreck at your back. This at least ensures a frontal attack.
4. Try to fend off the shark with something in your hand, be it a rock, your camera, a piece of wreckage, or your spear. A shark billy (equipped with points or short nails at its end to avoid sliding off the shark's skin) is best, but use it only to fend off the animal and ensure a distance between you. Do not strike at the shark.
5. Prodding it on the snout, eyes or gills is best.
6. Try not to wound it — it may become angry.
7. Avoid using your bare hands if possible — the animal's skin will rip them and the bleeding will compound problems by exciting him.
8. Ensure that the shark has an escape open to him. Putting him in the position where escape is via yourself is very unwise.
9. Powerheads can be used if the situation is right. This requires expertise

in its use as well as accuracy, and is only effective against a single shark. Using it in a school can easily precipitate a frenzy.

Features of a shark bite

Almost invariably the victim is swimming on the surface, not diving; there is only one shark and the attack occurs without any warning. The injury may consist of a parabolic wound, huge ragged wounds, limb amputations, major or minor lacerations and skin abrasions. Over 70 per cent of attacks involve the lower limbs only.

These injuries cause:
— haemorrhage,
— shock.

Management of shark bites

Action:
1. Get the victim out of the water.
2. Shout for someone to summon emergency trained help.
3. Lay the victim flat on his back.
4. Stop the bleeding: (AIDS awareness!)
    (a) digital pressure,
    (b) pressure bandage,
    (c) tourniquet.
5. Control shock:
    (a) ensure a clear airway,
    (b) ensure proper ventilation,
    (c) ensure circulation,
    (d) administer 100 per cent oxygen by mask if available,
    (e) elevate non-injured limbs to 30 degrees above the horizontal,
    (f) splint injured limbs,
    (g) cover the victim with a towel, blanket or space blanket,
    (h) set up two or three intravenous lines. Use Ringer's lactate and Haemaccel, then blood,
    (i) do not transfer the victim to hospital until shock is controlled.
6. Keep the crowds at bay.
7. Do not forget about the tourniquet!

Discussion of shark bite management
There are only three primary things to do:
1. *Get the victim out of the water.* This is critical for survival and must be done with the greatest speed possible. Do not waste time trying to ventilate the victim in the water by mouth-to-mouth respiration. He or she is busy bleeding all the oxygenated blood into the sea. *Just get the victim out.*
2. *Stop the bleeding.* The victim must be placed lying on the back in a flat or slightly head-down position on a firm place clear of the water or on the boat. The victim has lost blood, is shocked as a result, and may be

near-drowned. Uninjured limbs should be elevated 30 degrees above the horizontal.

(a) *Pressure bandages* are the first method to be used. Pack the wound with anything – a towel, shirt, overalls or pressure dressings from a *Shark Attack Pack* (see below), then apply pressure. In most cases, this will staunch the flow of blood. Finger pressure over the femoral artery in the case of a leg, or the brachial artery in the case of an arm will help while the pack is being fitted.

(b) If a big artery is seen spurting, it may be tied off with whatever is at hand – fishing-line, string, or a shoe lace.
Do not worry about sterility at this stage.

(c) *Tourniquets* should be used on limbs if bleeding persists despite firm packing and pressure. A limb can survive without its blood supply for 2 to 3 hours. The tourniquet should be wide and flat to distribute pressure over a reasonable surface area. Tight ropes and rubber hoses tend to pressure-injure underlying tissue. Do not forget to inform the rescue service that a tourniquet is in place. Attach a prominent label to the victim, clearly reading:

TOURNIQUET APPLIED
TO R/L LEG/ARM AT_____AM/PM_____DATE

Tourniquets are potentially dangerous and must be removed after 2 hours maximum. The surgeon who will be doing the definitive repair will not thank you for destroying normal tissue around the wound by cutting off its blood supply – nor will the victim.

3. *Control the shock.* If there are a few people available, while bleeding is being controlled by one person the others should:
(a) Ensure a clear airway.
(b) Ensure proper ventilation.
(c) Ensure circulation.
(d) Administer 100 per cent oxygen by mask, if available.
(e) Cover the victim with a towel, blanket or space blanket.
(f) Summon emergency help.
(g) Keep the crowds at bay.
The above is basic CPR. (See pp 175-182.)

Then: It is essential to replace some of the blood volume to alleviate shock. Haemaccel and Ringer's lactate intravenous infusions should be set up simultaneously.

Haemaccel is an efficient plasma expander and should be used when severe bleeding has occurred (maximum initial dose Haemaccel 1 500 ml, thereafter alternate with blood 1:1). The Ringer's lactate is a solution containing a mixture of salts for intravenous use. The idea is to replace lost blood volume so that the blood pressure can be improved until blood itself can be administered.

Under no circumstances should the victim be moved until an intravenous line has been established, bleeding is controlled, respiration and circulation are restored, and shock has improved. Do not rush a shocked, bleeding victim to hospital. He will die.

Do not forget about the tourniquet!

It is recommended that all diving groups possess a shark attack pack and are trained in its use. A paramedical training is a great asset when disasters such as near-drowning and marine animal injuries occur.

Shark attack pack

1 x non-return airway
2 pairs rubber gloves } HIV protective wear
2 x full-length plastic aprons } for CPR
2 x goggles } operators
2 x 1 litre Ringer's lactate solution
3 x 500 ml Haemaccel
3 only IV administration sets with blood filters and 18 gauge needles
3 only 16 gauge IV cannulae
1 only Butterfly needle 21 gauge
2 only Plastic syringes 10 ml
1 only Plastic syringe 50 ml
5 only Disposable needles 21 gauge
5 packs Alcohol swabs
1 only Adhesive tape reel 2.5 cm wide
4 only 25 cm x 50 cm Trauma Pads − sterile
4 only Crepe bandages 15 cm
1 only Crepe bandage 10 cm
5 only Steripad dressings 12.5 cm x 10 cm
1 only Esmarch's bandage 10 cm (tourniquet)
2 only Artery forceps, disposable 10 cm
1 only Aluminium foil blanket (space-blanket)

The artery forceps are used to clamp off obvious bleeders. The use of the shark pack is a more advanced form of primary aid and requires paramedical training or a doctor on site.

The importance of not moving a shocked victim until blood pressure has improved and is stabilised cannot be overstressed. Do not be persuaded by anxious and untrained bystanders or even ambulance people who are not paramedics to move a shark victim. Most deaths from shark bites occur because of inadequate attention to stopping haemorrhage, and then moving a shocked victim. If you are not paramedically trained, stop the bleeding, ensure easy breathing and circulation, give oxygen if available and *wait* for a qualified person to give intravenous assistance. Injured limbs may be splinted for support.

Barracuda

The incidence of attack by barracuda is much less than that by sharks. There are around 20 species of barracuda, but only one bites divers – the great barracuda *(Sphyraena barracuda)*. It reaches a size of about 1.5 metres although monsters of over two metres have been described. They usually make only one strike and their bite is a straight or V-shaped wound as they have nearly parallel rows of teeth.

Management of injury is identical to that for shark bites.

Moray Eels

Attack by a moray eel is invariably due to a diver poking where he or she shouldn't. Commonly found in coral reefs and even in temperate water, they reach a size of up to 3 metres. When accustomed to divers, they can become 'tame', welcoming a scratch on the head, but if threatened, startled or cornered, they are vicious and savage. They have narrow jaws with sharp pointed teeth. Once they have bitten, they tenaciously maintain their grip like terriers, lacerating the tissue. Their skin is extraordinarily tough so attempting to free oneself with a knife is going to be quite a performance. Treat them as you would a watchdog. Approach with caution and then stay clear.

Management of a bite follows the treatment of shark bites.

Grouper (Sea Bass, Garrupa)

These are the biggies. They reach a size of over 3.5 metres with a mass of 300 kilograms. Curious, non-aggressive, but bold, they cause diver injury through diver stupidity. When attacked or annoyed their large mouths cause ragged lacerations with extensive bruising, and ramming with their huge heads causes extensive internal organ injuries.

Management of bites is according to that for shark bites, but remember that severe internal invisible injury may have occurred as a result of ramming.

Killer Whales

These beautiful mammals live throughout the oceans of the world. They are the largest of the dolphins and probably the most intelligent. Previously described as ferocious killers, they are not now believed to be deliberate man-eaters. But they are flesh eaters, hunting seals, walrus, squid, fish, and even other whales with power and speed. They can bite a seal in half with their massively powerful jaws, so do not let them think that you are a new kind of seal in your eight-millimetre expanded neoprene. Stay clear of killer whales.

Others

The above are just some of the biters of the sea. There are plenty of others who are quite willing to oblige an incautious diver. For example, manta rays, seals and sea-lions, needlefish, saltwater crocodiles, and snoek *(Thyrsites atun).*

Marine Animals That Sting

This is a huge group. There are thousands of stingers out there, some simply causing itchy skin irritations and others that kill in minutes. Some stay put, such as coral; others hide, such as the stonefish; some flagrantly expose themselves, such as the zebra fish; some are long and thin, such as the sea-snake; some are flat, such as the stingray, and others just hang around, such as blue-bottles and sea-wasps.

Basically there are two groups. Man is very proud of his arthritis-prone spine so he has divided stingers into:
— animals without spinal columns — Invertebrates
— animals with spinal columns — Vertebrates

Stingers Without Spinal Columns — Invertebrates

Since there is no spine, zoologists with a passion for order looked for something else. This brings us to the first group. They all have hollow guts. You can't call a whole group of creatures hollowguts, so to be fancy they are called *Coelenterates* which is the same thing — *coele* being Greek for hollow and *enteron* being Greek for gut.

1. Coelenterates

When a hollow gut is your licence to join a club of spineless creatures, an amazing variety of members turn up. This group of stingers includes:
(a) *Hydroids.* These hollowguts look like disguised versions of the mythical monster Hydra. They have stinging tentacles round their mouths. Some stay put during their mature life and build a limestone shelter around themselves — these are the fire corals which only look like coral as they are really hydroids.

   Others have long plume-like tentacles disguised as feathers — these are the *Pennaria* or fire ferns. As mentioned previously, some just float around — these are the *Portuguese men-of-war* or blue-bottles. There are thousands of others but these illustrate the type.
(b) *Scyphozoa.* This group of hollowguts is also unable to speak English and gets its name from the Latin *scyphus*, meaning a deep hollow cup,

and the Greek *zoa,* meaning an animal. They also have the unpleasant habit of discharging their sex organs into their intestines. Included in this group are the inverted hollowcups of the jellyfish and the feared and deadly sea-wasp *(Chironex fleckeri).* Their stinging tentacles are grouped around the edge of the inverted bell.

(c) *Anthozoa.* Once again *zoa* appears, so these are animals too. *Anthos* from the Greek means flower, therefore these are the flower animals. Not surprisingly, the sea anemones belong to this group. Less obviously, the stony corals and the soft corals also belong to the hollowgut flower animals.

How do these animals sting? All of these groups have stinging cells (nematocysts) which are found mostly on their tentacles. These cells are capsules filled with venom and each possesses a hollow needle-like tube. On contact with the tentacles, the sharp tip of the tube is everted, penetrates the skin of the diver, and injects the venom. Contact with fire coral, jellyfish, a blue-bottle or an anemone results in thousands of these tiny intradermal injections. The result depends on the organism, individual sensitivity, and the area of the sting.

The hydroids usually only cause skin reactions at the site of the sting — although the Portuguese man-of-war can cause great pain. Death is not usually a feature of hydroid stings.

The effects of contact with scyphozoans vary from a very mild prickle in the case of many jellyfish to violent agony, loss of consciousness and death within a minute in the case of the sea-wasp, which is the most venomous marine animal known.

The anthozoans, such as some of the anemones, can cause severely painful stings which later break down and ulcerate.

The *sea-wasp* is patently the real problem in the whole group of coelenterates so let's look at it in more detail. The bell-shaped body can grow up to 20 centimetres across. Its tentacles are attached to the lower edge of the bell at four points and there may be as many as six tentacles growing up to three metres in length at each point. The sea-wasp is usually found in shallow, sheltered waters such as protected coves and bays. Swimming is achieved by expulsive movements of water by the bell and a rate of four knots can be reached, which easily beats any diver.

The sting is excruciatingly painful, causing the victim to scream. Pain then worsens, and the victim may lose consciousness and drown. Children and people with respiratory or cardiac disease may die within 30 seconds.

Locally at the site of the sting, numerous crossing and irregular red or purple lines develop within seconds. If the victim lives, these later form large welts which break down and form ulcerating sores during the next week.

General effects with absorption of the venom are threefold:
— terrible and shocking pain;
— depression of heart and circulatory function;
— depression of breathing and brain function.

Agony dominates a picture of progressive heart failure, inability to breathe, paralysis, generalised muscle cramps, rigidity of the abdomen, vomiting, frothing at the mouth, constriction of the throat, delirium, convulsions, and finally death. Remember that all this is occurring in the sea.

Management of sea-wasp stings
(a) Get the victim out of the water as fast as possible.
(b) Apply a tourniquet, rope, string or any ligature *above* the sting if it is on an arm or leg.
(c) Pour vinegar over the stings and pieces of tentacle. If vinegar is unavailable, alcohol or any spirits will help. This *inactivates* the venom and must be done before any attempt is made to remove the tentacles, still loaded with active nematocysts, which will worsen the condition of the diver and even poison the rescuer.
(d) Scrape off the inactivated tentacles with a knife. Drying them with powder makes this easier.
(e) Apply more vinegar to the area as a poultice. This can help by breaking down venom in the skin.
(f) Rescue breathing or CPR must be given if needed (see under drowning).
(g) Summon medical aid:
  — morphine will help the pain;
  — sea-wasp antivenin must be given if available and the condition is worsening.
(h) Transfer to hospital when shock is stabilised.
(i) Do not forget to release the tourniquet (maximum two hours).
The management of stings from the other coelenterates is along similar lines if severe, except that antivenin is not given.

Fire coral presents a particular problem. Stinging may occur. The sharp edges of the calcified shell can lacerate. These wounds almost always become infected and healing is slow.
  All coral injuries should be:
(a) thoroughly cleaned as soon as possible;
(b) washed with an antiseptic;
(c) treated with local antibiotic ointments;
(d) kept dry: further diving invariably results in a spreading infection or abscess formation.

2. Molluscs

The second group of invertebrates are the softies. These are the *molluscs* (from the Latin meaning soft). They may be soft bodied but there is nothing soft about the venom of their poisonous members. They are named according to their feet.
  This group includes:
— octopuses — called *cephalopods* (feet on head);
— cone shells — called *gastropods* (feet on stomach).

(a) *The octopus*

Your average octopus is a shy and retiring creature and its bite, though painful, is usually uneventful. In Australia lives a little relative, the blue-ringed or spotted octopus. It is small (about 20 centimetres across), bright orange or brown, and has bright blue markings. Its name is *Octopus maculosis*, and its bite can kill. It bites with its parrot-like beak and its saliva contains the venom, which is a nerve poison. Other softies amongst the cephalopods are cuttlefish, squid, and the nautilus, but these are not poisoners.

(b) *Cone shells*

The cone shells are cousins of the land snails and, like them, have a single spirally coiled shell, a distinct head with two or four tentacles, two eyes, and a fleshy foot (as they 'walk' on their bellies they are called gastropods). Cone shells have their shells conically shaped, are often very decorative, and all of them are venomous. Some species of the 400-odd types can be lethal.

The system is ingenious. Venom is stored in a venom bulb within the body. Before stinging, the venom passes along a venom duct to a tapering set of spiral teeth much like the drilling end of a borehole drill. These teeth lie inside the shell. To sting they are moved out (like grandpa's teeth), grasped by a trunk-like 'nose' (proboscis) and rammed into the victim.

Cone shells and the blue-ringed octopus both produce a poison that attacks the nervous system. The effects of their stings are similar.

It should be kept in mind that virtually all the poisoners of the sea, irrespective of whether they are invertebrates or fishes, use nerve poison as their weapon. Anticipate paralysis and respiratory failure in any stung diver, irrespective of the stinger.

Locally, the bite may be painless, numb, burning or very painful.

Generally, numbness and tingling start at the wound and then spread over the whole body after ten minutes. The lips and mouth are particularly numb. Paralysis of muscles may occur, ranging from mild weakness to total body paralysis. Speech and swallowing become difficult. In severe cases, paralysis of the breathing muscles causes death. If the victim lives six hours, survival is probable. After 24 hours the diver will be better.

Management: There are no antivenoms for the molluscs. The emphasis is on artificial respiration to keep the victim alive over the first hours. This means rescue breathing for extended periods if in a remote area, or until the victim can be placed on a hospital respirator.

3. Echinoderms

The third group of invertebrates that sting divers are the prickly-skins or *echinoderms.* They get their name from the Greek *echino,* meaning a hedgehog or sea-urchin, and *derm* meaning skin. They are a neat group in that they are radially symmetric. Included in this clan are starfish, sea-urchins and sea-cucumbers. The sea-cucumbers are fine, it is the starfish and sea-urchins that have stingers among them.

(a) *Starfish*
Usually, only one starfish is problematic to divers. This is the crown of thorns. Officially named *Acanthaster planci,* it has caused massive overgrowth and destruction of the Indo-Pacific coral, but this is apparently something it does from time to time as a cyclical event. It is big, over 60 centimetres in diameter, has about 16 arms and is covered with 6-centimetre sharp, thick and venomous spines covered in slime. These may break off after penetrating the skin.

(b) *Sea-urchins*
There are a large number of different sea-urchins, some with long spines (over 30 centimetres) and some with short ones. Some are very venomous and some less so. The sea-urchins have another, more venomous, stinging system aside from venomous spines. Delicate, long, stalk-like appendages called pedicellariae project between the spines. Each of these has a swollen end equipped with a set of jaws and a poison bag. Contact causes these pedicellarial jaws to close and venom to be injected. And these jaws do not let go as long as the prey moves. As a diver stung by them is far too powerful for them, they break off and continue to poison the diver. Pedicellarial venom is more potent than that of the spines.

The Japanese variety called *Toxopneustes elegans* has long floral pedicellariae wafting beyond the spines. Contact with this urchin can kill.

Presentation of starfish and sea-urchin stings. The presentation of a sting from the crown of thorns and most sea-urchin spines is similar and is usually local only.

Local effects are immediate severe burning pain, and spines are seen in the skin. The area around the wound becomes numb. Infection is common and a spreading inflammation then occurs around the site with pain and aching.

General effects involve a nerve poison once again, and it is the delicate pedicellariae that work this effect with their exotic venom. The severe local burning pain is followed by weakness, faintness and numbness, with progressive muscular paralysis. Speech and swallowing become difficult, and progression to respiratory paralysis may lead to death. The pain usually disappears after about one hour, but paralysis may last for over six hours. Note that this sequence of events is very similar to the effects from sea-wasp, blue-ringed octopus and cone shell stings.

Management. First aid is directed at the local injury and the generalised problems.
(a) It is difficult to remove sea-urchin spines. They break off very easily and usually will be absorbed within a few weeks anyway. Sometimes

they become infected and medical help and antibiotics will then be needed.

(b) The venom of these spines and pedicellariae is *heat-sensitive,* and application of heat to the area will inactivate the poison. Treat the sting with water at 50°C. Do not scald the victim, who is already in pain. Heating is the most effective way of destroying the venom.

(c) Alcohol may now be applied. It is antiseptic and also inactivates pedicellariae, which can now be removed if visible.

(d) Oral antihistamines may provide some relief and pain-killers by mouth can assist pain.

(e) Any signs of paralysis or difficulty with breathing may mean that rescue breathing will be needed, so *keep a watchful lookout.* Don't put the diver to bed quietly to suffocate in peace while the rest of the party sing songs and play guitars.

4. Annelids

The fourth group of stingers consists of the segmented worms or *annelids.* They have long, segmented bodies and work their mischief in two ways:
— the bite is inflicted using biting jaws;
— the sting is inflicted using bristles on each segment.
The bite or sting causes a painful local reaction which is handled with hot water, antiseptics and pain-killers. Bristles can be removed using sellotape or adhesive tape.

5. Porifera

These are the sponges and there are thousands of species of these simple animals. A few can cause painful skin irritations following contact with the surface of their fibrous outer skeletons. Again, management is along general lines.

General approach to sea-stingers

The average diver will not remember the technicalities of nomenclature nor the stinging methods used by the invertebrates. It is also common for the victim to be unable to identify the exact species of stinger involved. Unfortunately, the stingers couldn't care less and will continue to injure divers, whose buddies will be presented with a potentially lethal problem. A practical, simple, easy-to-remember approach is therefore necessary.

If the stinger has spines (starfish, urchin or fish), there will be a puncture wound: use hot water.

If the stinger has no spines, there will be welts or a rash: use vinegar or alcohol.

Example
• Pete Muckitt was diving with Charlie Crumpet at the sunken temple near Trincomalee in Sri Lanka. The water was warm and Pete had

decided not to bother with his wet suit. Clad only in borrowed underpants, Pete explored the shattered temple, squeezing between broken columns and peering under fallen plinths. Excruciating pain suddenly lashed at his bare back. Yowling in agony into his regulator, he crawled from under the ruins and made for the surface. Charlie, seeing Pete kicking frantically above him, followed, and at the surface helped the screaming Pete aboard the boat. Pete was thrashing in pain and had no idea as to what had happened, but a purpling mark on his bare back told Charlie that Pete had been stung. But by what? What to do?

This is the type of problem that may occur. The absence of a major wound excludes a large biting animal and the presence of intolerable pain indicates a stinger.

What did Charlie know? He knew that stingers use nerve poisons and that paralysis and respiratory arrest were possibly on the way. He knew that heat, alcohol, and vinegar were treatments for stings. He knew that antihistamines and oral pain-killers might help.

What did Charlie do? He tried the lot. While waiting for water to heat on the boat's stove, he poured Pete's vodka over the welt. He followed this with cold vinegar, then applied hot (45°C to 50°C) water compresses to Pete's back for 30 minutes. He gave Pete an antihistamine and two pain-killers and watched for any sign of weakness or paralysis. As the boat returned home, he radioed for medical assistance.

This would be a reasonable approach to any sting. Without knowing anything about the cause, it is possible to render effective assistance. It would even help with vertebrate stings, because stinging fish also use spines to sting and their venoms are destroyed by heat too.

Stingers With Spinal Columns — Vertebrates

Up to now we have examined some aspects of the stingers without spinal columns. When a spinal column is allowed as ticket of admission into the stingers' club, a whole host of horrible members enrol. Stingrays, scorpionfish, ratfish, catfish, weevers, toadfish, rabbitfish and stargazers make up only a portion of the horde of noxious fish waiting for a diver. The interesting thing is that the more venomous and spiky the demon fish, the more indolent and less aggressive it becomes. Who needs to attack when your first defence is a knockout? The venom effects can be lethal, but specific treatment is largely unknown.

Like sea-urchins, stinging fish use spines to sting. The spines form part of the dorsal, pelvic or anal fins, or are just in front of the dorsal or pectoral fins. In the case of the stingray, the sting is in the tail. Venom glands are commonly placed on either side of the base of the stinging spine, or around the spine. The spines may be sharp and needle-like, or have backward-facing barbs, causing extensive laceration of tissue on withdrawal of the spine. The spine is covered by a sheath which is pushed back when the spine enters the victim. This compresses the venom gland and injects the poison.

Stinging fish are generally recluses, and contact with them usually occurs inadvertently because they are hidden by burying themselves in sand, or camouflaged. The lionfish is the exception. It has beautiful, lacy dorsal and pectoral fins, but within the fancy finwork are the venomous spines. Contact also occurs when stinging fish are netted or caught. These fish must never be handled!

The two most important stinging fish are the stingrays and the scorpionfish.

Stingrays

There are many different species of stingray and they are commonly found in shallow water partially buried in the sand, ready for an incautious diver to step on them. Some have the tail sting very close to the body, making it difficult for them to use it, but others have the sting well placed down the tail enabling them to lash and sting very viciously. Their sting is long and barbed and dangerous.

Scorpionfish

Scorpionfish are the most poisonous fish known. They can be divided into three groups, using their venomous spines as a distinguishing character:
- *Zebra fish (Pterois)*, also called lionfish or turkeyfish, have long, delicate venomous spines. They are showy and indifferent to visitors, but a hazard in coral reefs.
- *Scorpionfish proper (Scorpaena)* have fairly thick spines. They rely on camouflage and blend their shape and colouring to the crevices, rocks and seaweed in which they lurk.
- *Stonefish (Synanceja)* have very heavy venomous spines, covered in warty, thick sheaths. They are well camouflaged, lie quietly in sheltered rocky niches and are difficult to see. Their poison is the most dangerous of all.

The known venoms of stinging fish are heat-labile, that is, they are destroyed by heat. They cause intense pain on contact, which may be so severe that the victim screams, thrashes around, and even loses consciousness. The venoms are toxic to muscle, causing paralysis which includes the muscles of breathing so that respiratory failure occurs. The heart muscle may also be affected, leading to cardiac failure.

The result is a diver screaming, writhing and vomiting in pain, losing consciousness and possibly drowning, developing a progressive paralysis which involves breathing and stops heart action and, should the diver survive, infection and gangrene of the area can occur.

Management of stinging fish injuries

Management of venomous fish stings has three dimensions – the control of pain, venom effects, and later infection.

1. Rescue the victim from the water.
2. Lay the victim flat on the ground.
3. Try to irrigate the wound with cold sea water (or saline solution if available) to rinse out some of the poison. Remember that some of the venom-producing sheath may also be in the wound and continue to poison the diver.
4. While the wound is being cleaned, fresh water must be heated as quickly as possible.
5. Immerse the limb in water at 50°C (as hot as bearable without scalding) for 30 to 60 minutes. The addition of Epsom salts to the water has been reported to be useful. If done quickly, heating rapidly destroys the venom and pain relief is dramatic. Wounds on the head and trunk should be treated with hot-water compresses.
6. Tourniquets have been used to try to stop generalised absorption of the venom, but their use is questionably effective.
7. Injection of local anaesthetic (2% lignocaine or xylocaine) into the area around the wound may help the pain.
8. Once the above has been done, keep a sharp lookout for respiratory and cardiac failure. If necessary, CPR must be done.
9. Call for medical help. The wound must still be properly cleaned and dressed, lacerated wounds may need suturing, antibiotics may be needed and, in severe cases, hospitalisation may be indicated.
10. Remember that the victim is frightened, and in very great pain and distress. Be calm and reassuring.
11. Stonefish antivenin. If available, this should be given in all cases of stonefish sting.

Sea-snakes

These highly venomous animals are true reptiles. They are air breathers, have lungs, no fins, and use their flattened tails as paddles for swimming, together with undulating sideward movements of their bodies. There are about 50 species of sea-snakes. Although generally regarded as docile, they can become aggressive during the mating season, when stepped on, and when caught on a line or netted. They are far more venomous than land snakes. The venom causes:

— nerve poisoning with paralysis;
— muscle-tissue breakdown;
— blood cell destruction.

The only good thing is that sea-snake fangs are short and are easily torn out, so that only just over half of bitees are poisoned.

Sea-snakes are most commonly found in shallow water near river mouths where the water is turbid. A wader stepping on a snake may not even know that he has been bitten, as the bite is usually painless. This can be very awkward because serious illness is on the way. Depending on the site, the species of sea-snake, the amount of venom injected and the victim's characteristics, there is a period of time from 10 minutes to hours before anything is noted.

The victim becomes restless and a little excitable. As the muscle-toxin component works, the tongue becomes 'thick' and generalised body aches and stiffness appear. Drooping of the eyelids is an early sign and spasm of the jaw muscles or lockjaw occurs. The nerve-toxin causes an ascending paralysis, starting in the legs and working up to the neck. Speech becomes difficult, swallowing an effort, and vomiting may occur. The blood-toxin causes breakdown of red blood cells with progressive shock. The destruction of muscle cells and red blood cells causes the urine to become red-pink and kidney failure can occur. Finally, convulsions, coma, cardiac failure, and respiratory failure lead to death.

Management
1. The victim must lie down and remain absolutely quiet. No walking, effort, or any exertion must be allowed. Splint the limb.
2. A tourniquet must be applied above the puncture wound. It must be released after two hours.
3. Obtain medical help urgently.
4. Rescue breathing or CPR as needed.
5. Sea-snake antivenin should be used if available, otherwise polyvalent serum with Krait (Elapidae) fraction may be used.
6. If possible, the snake should be kept for identification.

A point of importance
The above discussion describes the invertebrates and vertebrates capable of inflicting a paralysing sting, such as the blue-ringed octopus, sea-wasp, stonefish and sea-snake. It is all very well reading about these afflictions, but always remember that a paralysed victim can hear and see. The victim cannot move, or even breathe, but is conscious and can hear you and see you. It is absolutely imperative that you remember this and continually give reassurance and explain what you are doing. If you are in a state of uncontrolled excitement and wildly discuss what is happening, just remember that the victim, too, is aware of what you are saying and what he or she may then feel is beyond description. While you are performing mouth-to-mouth resuscitation and onlookers are saying that it's too late and that he's gone, he may be conscious and terrified and desperately praying that you do not listen and stop your possibly life-saving efforts.

Marine Animals That Are Poisonous To Eat

Most divers love a good seafood meal, whether it be curried crayfish, mussels moutarde, barbecued bonito or pickled parrot-fish. Under the right circumstances almost any seafood can be toxic or even lethal.

Most poisonings are relatively rare. Who in their right minds would eat sea-urchin eggs? It has been done, with splendid vomiting and diarrhoea. Sea-cucumbers can be bought in the East. If you buy them in the street, you purchase Trepang, but at a restaurant at ten times the price you can enjoy *Bêche-de-mer* which is the same thing and proves how expensive French lessons can be. In any event, eating sea-cucumbers can kill you.

There are some poisonings that are important either because they are common or because they can affect whole communities. These are:
— shellfish poisoning
— ciguatera
— tetrodotoxin
— scombroid

Shellfish Poisoning

You may poison your guests in three ways with a good shellfish dinner.

1. Gastroenteritis

Gastroenteritis follows the eating of shellfish contaminated by bacteria (off or rotten). Nausea, vomiting, diarrhoea and cramps occur, lasting a day or two. Treatment is dietary restriction, lots of fluids, antiemetics and anti-diarrhoeals.

2. Allergic reactions

People who have previously eaten shellfish may develop acute allergic reactions on their second or subsequent meal. This can present as a violently itchy and spreading red rash with large welts; as an acute episode of asthma; or as a sudden episode of collapse due to circulatory shock. The last two can kill, so this is a potentially serious problem.

Management
1. Itching and rashes can generally be controlled by the use of antihistamines.
2. Acute breathing difficulties due to sudden severe asthma, or sudden circulatory collapse and shock are medical emergencies. *A doctor or emergency paramedic service must be summoned.*
3. *If the diver is in a remote place with no recourse to any medical help:*
   (a) Inject adrenaline 1:1000 *subcutaneously* at a dose of 0.01 ml/kg body mass, *very slowly over five minutes.* Draw back on the syringe before injecting to ensure that a blood vessel has not been entered by the needle. Do not inject adrenaline into a blood vessel! An automatic adrenaline injector with a concealed spring-activated needle is now available (EpiPen).
   (b) Monitor the pulse continuously. It will become forceful and accelerate as the injection is given. If it rises above 120 beats per minute, stop injecting and wait until the pulse settles.
   (c) Watch the diver's face. It will become extremely pale due to the vasoconstrictive effect of adrenaline.
   (d) Monitor respiration continuously. Be prepared for CPR.
   (e) Inject 100-200 mg of hydrocortisone intramuscularly into the upper outer quadrant of the buttock muscle.
      Adrenaline and hydrocortisone are emergency life-saving drugs and may only be considered when it is impossible to get any trained help. These medications are being given without expert opinion and offer only a hope of success in extreme circumstances.
   (f) Administer CPR if breathing and heart function fail.

3. Paralytic shellfish poisoning (PSP)

This is a potentially lethal disease occurring during red tides which are caused by the sudden and massive proliferation of a tiny plankton organism called a dinoflagellate. The commonest dinoflagellates causing this sudden bloom revel in the names of *Gonyaulax catanella* and *Gonyaulax tamarensis.*

Fish eating these organisms may die, causing a mass death of fish. Molluscs, however, simply store the contaminating *Gonyaulax* and pass it on to the person who eats them. This can cause an epidemic of PSP at the time of the red tide and even for some time afterwards, as the poison may be retained by the molluscs for several months after a flush of red tide. The poison is a nerve toxin (saxitoxin) and, like so many marine venoms, causes a progressive paralysis which can affect the respiratory muscles and lead to death by suffocation.

Management of PSP
(a) The use of emetics to induce vomiting will reduce the amount of toxin absorbed.
(b) When signs develop, medical help must be sought.

(c) Mouth-to-mouth rescue breathing is necessary if breathing stops. *This may have to be continued for hours.*

(d) Monitor the pulse and heart beat continuously. Be ready to administer CPR.

(e) Remember that the victim is conscious and aware of what you are doing. Reassurance is *extremely* important.

Ciguatera Poisoning

Like PSP, this disease is transmitted to man by eating tainted fish products. With PSP, eating shellfish contaminated with the dinoflagellate *Gonyaulax* caused the problem. With ciguatera, another dinoflagellate called *Gambierdiscus toxicus* is believed to be the culprit. *Gambierdiscus* lives on brown seaweed. Herbivorous fish eat the seaweed and become contaminated. These fish may then be caught by man and eaten, and so the disease is passed on, or the herbivorous fish may be eaten by carnivorous fish which then become contaminated. Netting and eating these carnivorous fish will also cause the disease. The fish themselves are unaffected.

Most commonly reef fish, including file-fish, grouper, parrot-fish, surgeon-fish, trigger-fish, trunk-fish and wrasse, are the carriers. Moray eels are particularly poisonous when affected. The real problem arises when commonly eaten fish suddenly become poisonous. These include anchovies, herrings, barracuda and shad.

The disease starts within 12 hours of eating contaminated fish. Skin symptoms are typical. Cold feels hot and hot feels cold. Redness, itching, burning, and blistering of the skin may occur. Flu-like symptoms appear with muscle pains, aching joints, and headache. The muscle pains progress to severe weakness, tremors and paralysis. Diarrhoea and vomiting can occur. Eventually convulsions, coma and death occur in up to ten per cent of cases. Survival is a lengthy, painful process taking up to a year. Drinking alcohol can cause the features to reappear.

Management. The principles outlined for PSP apply. Don't eat reef fish, especially not their gonads and guts.

Tetrodotoxin Poisoning (Pufferfish Poisoning)

Why anyone would want to eat a pufferfish defies comprehension. Their very shape, with their large spines, should be enough to put off even the most avid piscivore. Characteristically, the Orientals have the capacity for exotic meals, but the puffer is surely their ultimate. In Japan the puffer is called *fugu*. Very highly trained and esteemed chefs prepare the fish for their gourmet clientele. The idea is just to cause numbness of the lips without further problems. Unfortunately, accidents do happen. Puffers, porcupine-fish and ocean sun-fish contain a deadly poison called tetrodotoxin in their skin, liver, gonads and gut. As usual, it is a potent nerve poison.

Poisoning commences with numbness around the mouth. If you had a lousy cook, your tongue and whole body will become numb. Twitching, progressive paralysis, difficulty with speech and swallowing, and convulsions occur. The diner is usually conscious all the while. Severe respiratory distress with a hypoxic blue colour and bleeding into the skin can occur. About 60 per cent of victims die.

Management. This is purely supportive, as for PSP and ciguatera.

Scombroid Poisoning

The name of this disease comes from the Latin *scomber,* meaning a mackerel. It occurs as a result of eating fish of the scombroid family and includes mackerel, tuna, albacore, swordfish and bonito. The muscle of all these fish is rich in the aminoacid histidine. Improper preservation or canning allows bacteria entrance to the flesh of the fish. These bacteria break the histidine down to a poisonous amine called saurine, which has many of the properties of *histamine.* From time to time one hears of the mass recall of canned tuna for this reason.

As histamine is the basic cause of allergic conditions, a pudding of allergic-type reactions occurs. The affected fish has a sharp peppery taste and should be given to your neighbour's cat. The features are a mixture of migraine, urticaria, asthma and gut irritation.

The victim develops an intense headache, with nausea and vomiting, an intensely itchy spreading rash, tightness of the chest with wheezing, palpitations, abdominal pain and diarrhoea, and circulatory shock can occur.

Management
(a) Induce vomiting as soon as possible unless the diver has already vomited or is very agitated by severe breathing difficulty.
(b) Antihistamines must be given, preferably by injection.
(c) Obtain medical help.
(d) *If medical help is absolutely unavailable,* adrenaline and hydrocortisone should be administered as detailed in allergic shellfish poisoning (p 234 above).

The condition can be avoided by prompt freezing or eating after catching the fish. *Do not* allow your mackerel catch to stand in the sun all day.

Marine Animals That Shock

A number of fish, including catfish and electric eels in fresh water, and stargazers and electric rays in sea water, possess voltage-generating electric organs.

The electric ray, like other rays, has a flattened disc-shaped body, but the tail is fish-shaped rather than whip-like. The electric organs are situated on either side of the front of the disc, the lower surface of the fish being electrically negative and the upper surface positive. Depending on the species, a voltage of 8 to 220 volts can be generated. Contact with a diver may result in short-lived incapacity, but rapid recovery invariably occurs.

The electric eel is the most advanced battery known. It is a South American river fish, but is an air breather, having to surface from time to time to breathe. About 1.2 metres long, it can generate a voltage of 370 to 550 volts at 40 watts which can easily knock a man out. The output lasts 0.002 seconds at a frequency of 400 per second. A steady output at this rate can be maintained for 20 minutes. Given a five-minute break, the output can be repeated. Eat your heart out, Duracell.

Underwater Explosions

A diver may be exposed to an underwater explosion for several reasons:
- underwater mining,
- underwater salvage,
- accidental exposure to unexploded ordnance on a sunken wreck,
- sabotage,
- war.

Whatever the reason, an explosion under water is extremely dangerous for a diver in the vicinity. An underwater blast is far more vicious than an equivalent explosion on the surface.

The following occurs:
1. An underwater explosion is triggered.
2. This results in the sudden formation of a large gas bubble which is under very great pressure and is very hot.
3. The pressure and heat cause immediate expansion of the size of the bubble. A very rapidly moving pressure wave is forced through the water. This first pressure wave (primary wave) is called the *short pulse*.
4. All liquids are incompressible and water is no exception. The surrounding water opposes the expanding bubble, tending to recompress it. A series of oscillating increases and decreases commences, each increase causing another, but progressively weaker, pressure wave.
5. The pressure waves move very rapidly near the centre of the explosion then slow down as distance increases. Eventually they reach the speed of sound and behave like sound in water, losing energy inversely to the square of the distance travelled.

   What does all this mean? In simpler terms, a series of high-speed pressure waves follow one another from a central high-pressure source of expanding gas. As distance increases, energy decreases, but because water is denser than air, the pressure waves move further in water than they do in air. They are reflected from the surface and from the bottom if it is solid. A soft sandy bottom will absorb some of the force. Reflected waves then add their force to other pressure waves, increasing their power and effect. At the surface, some of the reflected waves may move in the opposite direction to oncoming waves and reduce their effect.

6. Depending on the force and depth of the explosion, a well-described series of events takes place at the surface.

   (a) If the detonation is large or shallow enough, the surface water is torn or *shreds* and then bulges up. This bulge is called the *dome*.

   (b) Next comes a rapidly widening ring of dark water due to the advancing pressure waves. This is termed the *slick*.

   (c) Finally the ascending gas reaches the surface and breaks through, causing a gout of water to spray into the air. This is the *plume*.

If the explosion is deep or small, the above may not occur.

What happens to a diver in range of these pressure waves?

When a diver is in the water on a normal dive, he or she is unaware of the increased pressure on the arms and legs. As these are technically fluid systems, without any gas spaces, pressure is transmitted directly through them from the water. What the diver may be aware of are the air spaces:

— ears and sinuses,
— lungs and airways,
— abdomen.

When the pressure wave reaches the diver, the pressure is transmitted through tissues with little or no effect, being a fluid-to-fluid transmission. As the pressure wave reaches the lining of air spaces, destruction commences. Shredding and pluming occur, as at a water surface. The membranes and tissues of the ears, sinuses, airways, lungs and gut are simply torn to pieces.

This is very different from an explosion on land, where damage is caused by flying bits of bomb casing, shrapnel and debris hitting the victim. In water, movement of these solid objects is greatly impeded by the water resistance and they do not travel far. The pressure wave does the killing.

Management of underwater blast injuries

Prevention

1. Do not dive where explosives are being used.

2. If work with explosives must be done, protective clothing, shields and air-containing suits should be worn. The air causes reflection of the pressure waves and shredding of the first water-air interface, which happens to be the suit and not a lung.

3. If the diver is at the surface, he or she should try to get the air spaces out of the water. This means the head, chest and abdomen. At best the diver should lie on some floating material, and at worst should float on the back to try to minimise the injury. Remember that near the surface and the bottom reflection may augment the force of oncoming pressure waves — these are not good places to be in.

Treatment
1. Externally, the diver may appear intact and the damage may initially seem relatively minor. Only later will a ruptured bowel or torn lung cause a critically ill diver. All victims of underwater blast must be hospitalised as an emergency, if only for observation.
2. No fluids or food should be given by mouth in case penetration of the gut has occurred.
3. CPR and oxygen may be required.
4. Use 100 per cent oxygen by mask if lung injury has occurred.

The Management of an Unconscious Diver

'What do I do when a diver is found unconscious? How do I know what caused it?' The problem is a prickly one because the diver may be in water; may be breathing a complex gas mix; and may be exposed to cold or hot conditions, explosives, electricity and sea creatures. To make matters worse, divers may have a heart attack or a stroke under water. Whatever the primary cause for loss of consciousness, bends and a burst lung with arterial gas embolism hover during the rescue ascent.

Causes

It is vital to have a systematic approach to the causes. Be methodical. Don't give a perfect performance of CPR at the surface and forget that the diver has just missed all the required in-water decompression stops.

1. *What has the diver inhaled?*
   Water: Near-drowning
   Oxygen: Hypoxia or oxygen toxicity
   Nitrogen: Nitrogen narcosis
   Carbon dioxide build-up: Carbon dioxide toxicity
   Carbon monoxide: Carbon monoxide poisoning
   Foreign material: Dentures or vomit
2. *Is the diver injured?*
   Head injury
   Explosion
   Electricity
   Marine animal bite
   Marine animal sting
3. *Where did the diver lose consciousness?*
   On descent:
       Chest or helmet squeeze
       Any of the causes in 1 and 2 above
   At the bottom:
       Any of the causes in 1, 2 and 3 above
   On ascent:
       Acute decompression illness including arterial gas embolism

242 The Management of an Unconscious Diver

Blackout of ascent (in breathhold divers)
Any of the causes in 1, 2 and 3 above
Immediately on return to the surface:
Arterial gas embolism
Bubble formation with acute decompression illness
Any of the causes in 1, 2 and 3 above, except narcosis
Later after surfacing:
Acute decompression illness
Arterial gas embolism
Any of the causes in 2 above
4. *What is the diver's temperature?*
Hypothermia
Hyperthermia
5. *What equipment was the diver using?*
Scuba
Rebreather
Surface supply
Standard diving suit
6. *Any other medical problems?*
Heart attack
Stroke
Diabetes
Low blood sugar
Epilepsy

The final presentation may be multiple, e.g. a marine animal bite or sting causing near-drowning, followed by a missed decompression stop and bends as a result of a hasty rescue attempt, plus lung damage and arterial gas embolism due to inadequate regard to exhalation during the rapid ascent to save the diver's life.

Management

Going through lists of causes takes time and a cool head. In an emergency situation, time is a luxury and a cool head a rarity. Consider the inverted triangle of the 7 Bs.

Is the diver:

Below water?
Breathing?
Bleeding?
Beating?
Burst?
Bent?
Bit?

Whatever the primary and secondary causes, effectively handling the Bs can save the victim.

1. Below water

The first step is instinctive – the diver must be returned to the surface. Getting the diver there requires understanding. The danger is inducing pulmonary barotrauma of ascent. If the diver is convulsing, wait for the convulsion to pass. A return to the surface may be lethal if exhalation is inadequate. Dump the victim's weight belt. Commence a deep diver rescue ascent, ensuring that the diver's head is extended well back to allow exhalation of expanding air. Be calm! Do not perform an uncontrollably fast ascent (see p 149).

2. Breathing and beating

These are considered together, because their restoration is rescue breathing and external cardiac massage – together, cardiopulmonary resuscitation (CPR). (AIDS warning!)

Take a moment to look at the victim's colour before beginning resuscitation. Is the victim:
- a blue unconscious diver (hypoxic);
- a white unconscious diver (oxygen toxic, in shock or hypothermic);
- a red unconscious diver (carbon dioxide, carbon monoxide toxic, or hyperthermic).

Start CPR if necessary (see pp 175-182).

3. Bleeding

Bleeding is listed before beating in the triangle of Bs because if the victim is bleeding, he must be beating. Don't perform CPR if arterial blood is spurting from a gaping wound. *Pack and apply pressure.* (AIDS warning!) Rescue breathing and controlling bleeding should be done simultaneously if two or more helpers are available. If you are alone, control massive bleeding as quickly as possible, then start rescue breathing if required (see pp 178-179).

4. Burst

If unconsciousness occurred during ascent or very soon after surfacing, the diver *must* be considered to have arterial gas embolism. This means urgent transport to a recompression facility (see p 122).

5. Bent

A bent-only unconscious diver will very rarely be in the water. Bends occur after ascent unless the dive was so prolonged or deep that instant acute cerebral decompression illness developed. In nearly all cases the diver will be at the surface, and several minutes will have passed. Urgent transport to a recompression facility is needed (see pp 136-137).

6. **Bit**

A major bite, such as a shark or barracuda bite, will be obvious. Check for the mark of the poisoner — look for welts, discoloured streaks and tentacles on exposed areas, urchin spines in any area (spines penetrate suits and fins), and the puncture wounds of scorpionfish. Apply vinegar to welts and hot water to puncture stings (see p 231).

Contact a diving physician urgently.

Having controlled breathing, bleeding, beating, bursting, bending and bitten, now consider the causes. Speak to the victim's buddy. Get *exact* details of the dive profile, any previous dives, behaviour during the dive, contact with animal life, explosives, injury or electricity. Check the victim's equipment and make a list. Measure the air pressure remaining in the scuba cylinder. Did the victim run out of air? Was the air supply contaminated with carbon monoxide as a result of careless or inadequate filtration? Was he using pure oxygen or a gas mix? Was the victim using a contents gauge and a depth gauge? Did the victim have a buoyancy device? Was it inflated, causing an uncontrolled ascent? Was the weight belt too heavy? Was the victim familiar with the equipment used? When was the victim's last medical? Was the victim taking any medication? Write a full report for the doctor to read (see p 258).

ONSET OF UNCONSCIOUSNESS					
	DESCENT	BOTTOM	ON ASCENT	AT SURFACE	AFTER DIVE
N_2 NARCOSIS	X	X			
HYPOXIA	X	X	X		
O_2 TOXICITY	X	X	X		
CO_2 TOXICITY	X	X	X		
CO POISONING	X	X	X	X	
WATER INHALED	X	X	X	X	
FOREIGN MATTER	X	X	X	X	X
PUL. BAROTRAUMA			X	X	X
DECOMP. ILLNESS			X	X	X
SQUEEZE	X				
MARINE STING				X	X
MARINE BITE	X	X	X	X	X
SEA-SNAKE					X
SEAFOOD					X
HYPOTHERMIA		X	X	X	
HEAD INJURY		X	X	X	X
ELECTROCUTION		X			
EXPLOSION		X	X	X	
OTHER MEDICAL	X	X	X	X	X

UNCONSCIOUSNESS ON DESCENT USING SCUBA	
N$_2$ NARCOSIS	DEEP AIR DIVE; WRONG NITROX MIX
HYPOXIA	CYLINDER EMPTY; FAULTY REGULATOR; WRONG MIX
O$_2$ TOXICITY	PURE OXYGEN; NITROX; HELIOX; TRIMIX
CO$_2$ TOXICITY	AIR CONTAMINATION; TIGHT GEAR; DENSE NITROX
CO POISONING	AIR CONTAMINATION
WATER INHALED	PANIC; ALCOHOL; EQUIPMENT PROBLEM; COUGHING
FOREIGN MATTER	DENTURES; VOMIT
SQUEEZE	RAPID NEGATIVE DESCENT WITH REGULATOR FAILURE
MARINE BITE	SHARK; BARRACUDA; GROUPER; ETC.
OTHER MEDICAL	EPILEPSY; DIABETES; HEART ATTACK; STROKE

UNCONSCIOUSNESS AT BOTTOM USING SCUBA	
N$_2$ NARCOSIS	DEEP AIR DIVE; WRONG NITROX MIX
HYPOXIA	CYLINDER EMPTY; FAULTY REGULATOR; WRONG MIX
O$_2$ TOXICITY	PURE OXYGEN; NITROX; HELIOX; TRIMIX
CO$_2$ TOXICITY	AIR CONTAMINATION; TIGHT GEAR; DENSE NITROX MIX; STRENUOUS EXERCISE; SKIP BREATHING
CO POISONING	AIR CONTAMINATION
WATER INHALED	PANIC; ALCOHOL; EQUIPMENT PROBLEM; COUGHING
FOREIGN MATTER	DENTURES; VOMIT
MARINE BITE	SHARK; BARRACUDA; GROUPER; ETC.
OTHER MEDICAL	EPILEPSY; DIABETES; HEART ATTACK; STROKE
HEAD INJURY	WRECK, CAVE DIVING
HYPOTHERMIA	ALCOHOL; INADEQUATE INSULATION; ICE DIVING
ELECTROCUTION	CONTACT WITH UNDERWATER CABLES; WELDING
EXPLOSION	EXPLOSIVES IN WRECKS; SETTING EXPLOSIVES

UNCONSCIOUSNESS ON ASCENT USING SCUBA	
ARTERIAL GAS EMBOLISM	INADEQUATE EXHALATION; TIGHT GEAR; RAPID ASCENT; ASTHMA; RESPIRATORY INFECTION; PATENT FORAMEN OVALE
TENSION PNEUMOTHORAX	INADEQUATE EXHALATION; TIGHT GEAR; RAPID ASCENT; ASTHMA; RESPIRATORY INFECTION
ACUTE DECOMP-RESSION ILLNESS	RAPID ASCENT WITH SUBSTANTIAL GAS LOAD AND MISSED DECOMPRESSION STOPS
HYPOXIA	CYLINDER EMPTY; FAULTY REGULATOR; WRONG MIX
O_2 TOXICITY	PURE OXYGEN; NITROX; HELIOX; TRIMIX
CO_2 TOXICITY	AIR CONTAMINATION; TIGHT GEAR; DENSE NITROX MIX; STRENUOUS EXERCISE; SKIP BREATHING
CO POISONING	AIR CONTAMINATION
WATER INHALED	PANIC; ALCOHOL; EQUIPMENT PROBLEM; COUGHING
FOREIGN MATTER	DENTURES; VOMIT
MARINE BITE	SHARK; BARRACUDA; GROUPER; ETC.
OTHER MEDICAL	EPILEPSY; DIABETES; HEART ATTACK; STROKE
HEAD INJURY	WRECK, CAVE DIVING
HYPOTHERMIA	ALCOHOL; INADEQUATE INSULATION; ICE DIVING
EXPLOSION	TOO SHORT FUSE AFTER SETTING EXPLOSIVES

UNCONSCIOUSNESS AT THE SURFACE USING SCUBA	
ARTERIAL GAS EMBOLISM	INADEQUATE EXHALATION; TIGHT GEAR; RAPID ASCENT; ASTHMA; RESPIRATORY INFECTION; PATENT FORAMEN OVALE
TENSION PNEUMOTHORAX	INADEQUATE EXHALATION; TIGHT GEAR; RAPID ASCENT; ASTHMA; RESPIRATORY INFECTION
ACUTE DECOM-PRESSION ILLNESS	RAPID ASCENT WITH SUBSTANTIAL GAS LOAD AND MISSED DECOMPRESSION STOPS
CO POISONING	AIR CONTAMINATION – PERSISTING EFFECT
WATER INHALED	PANIC; ALCOHOL; STRONG CURRENTS; COUGHING
FOREIGN MATTER	DENTURES; VOMIT
MARINE BITE	SHARK; BARRACUDA; GROUPER; ETC.
MARINE STING	FOLLOWING VERTEBRATE OR INVERTEBRATE STINGS
OTHER MEDICAL	EPILEPSY; DIABETES; HEART ATTACK; STROKE
HYPOTHERMIA	ALCOHOL; INADEQUATE INSULATION; ICE DIVING
HEAD INJURY	COLLISION WITH BOAT, ROCKS
EXPLOSION	TOO SHORT FUSE AFTER SETTING EXPLOSIVES

UNCONSCIOUSNESS LATER AFTER SCUBA DIVING	
ARTERIAL GAS EMBOLISM	OCCURS IMMEDIATELY OR VERY SOON AFTER DIVING
TENSION PNEUMOTHORAX	OCCURS VERY SOON AFTER DIVING
MEDIASTINAL EMPHYSEMA	COMPRESSION OF HEART AND LUNG FUNCTION; OCCURS SOON AFTER DIVING
ACUTE DECOMP- RESSION ILLNESS	MAJORITY OCCUR WITHIN 30 MINUTES AFTER DIVING
MARINE BITE	SHARK; BARRACUDA; GROUPER; ETC.
MARINE STING	FOLLOWING VERTEBRATE OR INVERTEBRATE STINGS
SNAKE BITE	OCCURS SOON AFTER DIVING; BITE MAY BE PAINLESS
OTHER MEDICAL	EPILEPSY; DIABETES; HEART ATTACK; STROKE
HEAD INJURY	MAY BE DELAYED AFTER HEAD INJURY UNDER WATER
SEAFOOD	INGESTION OF POISONOUS OR CONTAMINATED SEAFOOD

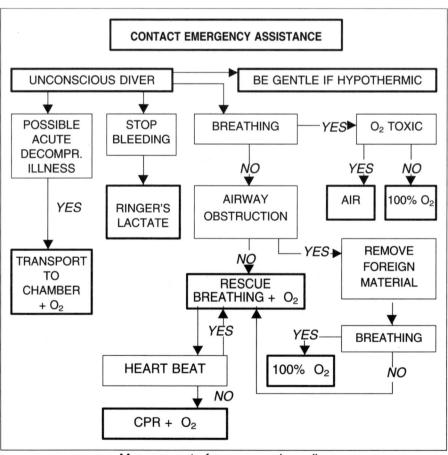

Management of an unconscious diver

Emergency Diver Rescue Protocol

1. **Take control of the situation**

   (a) Ensure that the rescued victim and the rescuers are in a safe place on the shore or in the boat.
   (b) Determine whether anyone at the site is CPR-trained.
   (c) Check the victim's airways, breathing, circulation and injuries.
   (d) Apply pressure and pack any wounds to control bleeding and commence CPR if required.
   (e) Appoint an assistant (preferably two if available) and a contacting person who will summon trained help.
   (f) Determine whether the victim belongs to a diver rescue service and obtain the contact number.

2. **Information to be delivered by the contacting person to the rescue service, hospital, diving physician or nearest hyperbaric facility, depending on circumstances**

   (a) Name, sex, age, home address and telephone number of the victim.
   (b) Name of the contacting person.
   (c) Contacting person's telephone number and area code.
   (d) Exact geographic site of victim:
       — remote: nearest town, village, landmarks
       — urban: suburb, street number, nearest cross street.
   (e) Approximate cause, nature and severity of emergency:
       — hyperbaric
       — non-hyperbaric
   (f) Victim's membership particulars with a diver rescue service.

3. **Give pre-travel advice to contact**

   (a) Keep calm and relay the information clearly and accurately.
   (b) Check victim's exact particulars with the diver rescue service's

central register if victim is a member (any known illnesses or therapy?).

(c) Ensure someone stays at contact telephone number.

4. On-site management if no paramedic is available

(a) Victim fully conscious:
   - Reassure.
   - Lie flat *(no Trendelenburg)*.
   - Encourage oral fluids − 150 ml of water per hour. Do not give oral fluids if abdominal or chest trauma has occurred.
   - Use 100 per cent oxygen by face mask if available.

(b) Victim unconscious and breathing:
   - Lie flat in left lateral rescue position to avoid inhalation of vomit.
   - Ensure clear airways and support chin.
   - Use 100 per cent oxygen by face mask if available.
   - Monitor pulse and breathing.
   - Be ready to perform CPR. (AIDS warning!)

(c) Victim receiving CPR:
   - Continue CPR until help arrives
   - Use 100 per cent oxygen if available − use an Ambubag if available. Otherwise the worker administering rescue breathing should inhale oxygen from a face mask before each mouth-to-mouth breath to the victim. An assistant can hold the mask for the worker in charge of airway and breathing.

(d) Definite victim of marine animal sting:
   - Injury caused by stinging spines: Immerse limb in hot water or apply hot packs (as hot as helpers can reasonably bear). Do not scald the victim.
   - Sting not caused by spines: Pour vinegar on to wound and apply hot vinegar poultice.
   - Watch victim carefully. Be prepared to commence prolonged rescue breathing at any time.

(e) Definite victim of sea-snake bite:
   - Immobilise affected limb and keep limb below level of heart.
   - Victim must lie absolutely still. *No walking.*
   - Apply tourniquet above wound on limb bites. Note the time. The contact person must inform the diving medical officer, ambulance paramedic or hospital that a tourniquet has been applied, notify them of the time and request advice on how long to maintain it. It *must* be removed after two hours maximum in any event.
   - Keep victim warm and give fluids. No alcohol.
   - If possible, keep snake for identification.

5. **On-site action if paramedically trained**

(a) Ensure access and safety of site.

(b) Control airways, breathing, circulation and bleeding.

(c) Administer 100 per cent oxygen.

(d) Perform field neurological assessment.

(e) Assess possibilities:
  - hyperbaric disease:
    acute decompression illness
    pulmonary barotrauma
    AGE
  - non-hyperbaric disease:
    near-drowning
    trauma
    marine animal bite, sting
    hypoxia
    oxygen toxicity
    carbon dioxide toxicity
    carbon monoxide toxicity
    hypothermia
    hyperthermia
    electrical injuries or explosives
  - medical history: heart disease, hypertension, diabetes or hypoglycaemia (assess using finger prick Dextrostix), epilepsy, medicines, drugs, alcohol, date of last diving medical.

(f) Establish IV line:
  (i) Use Ringer's lactate and Haemaccel for trauma (maximum dose Haemaccel 1500 ml, thereafter alternate with blood 1:1). Rate to depend on degree of blood loss and shock.
  (ii) Use Ringer's lactate for acute decompression illness and AGE. Request advice from diving physician re possible use of Dextran 40 (Rheomacrodex) — 500 ml in first half-hour then 1000 ml over an 8-hour period (maximum total dose 2 g/kg bm).
  (iii) Use 5% glucose in non-diving, non-trauma cases. With hypoglycaemia confirmed with glucose stick on finger-prick blood, infuse 50 ml of 50% glucose into the IV line.

(g) Drugs:
  - Very limited use in hyperbaric disease.
  - No sedatives e.g. Valium, without permission from diving medical officer (DMO).
  - No aspirin or anticoagulants (heparin) with spinal or vestibular bends or pulmonary barotrauma. These may precipitate bleeding and worsen the victim's condition.
  - No steroids (Decadron, Dexamethasone) without permission from DMO. These can worsen acute spinal and cerebral decompression illness.

- Ascorbic acid (Vitamin C) 1 000 mg may be given orally.
- With non-hyperbaric disease drugs as per EMA protocol.

(h) Urine output: Monitor volume and, if trained, insert a urinary catheter if victim is unconscious or urinary retention is present.

6. Evacuation of victim

(a) Check geographic site of victim: physical altitude, travel distance, road access, nearest fixed-wing landing strip, helicopter access.

(b) Choose the most practical transport mode depending on accessibility, travel time, distance and urgency.
Options:
   (i) *Road transport.* Travel time is longer. Costs are less. If a one-man chamber is anticipated, there must be room for the chamber plus the operator in the vehicle.
   (ii) *Helicopter.* Travel time is short. Costs are high. Low flying is possible without pressurisation. If a helicopter and chamber are needed, the chamber must fit inside the helicopter.
   (iii) *Fixed-wing aircraft.* Travel time is short. Costs are high. A landing field is needed. If a fixed-wing aircraft without a chamber is used, it must be a pressurised or low-flying aircraft.

(c) Check the address and telephone number of the nearest hospital, ambulance service and police station.

(d) Notify DMO — request advice and ask whether doctor wishes to travel to victim.

(e) Notify nearest recompression facility.

(f) Prepare a detailed report. Obtain exact details from the victim or his buddies regarding the circumstances of the dive, previous dives, all equipment used, hazards encountered and rescue techniques used.

(g) Ensure that *all* the equipment used by the diver has been collected for expert assessment and analysis. These must be delivered to the responsible authority, hospital, facility or, in the event of death, the police.

7. Use of one-man chamber

Use with extreme caution and after discussion with DMO.

(a) Indications:
   (i) Acute skin or limb decompression illness.
   (ii) Acute severe decompression illness only if DMO advises. The therapeutic schedule will have to be aborted if the victim vomits with inhalation of vomit or becomes confused or loses consciousness during pressurisation.
   (iii) Carbon monoxide poisoning.

(b) Contraindications:
   (i) Unconscious or confused hyperbaric victim.

      (ii)   Pneumothorax.

(c) Method

    Check:

      (i)   Chamber fully functional and hosing clean and grease-free.

      (ii)   Adequate HP air for blowdown and flushing at 18 msw.

      (iii)   Adequate oxygen for at least 3 hours under pressure.

      (iv)   Couplings to inlets:
- chamber-pressurise-using-air inlet coupling,
- face-mask-oxygen inlet coupling.

      (v)   Couplings to outlets:
- chamber exhaust,
- overboard oxygen dump,
- pneumofathometer.

      (vi)   Communications functional.

    Then:

Remove all IV lines from the victim − reconsider the need for a one-man chamber pressurisation schedule versus a rapid transportation to a hyperbaric facility using oxygen at surface pressure.

      (vii) Place the victim in the chamber after removing his or her shoes and all metal objects (including any watch, jewellery or coins). Explain what you are doing and reassure the victim. Instruct the victim on the need for middle ear equalisation during repressurisation.

      (viii) Open the oxygen supply and fit the oxygen demand mask to the victim's face. Ensure that the head straps are properly positioned and that the inlet and overboard dump are functional − ask the victim to breathe.

      (ix)   Close the hatch. Inform the victim that pressurisation will commence and request acknowledgement. *Note the time.*

      (x)   Begin slow pressurisation to 18 msw using *air*. Ensure that the hatch has a good seal. Watch the victim constantly and ensure that he or she is equalising adequately. If the victim cannot equalise, *stop* pressurisation and open the exhaust valve until the victim signals relief. If the victim is still unable to equalise on recommencing pressurisation − exhaust the chamber, remove the victim, replace the IV lines and give 100 per cent oxygen by face mask.

      (xi)   With successful pressurisation to 18 msw:
- Note the time and start the stop watch.
- Inform the victim that pressurisation was successful and give reassurance.

      (xii) Use the therapeutic schedule as outlined in Table 5 US Navy or Table 61 Royal Navy. Observe all air breaks carefully.

      (xiii) Observe the victim constantly for any deterioration and request him or her to report any worsening or improvement.

      (xiv) Keep communications short and clear. Unnecessary chatter must be avoided. Keep coms from the chamber open constantly. Ensure coms to the victim is off except when the chamber operator is instructing the victim — the victim must not hear idle chatter or unguarded comments about his or her condition.

(xv) Keep a close watch on the chamber pressure. The victim's body heat will warm the chamber and the chamber pressure will begin rising (Amontons' Law). Use the exhaust valve to maintain 18 msw depth.

(xvi) Flush the chamber smoothly every 10 minutes by simultaneous slow partial opening of both air inlet and exhaust valves for 15 seconds. Ensure that the chamber pressure stays at 18 msw. *Do not violently pressurise plus vent.*

(xvii) Maintain a close watch for possible oxygen toxicity.

(xviii) Instruct the victim to hyperventilate chamber air if oxygen toxicity is suspected. *Do not bring a convulsing victim to surface pressure.* Wait for the convulsion to pass before commencing ascent.

(xix) Evacuation must commence when the victim is stable at 18 msw. Transport the victim to the appropriate facility — decompression unit or hospital. Notify the facility of your ETA, the condition of the victim, treatment given and anticipated requirements. Monitor the victim continuously en route to the facility.

(xx) At the decompression facility, the DMO will decide:
   — whether to continue with the 18 msw table;
   — whether to transfer the victim under pressure into a therapeutic chamber for further hyperbaric treatment.

(xxi) Prepare a full written report about the event (see p 258).

Neurological Assessment

The following protocol is a guide when a neurological assessment is required, whether following a head injury, suspected stroke, coma, or acute decompression illness. In the event of any abnormality being elicited in a diving-related case, the victim must be regarded as a case of acute decompression illness. Immobilise the neck and spine if trauma is suspected. With practice, this assessment can be completed in ten minutes and should be repeated at one-hourly intervals thereafter.

A Diving Medical Officer must be notified in all cases.

NEUROLOGICAL ASSESSMENT

Tick the appropriate block in each section.
NOTE: If the diver is unconscious, perform a modified assessment as follows:
1. Consciousness only (Section 1).
2. Pupil light reflex and equality of pupil size (Section 2).
3. Muscle tone (Section 10).
4. Limb reflexes (Section 13).

1. C.O.M.A. (Consciousness, Orientation, Memory, Arithmetic)						
CONSCIOUSNESS	YES		NO		SEIZURES	
ORIENTATION Time	YES		NO		Ask the diver: 'What is the time?' 'What day is it?'	
Place	YES		NO		Ask the diver: 'Where are you?'	
Person	YES		NO		Ask the diver: 'What is your name?'	
MEMORY Immediate	YES		NO		Ask diver to repeat: 11, 3, 79, 8	
Recent	YES		NO		Ask the diver: 'Where are you staying?', 'What did you last eat?'	
Remote	YES		NO		Ask the diver: 'What is your phone no.?', 'Where do you work?'	
ARITHMETIC	YES		NO		Ask diver to subtract serial 7s from 100.	

2. EYES

SIGHT NORMAL IN BOTH EYES	YES		NO		Can count 2-4 fingers, one eye at a time. Can read this page.
PUPIL LIGHT REFLEX NORMAL	YES		NO		Are the pupils equal in size? Do they contract in a bright light?
ACCOMMODATION NORMAL	YES		NO		Are the pupils smaller on looking far, larger on looking close?
EYE MOVEMENTS NORMAL	YES		NO		Can both eyes follow a moving finger up, down, L and R? Check for any rapid abnormal jerking movements, up, down or sideways (nystagmus).

3. FACE

FACIAL MOVEMENTS NORMAL ON BOTH SIDES	YES		NO		Can close/open eyes, wrinkle forehead, smile, clench teeth tightly (feel that the jaw muscles do tighten)
FACIAL SENSATION NORMAL ON BOTH SIDES	YES		NO		Can feel a light touch on both sides of chin, cheeks, nose and forehead.

4. HEARING AND SPEECH

HEARING NORMAL IN BOTH EARS	YES		NO		Can hear two fingers rubbed 50 cm from each ear in a quiet place.
SPEECH INTACT	YES		NO		Is there any huskiness? Are there any misplaced words or slurring?

5. TONGUE

TONGUE MOVEMENT NORMAL	YES		NO		Can put out tongue and move it L+R. Check for deviation to one side.

6. TASTE AND SMELL

TASTE NORMAL	YES		NO		Can taste sweet: sugar. Can taste salty: salt. Can taste sour: lemon.
SMELL NORMAL	YES		NO		Can smell coffee, garlic, vinegar, with each nostril.

7. SWALLOWING REFLEX

SWALLOWING NORMAL	YES		NO		Watch the larynx move up and down as the diver swallows.

8. MUSCLE POWER

SHOULDER MOVEMENTS EQUAL AND NORMAL	YES		NO		Press down on the diver's shoulders and ask the diver to shrug. Look for equal power.
GRIP	YES		NO		Can firmly grasp two of your fingers. Check that R+L grip are more or less similar.
ARMS	YES		NO		Can pull and push against resistance with both arms and with similar power.
LEGS	YES		NO		Can lift, part, and push legs together against resistance.

9. *RANGE OF MOVEMENTS*

Check that the diver can move all limbs equally and easily in all directions — up, down, outwards and inwards. Check that each joint can be fully flexed and extended.

SHOULDERS	YES	NO		
ELBOWS	YES	NO		
WRISTS	YES	NO		
HIPS	YES	NO		
KNEES	YES	NO		
ANKLES	YES	NO		
SPINE	YES	NO		

10. *MUSCLE TONE*

SPASTIC	YES	NO		Are one or more limbs very stiff or fixed in flexion or extension?
FLACCID	YES	NO		Are one or more limbs very floppy when lifted and allowed to drop?

11. *SENSORY FUNCTION*

Use: Cotton wool ball for light sensation; Point of pin or injection needle for sharp sensation; Back of pin or injection needle for dull sensation; Tuning fork (middle C) for vibration sense
ARE ALL MODALITIES OF SENSATION INTACT IN:

HANDS	YES	NO		Back of hands; Base of thumbs; Base of 5th fingers
ARMS	YES	NO		Back of arms; Front of arms.
TORSO	YES	NO		Back of torso; Front of torso
LEGS	YES	NO		Front of legs; Back of legs.
FEET	YES	NO		Tops of feet; Soles of feet.

12. *COORDINATION (cerebellar function)*

POINT ORIENTATION (Test both hands)	YES	NO		Using an index finger, the diver can touch an object in front of him.
FINGER-NOSE TEST (Test both hands)	YES	NO		The diver can rapidly touch his nose then your finger held in front of him/her.
GAIT NORMAL	YES	NO		Check for wobbly legs, unsteadiness, stagger, or walking heel-to-toe.
BALANCE (RHOMBERG) (Normal answer is NO)	YES	NO		The diver sways when standing with eyes shut, arms crossed, and feet together.

13. LIMB REFLEXES
Use a patellar hammer or a blunt object.
Test both sides

KNEES	YES		NO			With the knee flexed and relaxed, tap the tendon below the kneecap. The lower leg should jerk up.
ANKLES	YES		NO			Pull the foot upward and tap the Achilles tendon. The foot should jerk down.
BICEPS	YES		NO			Rest the diver's arm on his/her lap. Place your free thumb in front of the diver's elbow and tap your thumb. The lower arm should jerk up.
TRICEPS	YES		NO			Rest the diver's arm on his/her lap. Tap the tendon just above the elbow. The lower arm should jerk down

BABINSKI RESPONSE
This is an abnormal reflex. It indicates brain damage. Run a blunt object up the soles of the feet. A normal response is curling down of the toes. A Babinski response is an upward movement of the big toe with the other toes fanning out.

BABINSKI RESPONSE	YES		NO	

FINAL ASESSMENT
Note all abnormal findings here:

_____

_____

_____

_____

_____

_____

_____

_____

_____

_____

_____

_____

_____

_____

_____

_____

_____

_____

Diving Accident Report Form

DIVING ACCIDENT REPORT FORM
1. PERSONAL INFORMATION
Name of victim
Address
Telephone: Work   Home:
Date of birth: Sex: Age:
Illnesses injuries or operations in the past 5 years:
Health problems in past 3 months:
Names and addresses of doctors consulted:
Smoking: No. per day: Years smoking:
Previous smoking history: Never:
2. WOMEN ONLY
At the time of the diving incident:
Menstruating: Pregnant: Using oral contraceptives:
3. DIVING EXPERIENCE
Type of diving qualification: NAUI   PADI   SSI   YMCA   SAUU   Other
Date of latest qualification: Certification No.:
School at which trained: Tel. No.:
Certification level: Openwater 1   Openwater 2
Advanced diver   Dive master   Instructor
SAUU one star   SAUU two star   SAUU three star
Speciality qualifications (e.g. ice, cave, wreck)
Other:
Total number of dives logged: Date of most recent diving medical:
Name & address of that diving physician:

Diving Accident Report Form 2

4. TYPE OF DIVE

Sea water:	Fresh water:	Surf entry:
Boat:	Altitude:	Cave:
Night:	Wreck:	Kelp:
Ice:	Deep:	No decompression:
Decompression:	Other:	Water temp.:

Was the diver experienced in this type of dive?   Yes   No

Solo dive:	Buddy system:	Trio diving

Names of divers in group and contact tel. nos.

Hazards: Entanglement   Entrapment   Live boating

5. TYPE OF DIVING INCIDENT

Decompression illness:	Pulmonary barotrauma:
Arterial gas embolism:	Squeeze:
Boating:	Drowning:
Near-drowning:	Marine bite or sting:

Other:

6. TIME AND PLACE

Date of diving incident:	Time of incident:

Location:

Time of first obtaining help:

Time when definitive treatment was begun:

7. DETAILS OF CONTACTS HELPING AFTER THE INCIDENT

Sea rescue:	Hospital:
Physician:	Diver rescue service:
Police:	Ambulance Service:

Dive leader or instructor:

Other:

8. DETAILS OF DIVING INCIDENT

    (a)   Previous dives on the diving trip:

              Number of consecutive days of diving:

              Dive profiles of previous dives:

DATE & TIME	DEPTH	BOTTOM TIME	ASCENT TIME	DECOMPRESSION (depth/minutes)

				Diving Accident Report Form 3
DATE & TIME	DEPTH	BOTTOM TIME	ASCENT TIME	DECOMPRESSION (depth/minutes)

(b)   Dive on which the incident occurred:

Dive leader's name and address or contact telephone number

Time dive began   Time of surfacing

Max. Depth   Time at bottom   Ascent time

First dive of day   Y/N   Repetitive dive (how many?)

Any decompression obligations?   Y/N   Stops actually done

Decompression stops missed

Required decompression stops (depth/mins)

Dive completed   Dive aborted

Safety stops performed Y/N

Altitude obligations?   Y/N   Altitude correction used

Surface interval before the dive   Residual nitrogen time at start of dive

Ascent (state rate in metres/min where applicable:

Normal   Fast   Assisted by buddy

Uncontrolled buoyant   Emergency

Narcosis   Vertigo   Coughing   Vomiting

Sneezing   Skip breathing   Buddy breathing

Octopus rig breathing   Out of air

Other problem

Dive plan:

Computer (state make of computer)

Table (state table and schedule used)

Additional factors:

Flying between dives? Y/N   After dive? Y/N

If yes how long after?   Aircraft pressurised? Y/N

Alcohol: None   Night before dive   Predive

During dive   Postdive

Drugs or medicines used before the dive

Exercise predive   During dive   Postdive

Predive fatigue or hangover

Hot bath or shower postdive

Other symptoms before diving

9. EQUIPMENT USED

Suit: Wet   Thickness   Dry   Other

Cylinder size:

Date of last visual inspection of cylinder

Date of last hydraulic testing of cylinder

Cylinder air pressure: Predive   Postdive

Cylinder contents gauge   Depth gauge

Compressor operator's name

Compressor operator's registration number

Boat skipper's name

Boat skipper's ticket number

Weight belt: Mass   Own   Borrowed   Dumped

Dive watch: Own used   Buddy's used   None

Buoyancy vest: ABLJ   BC   None

Buoyancy inflation: CO_2 cartridge   Power   Oral

Second stage regulator   Octopus rig

Ropes, lines and tools used

Dive knife   Dive torch   Cyalumes

Equipment failure?

Predive equipment and signals check performed? Y/N

Predive buoyancy check performed (especially with borrowed weight belt)? Y/N

Any equipment fault found with predive check? Y/N

Comment on any equipment fault found

10. SYMPTOMS AND SIGNS EXPERIENCED AT THE DIVE INCIDENT

Before diving   On descent   At bottom

On ascent   Immediately after surfacing

Later after surfacing (state hrs/mins)

Tick below next to corresponding feature:

Confusion	Headache	Rash
Disorientation	Undue fatigue	Swelling
Dizziness	Numbness	Itching
Unconscious	Pins and needles	Chest pain
Convulsions	Weakness	Abdomen pain

		Diving Accident Report Form 5
Blurred vision	Difficulty standing	Arm pain R/L
Double vision	Difficulty walking	Leg pain R/L
Tunnel vision	Paralysis	Nausea
Blindness	Speech problem	Vomiting
Ringing in ears	Hoarseness	Coughing
Deafness	Skin mottling	Coughing blood
Ear pain	Squeeze	Breathless
Bleeding: Minor Moderate Major		Site
Fractures:		
Wounds:		
Death: At bottom	On surface	Later
Comments		

11. FIRST AID GIVEN

Mouth to mouth	CPR	Oxygen
Oral fluids	IV fluids	Drugs
Position: Lying flat	Head down	Sitting
Other first aid treatment		

12. DEFINITIVE TREATMENT

(a)   Recompression therapy Y/N

Site of chamber

Type of chamber: One man   Two man   Multiplace

Date recompression commenced   Time commenced

Delay between incident and recompression (days/hrs)

Therapeutic tables used

Chamber operator's name

Diving physician in charge of recompression

Result of recompression therapy: Complete relief   Partial relief   No relief

Recurrence of symptoms after recompression Y/N

Repeat recompression therapy needed Y/N

Residual problems or defects after treatment (describe)

Final result of therapy: Full recovery   Partial

Permanent disability   Death

(b)   Other therapy:

Attending doctor's name(s):

Hospital admission

Treatment received

Results of treatment

13. COMMENTS

Dated at   this   day of   19

Name

(Signature)

Medical Equipment for Divers

As major or minor injuries and ailments can occur at any time in the diving environment, it is important that divers be able to render assistance to themselves and others. A first aid certificate is an essential for any diver, and a diver rescue qualification is of immense value at times of need. Depending on the remoteness of the area, available professional medical help and facilities, and the type of injury or disease, the requirements of medical kits vary.

Dive bag medical kit

One waterproof container with:
- 1 bottle sun barrier cream
- 1 bottle postdive ear drops, e.g. 5% glacial acetic acid in propylene glycol + dropper
- 1 small pack paracetamol or aspirin tablets
- 1 small pack adhesive bandages
- 1 small bottle 10% cetrimide solution
- 1 small pack cotton wool
- 1 bottle anti-seasickness tablets

Small dive boat medical kit

(maximum 30 minutes from shore help)
1. One small oxygen bottle with regulator, face mask and tubing.
2. One waterproof container with:
   - 3 small Standard Dressings (No. 7)
   - 3 large Standard Dressings (No. 9)
   - 2 triangular bandages
   - 2 crepe bandages 15 cm
   - 1 pack 75 mm x 75 mm gauze squares (individually wrapped)
   - 4 medium safety pins
   - 1 roll adhesive plaster
   - 1 small pack adhesive bandages
   - 1 pair scissors
   - 1 pair tweezers

- 1 tourniquet (Esmarch)
- 1 x 500 ml bottle vinegar or anti-sting solution or spray
- 1 bottle sun barrier cream
- 1 bottle postdive ear drops, e.g. 5% glacial acetic acid in propylene glycol + dropper
- 1 small pack paracetamol tablets
- 1 bottle antihistamine tablets
- 1 bottle anti-seasickness tablets
- 1 tube antihistamine ointment
- 1 bottle mercurochrome or iodine or antiseptic ointment
- 1 small pack cotton wool
- 1 pair rubber gloves
- 1 pair goggles
- 1 disposable plastic non-return airway for CPR
- 1 standard thermometer
- 1 low-reading thermometer

Medical equipment for diving expeditions in remote areas

Before leaving on a remote diving expedition:
1. Determine whether a doctor is available in the area. Obtain the doctor's name, address and telephone number.
2. Contact and inform the doctor about the expedition and request any special information relevant to the area (malaria, dysentery, medical facilities, etc.). Ensure immunisation against diseases such as cholera and typhoid if these are locally prevalent.
3. Choose an expedition medical leader before leaving. One member of the team should ideally have EMA training. See your own doctor before departing and discuss the expedition.
4. Ensure available radio or telephone contact with a diver rescue service and a diving doctor in case of serious problems.

Emergency medical box
The complexity and range of a medical kit in remote areas depends upon the medical training of the members in the group and on local endemic diseases. Intravenous infusions and injections, and the use of drugs such as adrenaline, morphine and atropine require special knowledge and training. If members of the group are medically or paramedically trained, the onus of providing and using advanced life-support equipment and drugs must rest with them and the level of their protocol training. In addition to the dive bag and small boat medical kits, provision should be made for the following items:
1. *Oxygen*
   At least two large cylinders of oxygen and administration sets are required on board or at the shore base. Until trained emergency help can arrive or be reached, oxygen is the mainstay of treatment in acute decompression illness, severe trauma, and shock.

2. *Trauma Pack*
    An adequate supply of equipment is necessary in case of major trauma.
    A kit such as one recommended for shark attacks is advised (see p 220).
3. *Oral medicines*
    The indications and use of oral medicines must be discussed with a
    doctor and a prescription obtained. A supply adequate for the group
    size must be provided. In general, oral medicines include the following:
    Pain-killer tablets
    Antiemetics
    Antidiarrhoeals
    Antispasmodics
    Antacid suspension
    Antibiotics (prior instruction in their use is essential)
4. *Ear/eye drops*
    Antiseptic and antibiotic drops

Physics

Over the past centuries, while the concept of pressure was being developed and extended, different workers used different standard measures in different countries. The result is that a diver is now pressurised by a variety of different units.

Pressure conversion factors

Commonly used approximations are shown in parentheses.

1 ATMOSPHERE
= 1 ATA
= 10.08 (10) metres sea water
= 33.07 (33) feet sea water
= 33.90 (34) feet fresh water
= 1.033 (1) kg/cm^2
= 14.696 (14,7) $lbs/inch^2$
= 1.013 (1) bar
= 101 (100) kilopascals, kPa
= 760 millimetres mercury, mmHg
= 760 Torr

Physical Laws in diving

There are six laws in all.
    Four involve gases only:
— Boyle's Law
— Charles's Law
— Amontons' Law
— Dalton's Law
    One involves gases and fluids:
— Henry's Law
    One involves fluids only:
— Archimedes' Principle

1. *Boyle's Law*

Robert Boyle was a bright lad who lived in the 1600s and went to Eton at the age of eight. Aside from being an alchemist and trying to turn lead into gold, he discovered that pressure and volume were related when he passed wind and the pain improved.

In a given gas system at constant temperature, the volume is inversely proportional to the absolute pressure.

P x V = K

or

P1 x V1 = P2 x V2

Problem

A 1-litre balloon at 110 metres is floating up to the surface. At what depth will its volume:

(a) double?

(b) quadruple?

Answers

(a) 110 metres   =   1 + 11 ATA = 12 ATA

Since P x V = constant,   P1 V1 = P2 V2

$$12 \times 1 = P2 \times 2$$

$$P2 = \frac{12 \times 1}{2} = \frac{12}{2} = 6 \text{ ATA}$$

Remember that there is always 1 ATA of air pressure.

So 6 ATA = 5 ATA + 1 ATA

5 ATA = *50 metres* (doubled)

(b) 110 metres =   11 ATA + 1 ATA = 12 ATA

$$12 \times 1 = P2 \times 4$$

P2 = 3 ATA

3 ATA = 1 ATA + 2 ATA

2 ATA = *20 metres* (quadrupled)

Note: Between 110 metres and 50 metres (60 metres of depth difference), the volume doubled. Between 50 metres and 20 metres, it quadrupled (only 30 metres difference).

The major volume changes occur between 10 metres and the surface.

2. *Charles's Law*

One century after Boyle, Jacques Alexandre César Charles came on the scene. He got tired of working as a clerk in the Ministry of Finance, so began filling balloons with hydrogen. He must have got a bang out of this, because he invented Charles's Law.

At constant pressure, the volume of a given mass of gas is directly proportional to its absolute temperature.

In Charles's Law, pressure is always constant.

$$\frac{V}{T} = K \text{ (constant)}$$

Temperature, like pressure, is always absolute in diving calculations. The lowest theoretical temperature possible is $-273°C$. At this temperature all molecules stop moving. All chemical activity stops.

Absolute zero	$0°A$	$=$	$-273°C$
	$0°C$	$=$	$273°A$
	$10°C$	$=$	$283°A$
	$25°C$	$=$	$298°A$
			etc.

You must *always* convert $°C$ into $°A$ in all calculations involving P, V, and T.

Although always quoted, Charles's Law is rarely used in sport diving, as pressures are rarely constant. It does have relevance in bubble growth with increased temperature, however, such as bends development with a hot bath after diving. The hot bath reduces nitrogen solubility in tissues, bubbles form, and Charles's Law then ensures that they increase in size.

3. *Pressure Law (Amontons' Law)*

For those who like names, the Pressure Law was described during the 1600s by Guillaume Amontons who invented a hygrometer and pioneered work on friction. The Pressure Law is sometimes called Amontons' Law. (Another piece of confusing trivia is that a scientist called Gay Lussac also described Charles's Law, but Charles won the name race.)

With the Pressure Law, VOLUME is the constant.

At constant volume, the pressure of a given mass of gas is directly proportional to the absolute temperature.

$$\frac{P}{T} = K$$

This law is of practical importance in diving, because divers use cylinders, storage tanks and chambers. For example, when a scuba cylinder is being filled, it heats up; or when it is left in the sun, its pressure increases. Similarly, when a decompression chamber is pressurised it heats up inside and cools down during depressurisation.

Boyle's Law, Charles's Law and the Pressure Law can all be combined into one formula:

$$\frac{P1 \ V1}{T1} = \frac{P2 \ V2}{T2}$$

This is the *Universal Gas Equation*.

Examples

- Mike goes to his local dive shop to have his scuba cylinder filled. He wants the cylinder filled to 200 ATA. Pete Muckitt does not put the cylinder in a tub of cold water to keep it cool. As the pressure in the cylinder increases, so does the temperature, up to 47°C. Mike then goes to Flounder-on-Sea, where the water temperature is 7°C and begins to scream and swear. What is the pressure in his cylinder? Which law are we using?

P1 = 200 ATA

V1 = K (constant) (for practical purposes, the volume of his cylinder does not change)

T1 = 47°C = 320°A

P2 = ?

V2 = K

T2 = 7°C = 280°A

$$\frac{200 \times K}{320} = \frac{P2 \times K}{280}$$

$$P2 = \frac{200 \times K \times 280}{320 \times K}$$

$$P2 = 175 \text{ ATA (Pressure Law: V is K)}$$

- Dr Parrotfish taps 1 litre of gas to analyse from a decompression chamber into a balloon. The chamber is baking in the sun and the temperature inside the chamber is 37°C. At the laboratory the temperature is 17°C. What is the volume of the sample, and which law are we using?

P1 = K

V1 = 1 litre

T1 = 37°C = 273 + 37 = 310°A

P2 = K

V2 = ?

T2 = 17°C = 273 + 17 = 290°A

$$\frac{K \times 1}{310} = \frac{K \times V2}{290}$$

$$V2 = \frac{290 \times K \times 1}{310 \times K} = \frac{290}{310} = 0.935 \text{ litre (Charles's Law)}$$

4. *Dalton's Law*

John Dalton was a Quaker, who lived in the eighteenth century and played bowls on Thursday afternoons. He also first described colour-blindness and the atomic theory. He was very interested in gas mixtures and, since laws were in vogue, he invented Dalton's Law.

In a mixture of gases, the total pressure is equal to the sum of the partial pressures of the individual gases in the mixture.

In a sample of air at sea-level, the total pressure is 1 ATA. This consists of approximately 80% nitrogen and 20% oxygen (ignoring traces of carbon dioxide, water and argon).

Total pressure = 1 ATA

Nitrogen = 80% = 0.8 ATA

Oxygen = 20% = 0.2 ATA

Total of nitrogen and oxygen = 0.8 + 0.2 = 1.0 ATA

Simple enough, but it can become tricky. For instance: A diver breathes a mixture of helium, nitrogen and oxygen. At 90 metres, the helium flowing through his demand valve has a partial pressure of 8 ATA. At the surface, the partial pressure of the nitrogen in his purged gas is 0.15 ATA. What is the percentage oxygen in the mix?

Answer

At 90 metres, the total pressure is:

9 ATA + 1 ATA = 10 ATA

His helium exerts a pressure of 8 ATA in his demand valve, i.e. 8/10 of the total *ambient* pressure or 80% of the mix is helium.

At the surface, nitrogen exerts a partial pressure (pp) of 0.15 ATA or 15% of 1 ATA. So 15% of the mix is nitrogen.

According to Dalton's Law:

$$ppHe + ppN_2 + ppO_2 = \text{total pressure}$$
$$80\% + 15\% + x = 100\%$$
$$x = 5\% \text{ oxygen}$$

Dalton's Law is important in:
1. calculating the proportions of various gases in a breathing mixture to avoid nitrogen narcosis or oxygen toxicity;
2. calculating the depth at which trace contaminants such as carbon monoxide become significant as toxic gases.

Example
• Nitrox Albert wants to dive to 140 metres. He knows that helium is expensive, so he wants to add some nitrogen to the mixture, equivalent to the nitrogen partial pressure at 30 metres breathing air. He also does not want the partial pressure of oxygen to be greater than 0.5 ATA at the bottom. What is his mix?

Answer

We must calculate the proportions of oxygen and nitrogen required. The rest is helium.

Oxygen:
The pressure at 140 metres is 14 ATA + 1 ATA = 15 ATA
This is his *ambient* 'atmospheric' pressure.
His oxygen partial pressure at this depth must be 0.5 ATA.

Expressed as a percentage: $\dfrac{0.5 \times 100}{15}$ = 3.33% oxygen

Nitrogen:
We want the ppN_2 to be the same as the ppN_2 at 30 metres on air, i.e. the *equivalent nitrogen partial pressure*.
In air, N_2 = 80%
At the surface its pp is 0.8 ATA
At 30 metres, its pp is 0.8 x 4 (3 ATA + 1 ATA) = 3.2 ATA
So we want 3.2 ATA of N_2 at 140 metres (15 ATA)

As a percentage: $\dfrac{3.2 \times 100}{15}$

= 21.33% nitrogen

Mix is: oxygen   :   3.33%
            nitrogen :   21.33%
            helium   :   100 − 24.66 = 75.34%

If the minimum ppO_2 safe to breathe is taken as 0.15 ATA, could Nitrox Albert breathe this mix at the surface?

Oxygen = 3.33%
At 1 ATA, the partial pressure of oxygen would be 0.033 ATA, and the mix would be fatal, as gross oxygen starvation (hypoxia) would occur. Up to what depth could he breathe the mixture?

The percentage oxygen in the mixture is 3.33%
This would exert a ppO_2 of 0.15 ATA

$$\text{at } \dfrac{0.15}{x} = \dfrac{3.33}{100}$$
$$x = \dfrac{15}{3.33} \text{ ATA}$$
$$= 4.5 - 1 \text{ ATA} = 3.5 \text{ ATA}$$
$$= 35 \text{ msw}$$

Note: Although the partial pressure of a gas varies with changes in depth, the percentage does not. Percentage is constant. Dalton's Law also explains the blackout of ascent in skin divers after hyperventilation.

5. *Henry's Law*
William Henry was a melancholic chap and, after inventing his law,

committed suicide at Pendlebury, Sept. 2, 1836.

At a constant temperature, the amount of gas that will dissolve in a liquid is proportional to the partial pressure of the gas over the liquid.

This law involves gases and liquids and refers to the dissolving of gases into liquids. In the diving sense, the liquid would be body tissues, and the gas would be the gas breathed, i.e. air or a mixture.

• At 1 ATA, Martin, a diver at Crankshaft Bay, has about 1 litre of gaseous nitrogen dissolved in his body. (He is said to be saturated with air-nitrogen at 1 ATA.) If he needed some abalone and scuba-dived to 20 metres (3 ATA), he would eventually reach equilibrium again and have 3 litres of nitrogen dissolved in his body (if he were not first arrested for fishing without a permit).

Time is needed for this absorption of nitrogen. The longer the dive, the more nitrogen is dissolved.

When he surfaces, the air he breathes is again at 1 ATA. The nitrogen dissolved in his body will then reverse its direction, i.e. out of his tissues and into the air via his lungs. If the pressure drop is too rapid, his tissues may have more nitrogen than they can hold in solution, and bubble formation then occurs, causing acute decompression illness. Henry's Law is also directly responsible for:

— nitrogen narcosis
— oxygen toxicity
— high pressure nervous syndrome.

During diving, the partial pressures of any gas increase with descent, and decrease on ascent. At depth, the gradient is gas to lungs to blood to tissues. On return to the surface, the gradient is tissues to blood to lungs to air.

6. *Archimedes' Principle*

In shrouded times, when the earth was flat and magicians and monsters prevailed, a fat man weighed a lot and a thin man didn't. Nowadays, with man standing on the moon, even weight is not what it used to be. As the moon's gravity is less than that of the earth, a fat man standing on its surface would weigh less, even though the total amount of blubber on his well-covered bones was the same. To put it another way, his mass is constant but his weight is dependent on gravity.

The Germans have introduced the term 'weight-force' to distinguish between mass and weight. Weight-force is the product of mass and gravity and is expressed in newtons.

Weight-force (G) = m x g newtons (N)
when m = mass in kilograms
g = local acceleration due to gravity in m/sec/sec.

Example

• Mike decides to step on to the scales at his local laundromat. He gets a reading of 65 kg. This is his mass. The local acceleration due to gravity is 9.812523 m/sec/sec. This means that if Mike were falling in this particular area he would accelerate by 9.812523 metres per second per second, that is, for every second he fell, he would travel 9.812523 metres per second faster than the previous second.

As G = mg

Mike's weight-force would be 65 x 9.812523

or 637.814 N

In English-speaking countries there is no word for weight-force and the word weight is loosely used to mean mass or weight-force. So, Mike would say he weighs 65 kg or that his 'weight' is 65 kg. To distinguish between mass and weight-force one looks at the units.

If the units are in kilograms, mass is meant.

If the units are in newtons, force is meant.

If Mike were on Jupiter with a gravity 12 times that of the earth, he would have a weight of 637.814 x 12 or 7653.77 N, but his mass would still be 65 kg. On the moon his weight would be 106.30 N and his mass would again be 65 kg.

Now, back in time to Archimedes, where 'weight' is expressed in kg so mass is the order of the day.

Eureka!

Around 250 BC, Archimedes invented the water screw. One day he displaced his mass in his bathtub and ran naked through the streets of Syracuse screaming 'Eureka! Eureka!' King Hieron II had just received a nice new golden crown. He wanted to know whether it was pure gold or mixed with silver. He gave the problem to Archimedes and the bath gave him the answer. He weighed the crown, then, immersing it in water, noted the amount of water displaced. He then weighed an identical mass of pure gold, and immersed that in water. If the two amounts of water displaced were the same, the crown was pure gold. I don't know the end of the story, so the crown's purity remains a secret forever. But the principle states:

Any object, wholly or partially immersed in liquid, is buoyed up by a force equal to the mass of liquid displaced.

Example

• Supposing a diver weighing 70 kg fully geared up steps off his boat into the water. If he displaces 75 kg of water, he will float, being 5 kg lighter than the mass of water displaced. He is *positively buoyant.* This makes descent difficult, but ascent easy. If he displaces 65 kg of water, he will sink, being 5 kg heavier than the mass of water displaced. He is *negatively buoyant.* This makes descent easy, but ascent difficult. If he displaces exactly 70 kg of water, he is *neutrally buoyant* and will neither sink nor float. He experiences a sense of weightlessness similar to an astronaut in zero gravity. He can descend or ascend with ease.

Suppose he decides to descend:
As he descends, Boyle's Law comes into operation. His neoprene sponge wet suit contains thousands of tiny gas bubbles which become compressed with the increasing pressure. This reduces his suit's volume and so decreases the mass of water displaced. The deeper he goes, the more negatively buoyant he becomes, and descent becomes easier and faster. Sport divers use a buoyancy compensator, which can be partially inflated at depth to counter this negative buoyancy, and to assist ascent if required.

Problem
Charlie takes his mother-in-law diving. He helps her tog up, and carefully places 16 kg of lead weights on to her weight belt. When she enters the water, her weight is 80 kg. She displaces 80 litres of sea water. Is he rid of her? (The density of sea water is 1.025 and density = mass ÷ volume.)
Answer
No. She is 2 kg buoyant. He should have used more weight.

Dive Tables

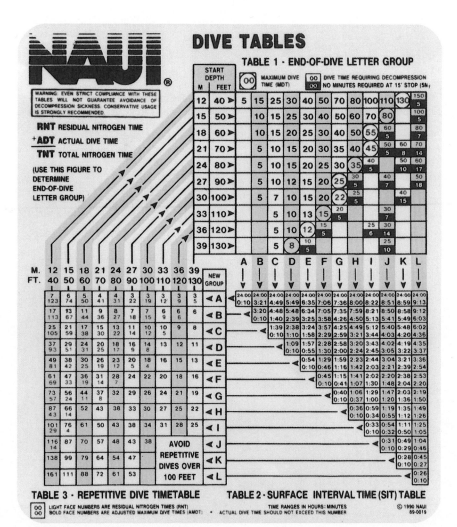

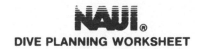

DIVE PLANNING WORKSHEET

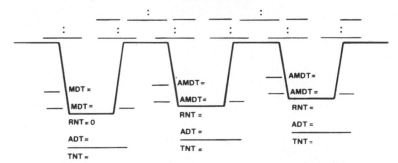

TERMS AND ABBREVIATIONS USED IN DIVE PLANNING

Repetitive Dive - Any dive made less than 24 hours after a previous dive.
ADT - Actual Dive Time - The time from the moment of descent until returning to the surface.
Letter Group - A letter symbol for the amount of Residual Nitrogen remaining in the body from previous dives.
SIT - Surface Interval Time - The time spent at the surface between dives.

RNT - Residual Nitrogen Time - The nitrogen remaining in the body from a dive or dives made within the past 24 hours.
AMDT - Adjusted Maximum Dive Time - The Maximum Dive Time for the depth of a dive minus the RNT.
TNT - Total Nitrogen Time - The sum of RNT and ADT. This figure is used to obtain a letter group after repetitive dives.

© **1990 NAUI**

REMEMBER

- Consider all dives made shallower than 40' (12m) as 40' dives.
- On any dive, ascend no faster than one foot per second.
- For maximum dive time, make all repetitive dives shallower than your previous dive.

US Navy Standard Air Decompression Table†

Depth (feet)	Bottom time (min)	Time to first stop (min:sec)	Decompression stops (feet) 50	40	30	20	10	Total decompression time (min:sec)	Repetitive group
40	200						0	0:40	*
	210	0:30					2	2:40	N
	230	0:30					7	7:40	N
	250	0:30					11	11:40	O
	270	0:30					15	15:40	O
	300	0:30					19	19:40	N
	360	0:30					23	23:40	**
	480	0:30					41	41:40	**
	720	0:30					69	69:40	**
50	100						0	0:50	*
	110	0:40					3	3:50	L
	120	0:40					5	5:50	M
	140	0:40					10	10:50	M
	160	0:40					21	21:50	N
	180	0:40					29	29:50	O
	200	0:40					35	35:50	O
	220	0:40					40	40:50	N
	240	0:40					47	47:50	N

* See No Decompression Table for repetitive groups

** Repetitive dives may not follow exceptional exposure dives

† Source: US Navy 1988

US Navy Standard Air Decompression Table

Depth (feet)	Bottom time (min)	Time to first stop (min:sec)	Decompression stops (feet) 50	40	30	20	10	Total decompression time (min:sec)	Repetitive group
60	60						0	1:00	*
	70	0:50					2	3:00	K
	80	0:50					7	8:00	L
	100	0:50					14	15:00	M
	120	0:50					26	27:00	N
	140	0:50					39	40:00	O
	160	0:50					48	49:00	N
	180	0:50					56	57:00	N
	200	0:40				1	69	71:00	N
	240	0:40				2	79	82:00	**
	360	0:40				20	119	140:00	**
	480	0:40				44	148	193:00	**
	720	0:40				78	187	266:00	**
70	50						0	1:10	*
	60	1:00					8	9:10	K
	70	1:00					14	15:10	L
	80	1:00					18	19:10	M
	90	1:00					23	24:10	N
	100	1:00					33	34:10	N
	110	0:50				2	41	44:10	O
	120	0:50				4	47	52:10	O
	130	0:50				6	52	59:10	N
	140	0:50				8	56	65:10	N
	150	0:50				9	61	71:10	N
	160	0:50				13	72	86:10	N
	170	0:50				19	79	99:10	N

* See No Decompression Table for repetitive groups

** Repetitive dives may not follow exceptional exposure dives

US Navy Standard Air Decompression Table

Depth (feet)	Bottom time (min)	Time to first stop (min:sec)	Decompression stops (feet)					Total decompression time (min:sec)	Repetitive group
			50	40	30	20	10		
80	40						0	1:20	*
	50	1:10					10	11:20	K
	60	1:10					17	18:20	L
	70	1:10					23	24:20	M
	80	1:00				2	31	34:20	N
	90	1:00				7	39	47:20	N
	100	1:00				11	46	58:20	O
	110	1:00				13	53	67:20	O
	120	1:00				17	56	74:20	N
	130	1:00				19	63	83:20	N
	140	1:00				26	69	96:20	N
	150	1:00				32	77	110:20	N
	180	1:00				35	85	121:20	**
	240	0:50			6	52	120	179:20	**
	360	0:50			29	90	160	280:20	**
	480	0:50			59	107	187	354:20	**
	720	0:40		17	108	142	187	455:20	**
90	30	1:20					0	1:30	*
	40	1:20					7	8:30	J
	50	1:20					18	19:30	L
	60	1:20					25	26:30	M
	70	1:10				7	30	38:30	N
	80	1:10				13	40	54:30	N
	90	1:10				18	48	67:30	O
	100	1:10				21	54	76:30	N
	110	1:10				24	61	86:30	N
	120	1:10				32	68	101:30	N
	130	1:00			5	36	74	116:30	N

* See No Decompression Table for repetitive groups

** Repetitive dives may not follow exceptional exposure dives

US Navy Standard Air Decompression Table

Depth (feet)	Bottom time (min)	Time tp first stop (min:sec)	50	40	30	20	10	Total decompression time (min:sec)	Repetitive group
100	25						0	1:40	*
	30	1:30					3	4:40	—
	40	1:30					15	16:40	K
	50	1:20				2	24	27:40	L
	60	1:20				9	28	38:40	N
	70	1:20				17	39	57:40	O
	80	1:20				23	48	72:40	O
	90	1:10			3	23	57	84:40	N
	100	1:10			7	23	66	97:40	N
	110	1:10			10	34	72	117:40	N
	120	1:10			12	41	78	132:40	N
	180	1:00		1	29	53	118	202:40	**
	240	1:00	2	14	42	84	142	283:40	**
	360	0:50	21	42	73	111	187	416:40	**
	480	0:50	55	61	91	142	187	503:40	**
	720	0:50		106	122	142	187	613:40	**
110	20						0	1:50	*
	25	1:40					3	4:50	H
	30	1:40					7	8:50	J
	40	1:30				2	21	24:50	L
	50	1:30				8	26	35:50	M
	60	1:30				18	36	55:50	N
	70	1:20			1	23	48	73:50	O
	80	1:20			7	23	57	88:50	N
	90	1:20			12	30	64	107:50	N
	100	1:20			15	37	72	125:50	N

Decompression stops (feet) span the 50 / 40 / 30 / 20 / 10 columns.

* See No Decompression Table for repetitive groups

** Repetitive dives may not follow exceptional exposure dives

US Navy Standard Air Decompression Table

Depth (feet)	Bottom time (min)	Time to first stop (min:sec)	70	60	50	40	30	20	10	Total decompression time (min:sec)	Repetitive group
120	15	1:50							0	2:00	*
	20	1:50							2	4:00	H
	25	1:50							6	8:00	I
	30	1:50							14	16:00	J
	40	1:40						5	25	32:00	L
	50	1:40						15	31	48:00	N
	60	1:30					2	22	45	71:00	O
	70	1:30					9	23	55	89:00	O
	80	1:30					15	27	63	107:00	N
	90	1:30					19	37	74	132:00	N
	100	1:30					23	45	80	150:00	N
	120	1:20				10	19	47	98	176:00	**
	180	1:10			5	27	37	76	137	284:00	**
	240	1:10			23	35	60	97	179	396:00	**
	360	1:00		18	45	64	93	142	187	551:00	**
	480	0:50	3	41	64	93	122	142	187	654:00	**
	720	0:50	32	74	100	114	122	142	187	773:00	**
130	10	2:00							0	2:10	*
	15	2:00							1	3:10	F
	20	2:00							4	6:10	H
	25	1:50							10	12:10	J
	30	1:50						3	18	23:10	M
	40	1:40						10	25	37:10	N
	50	1:40					3	21	37	63:10	O
	60	1:40					9	23	52	86:10	N
	70	1:40					16	24	61	103:10	N
	80	1:30				3	19	35	72	131:10	N
	90	1:30				8	19	45	80	154:10	N

Decompression stops (feet)

* See No Decompression Table for repetitive groups

** Repetitive dives may not follow exceptional exposure dives

US Navy Standard Air Decompression Table

Depth (feet)	Bottom time (min)	Time to first stop (min:sec)	90	80	70	60	50	40	30	20	10	Total decompression time (min:sec)	Repetitive group
140	10										0	2:20	*
	15	2:10									2	4:20	G
	20	2:10									6	8:20	I
	25	2:00								2	14	18:20	J
	30	2:00								5	21	28:20	K
	40	1:50							2	16	26	46:20	N
	50	1:50							6	24	44	76:20	O
	60	1:50							16	23	56	97:20	Z
	70	1:40							19	32	68	125:20	Z
	80	1:40						4	23	41	79	155:20	Z
	90	1:30						10	18	42	88	166:20	**
	120	1:30					2	14	36	56	120	240:20	**
	180	1:20					12	14	54	94	168	386:20	**
	240	1:10				10	26	32	78	124	187	511:20	**
	360	1:00			8	28	34	50	122	142	187	684:20	**
	480	1:00		9	32	42	64	84	122	142	187	801:20	**
	720	0:50	16	56	88	97	100	114	122	142	187	924:20	**
150	5										0	2:30	C
	10	2:20									1	3:30	E
	15	2:20									3	5:30	G
	20	2:10								2	7	11:30	H
	25	2:10								4	17	23:30	K
	30	2:10								8	24	34:30	L
	40	2:00							5	19	33	59:30	N
	50	2:00							12	23	51	88:30	O
	60	1:50						3	19	26	62	112:30	Z
	70	1:50						11	19	39	75	146:30	Z
	80	1:40					1	17	19	50	84	173:30	Z

* See No Decompression Table for repetitive groups

** Repetitive dives may not follow exceptional exposure dives

US Navy Standard Air Decompression Table

Depth (feet)	Bottom time (min)	Time to first stop (min:sec)	110	100	90	80	70	60	50	40	30	20	10	Total decompression time (min:sec)	Repetitive group
160	5												0	2:40	D
	10	2:30											1	3:40	F
	15	2:20										1	4	7:40	H
	20	2:20										3	11	16:40	J
	25	2:20										7	20	29:40	K
	30	2:10									2	11	25	40:40	M
	40	2:10									7	23	39	71:40	N
	50	2:00								2	16	23	55	98:40	N
	60	2:00								9	19	33	69	132:40	N
	70	1:50							1	17	22	44	80	166:40	**
170	5												0	2:50	D
	10	2:40											2	4:50	F
	15	2:30										2	5	9:50	H
	20	2:30										4	15	21:50	J
	25	2:20									2	7	23	34:50	L
	30	2:20									4	13	26	45:50	M
	40	2:10								1	10	23	45	81:50	O
	50	2:10								5	18	23	61	109:50	N
	60	2:00							2	15	22	37	74	152:50	N
	70	2:00							8	17	19	51	86	183:50	**
	90	1:50						12	12	14	34	52	120	246:50	**
	120	1:30				2	10	12	18	32	42	82	156	356:50	**
	180	1:20			4	10	22	28	34	50	78	120	187	535:50	**
	240	1:20			18	24	30	42	50	70	116	142	187	681:50	**
	360	1:10		22	34	40	52	60	98	114	122	142	187	873:50	**
	480	1:00	14	40	42	56	91	97	100	114	122	142	187	1007:50	**

Decompression stops (feet)

* See No Decompression Table for repetitive groups

** Repetitive dives may not follow exceptional exposure dives

US Navy Standard Air Decompression Table

Depth (feet)	Bottom time (min)	Time to first stop (min:sec)	110	100	90	80	70	60	50	40	30	20	10	Total decompression time (min:sec)	Repetitive group
180	5												0	3:00	D
	10	2:50											3	6:00	F
	15	2:40										3	6	12:00	I
	20	2:30									1	5	17	26:00	K
	25	2:30									3	10	24	40:00	L
	30	2:30									6	17	27	53:00	N
	40	2:20								3	14	23	50	93:00	O
	50	2:10							2	9	19	30	65	128:00	N
	60	2:10							5	16	19	44	81	168:00	N
190	5												0	3:10	D
	10	2:50										1	3	7:10	G
	15	2:50									2	4	7	14:10	I
	20	2:40									5	6	20	31:10	K
	25	2:40									8	11	25	44:10	M
	30	2:30								1	14	19	32	63:10	N
	40	2:30								8	14	23	55	103:10	O
	50	2:20							4	13	22	33	72	147:10	**
	60	2:20							10	17	19	50	84	183:10	**

* See No Decompression Table for repetitive groups

** Repetitive dives may not follow exceptional exposure dives

US Navy Standard Air Decompression Table

Depth (feet)	Bottom time (min)	Time to first stop (min:sec)	130	120	110	100	90	80	70	60	50	40	30	20	10	Total decompression time (min:sec)
200	5	3:10													1	4:20
	10	3:00												1	4	8:20
	15	2:50											1	4	10	18:20
	20	2:50											3	7	27	40:20
	25	2:50											7	14	25	49:20
	30	2:40										2	9	22	37	73:20
	40	2:30									2	8	17	23	59	112:20
	50	2:30									6	16	22	39	75	161:20
	60	2:20								2	13	17	24	51	89	199:20
	90	1:50					1	10	10	12	12	30	38	74	134	324:20
	120	1:40				6	10	10	10	24	28	40	64	98	180	473:20
	180	1:20		1	6	10	10	24	24	54	48	70	106	142	187	685:20
	240	1:20		6	20	24	18	36	42	60	68	114	122	142	187	842:20
	360	1:10	12	22	36	40	44	56	82	98	100	114	122	142	187	1058:20
210	5	3:20													1	4:30
	10	3:10												2	4	9:30
	15	3:00											1	5	13	22:30
	20	3:00											4	10	23	40:30
	25	2:50										2	7	17	27	56:30
	30	2:50										4	9	24	41	81:30
	40	2:40									4	9	19	26	63	124:30
	50	2:30								1	9	17	19	45	80	174:30

Decompression stops (feet)

* See No Decompression Table for repetitive groups

** Repetitive dives may not follow exceptional exposure dives

US Navy Standard Air Decompression Table

Depth (feet)	Bottom time (min)	Time to first stop (min:sec)	130	120	110	100	90	80	70	60	50	40	30	20	10	Total decompression time (min:sec)
220	5	3:30													1	5:40
	10	3:20												2	5	10:40
	15	3:10											2	5	16	26:40
	20	3:00										1	3	11	24	42:40
	25	3:00										3	8	19	33	66:40
	30	2:50									1	7	10	23	47	91:40
	40	2:50									6	12	22	29	68	140:40
	50	2:40								3	12	17	18	51	86	190:40
230	5	3:40													2	5:50
	10	3:20												2	6	12:50
	15	3:20											1	6	18	30:50
	20	3:10										2	3	12	26	48:50
	25	3:10										4	5	22	37	74:50
	30	3:00									2	8	8	23	51	99:50
	40	2:50								1	7	15	22	34	74	156:50
	50	2:50								5	14	16	24	51	89	202:50
240	5	3:50													2	6:00
	10	3:30												3	6	14:00
	15	3:30											1	6	21	35:00
	20	3:20										3	4	15	25	53:00
	25	3:10									1	4	6	24	40	82:00
	30	3:10									4	8	9	22	56	109:00
	40	3:00								3	7	17	15	39	75	167:00
	50	2:50							1	8	15	16	29	51	94	218:00

Decompression stops (feet)

* See No Decompression Table for repetitive groups

** Repetitive dives may not follow exceptional exposure dives

US Navy Standard Air Decompression Table

The decompression-stop columns span the depths 200 190 180 170 160 150 140 130 120 110 100 90 80 70 60 50 40 30 20 10 (feet). Only columns 150 ft and shallower contain data and are shown below.

Depth (feet)	Bottom time (min)	Time to first stop (min:sec)	150	140	130	120	110	100	90	80	70	60	50	40	30	20	10	Total decompression time (min:sec)
250	5	3:50															2	7:10
	10	3:40														1	7	16:10
	15	3:30														4	22	38:10
	20	3:30													4	7	27	59:10
	25	3:20												2	7	17	45	92:10
	30	3:20											2	7	10	24	59	116:10
	40	3:10										5	9	17	17	23	79	178:10
	60	2:40									10	10	12	22	36	45	164	298:10
	90	2:10					8	10	10	10	24	28	28	44	68	64	186	514:10
	120	1:50		4	8	10	10	10	16	24	24	36	48	64	94	98	187	684:10
	180	1:30		8	8	22	22	24	32	42	44	60	84	114	122	142	187	931:10
	240	1:30	9	14	21	22	22	40	42	56	76	98	100	114	122	142	187	1109:10
260	5	4:00															2	7:20
	10	3:50														1	9	19:20
	15	3:40												2	2	4	22	42:20
	20	3:30											1	4	4	10	31	67:20
	25	3:30											3	8	7	20	50	99:20
	30	3:20										2	6	8	11	26	61	126:20
	40	3:10									1	6	11	16	19	49	84	190:20
270	5	4:10															3	8:30
	10	4:00														1	11	22:30
	15	3:50													2	5	24	46:30
	20	3:40											2	3	4	11	35	74:30
	25	3:30										2	3	8	9	21	53	106:30
	30	3:30										3	6	12	13	27	64	138:30
	40	3:20									5	6	11	17	22	51	88	204:30

US Navy Standard Air Decompression Table

Depth (feet)	Bottom time (min)	Time to first stop (min:sec)	Decompression stops (feet) 200	190	180	170	160	150	140	130	120	110	100	90	80	70	60	50	40	30	20	10	Total decompression time (min:sec)
280	5	4:20																			2	2	8:40
	10	4:00																	1	2	5	13	25:40
	15	3:50																1	3	4	11	26	49:40
	20	3:50																3	4	8	23	39	81:40
	25	3:40															2	5	7	16	23	56	113:40
	30	3:30														1	3	7	13	22	30	70	150:40
	40	3:20													1	6	6	13	17	27	51	93	218:40
290	5	4:30																			2	3	9:50
	10	4:10																	1	3	5	16	29:50
	15	4:00																1	3	6	12	26	52:50
	20	4:00																3	7	9	23	43	89:50
	25	3:50															3	5	8	17	23	60	120:50
	30	3:40														1	5	6	16	22	36	72	162:50
	40	3:30													3	5	7	15	16	32	51	95	228:50
300	5	4:40																			3	3	11:00
	10	4:20																	1	3	6	17	32:00
	15	4:10																2	3	6	15	26	57:00
	20	4:00															2	3	7	10	23	47	97:00
	25	3:50														1	3	6	8	19	26	61	129:00
	30	3:50														2	5	7	17	22	39	75	172:00
	40	3:40													4	6	9	15	17	34	51	90	231:00
	60	3:00									4	10	10	10	10	10	14	28	32	50	90	187	460:00
	90	2:20					3	8	8	10	10	10	10	16	24	24	34	48	64	90	142	187	693:00
	120	2:00			4	8	8	8	8	10	14	24	24	24	34	42	58	66	102	122	142	187	890:00
	180	1:40	6	8	8	8	14	20	21	21	28	40	40	48	56	82	98	100	114	122	142	187	1168:00

US Navy Standard Air Decompression Table

NO-DECOMPRESSION LIMITS AND REPETITIVE GROUP DESIGNATION TABLE FOR NO-DECOMPRESSION AIR DIVES

Depth (feet)	No-decompression limits (min)	A	B	C	D	E	F	G	H	I	J	K	L	M	N	O
10		60	120	210	300											
15		35	70	110	160	225	350									
20		25	50	75	100	135	180	240	325							
25		20	35	55	75	100	125	160	195	245	315					
30		15	30	45	60	75	95	120	145	170	205	250	310			
35	310	5	15	25	40	50	60	80	100	120	140	160	190	220	270	310
40	200	5	15	25	30	40	50	70	80	100	110	130	150	170	200	
50	100		10	15	25	30	40	50	60	70	80	90	100			
60	60		10	15	20	25	30	40	50	55	60					
70	50	5	5	10	15	20	30	35	40	45	50					
80	40	5	5	10	15	20	25	30	35	40						
90	30	5	5	10	12	15	20	25	30							
100	25	5	5	7	10	15	20	22	25							
110	20			5	10	13	15	20								
120	15			5	10	12	15									
130	10			5	8	10										
140	10			5	7	10										
150	5			5	5											
160	5				5	5										
170	5				5											
180	5				5	5										
190	5				5											

Group Designation

RESIDUAL NITROGEN TIMETABLE FOR REPETITIVE AIR DIVES

Locate the diver's repetitive group designation from his previous dive along the diagonal line above the table. Read horizontally to the interval in which the diver's surface interval lies.

Next read vertically downward to the new repetitive group designation. Continue downward in this same column to the row which represents the depth of the repetitive dive. The time given at the intersection is residual nitrogen time, in minutes, to be applied to the repetitive dive.

* Dives following surface intervals of more than 12 hours are not repetitive dives. Use actual bottom times in the Standard Air Decompression Tables to compute decompression for such dives.

** If no Residual Nitrogen Time is given, then the repetitive group does not change.

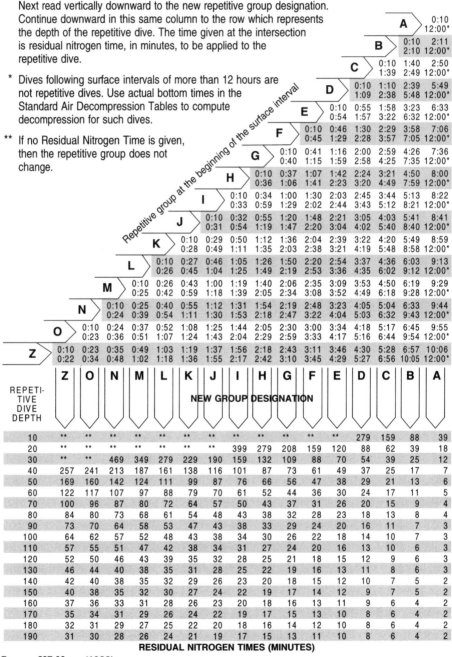

	Z	O	N	M	L	K	J	I	H	G	F	E	D	C	B	A
REPETITIVE DIVE DEPTH					NEW GROUP DESIGNATION										
10	**	**	**	**	**	**	**	**	**	**	**	**	279	159	88	39
20	**	**	**	**	**	**	**	399	279	208	159	120	88	62	39	18
30	**	**	469	349	279	229	190	159	132	109	88	70	54	39	25	12
40	257	241	213	187	161	138	116	101	87	73	61	49	37	25	17	7
50	169	160	142	124	111	99	87	76	66	56	47	38	29	21	13	6
60	122	117	107	97	88	79	70	61	52	44	36	30	24	17	11	5
70	100	96	87	80	72	64	57	50	43	37	31	26	20	15	9	4
80	84	80	73	68	61	54	48	43	38	32	28	23	18	13	8	4
90	73	70	64	58	53	47	43	38	33	29	24	20	16	11	7	3
100	64	62	57	52	48	43	38	34	30	26	22	18	14	10	7	3
110	57	55	51	47	42	38	34	31	27	24	20	16	13	10	6	3
120	52	50	46	43	39	35	32	28	25	21	18	15	12	9	6	3
130	46	44	40	38	35	31	28	25	22	19	16	13	11	8	6	3
140	42	40	38	35	32	29	26	23	20	18	15	12	10	7	5	2
150	40	38	35	32	30	27	24	22	19	17	14	12	9	7	5	2
160	37	36	33	31	28	26	23	20	18	16	13	11	9	6	4	2
170	35	34	31	29	26	24	22	19	17	15	13	10	8	6	4	2
180	32	31	29	27	25	22	20	18	16	14	12	10	8	6	4	2
190	31	30	28	26	24	21	19	17	15	13	11	10	8	6	4	2

RESIDUAL NITROGEN TIMES (MINUTES)

Source: US Navy (1988)

Therapeutic Tables

Royal Navy Recompression Therapy Tables

5516. Application of therapeutic tables

1. Different therapeutic tables are provided for different sets of circumstances and are applied as described in the preamble to each series.
2. Additionally there are some common factors, which are outlined below:
    (a) *Descent time.* Descent time, which varies between tables, is not included in the elapsed time.
    (b) *Elapsed time.* The timing of each table starts when maximum pressure is reached, and is given in hours and minutes opposite each step of the table.
    (c) *Stoppages.* The duration of stoppages is given, oxygen being breathed as indicated.
    (d) *Ascent.* The rate of ascent varies between tables, but with all tables the ascent becomes critical near the surface, where the rate of change of pressure is greatest. If, as the compression chamber nears the surface, air begins to escape round the door seal, compensation by admitting more compression air may be needed. In addition, the gauges may indicate that the surface has been reached when there is still some pressure in the chamber. If this occurs the chamber must continue to be vented at the established rate until pressure is equalised.
    (e) *Surfacing.* On arrival at the surface both patient and attendant must remain in the chamber for one minute in case of return of symptoms.

5517. Tables 52 to 55: Air recompression therapy

1. Tables 52, 53 and 55 are the air tables normally employed for therapeutic decompression. Table 54 may be employed instead of Table 55 when oxygen is available.
2. These tables are applied as described in Article 5516, but with the following modifications:

(a) *Rate of descent*
  (i)   In mild cases − at a rate of approximately 10 m per minute.
  (ii)   In serious cases − as fast as can be tolerated by the patient. This is normally of the order of 30 m per minute.
(b) *Ascent.* Ascent between stoppages is to take five minutes. This is not included in the stoppage times, but has been allowed for in the elapsed times.
(c) *Oxygen.* Both patient and attendant are to breathe oxygen as indicated in Table 54.

Table 52
Air Recompression Therapy

GAUGE DEPTH (metres)	STOPPAGES (hours (h) and minutes (min))		ELAPSED TIME (hours and minutes)	RATE OF ASCENT
50		30 min	0000-0030	5 minutes
42		12 min	0035-0047	between
36		12 min	0052-0104	stoppages
30		12 min	0109-0121	throughout
24		12 min	0126-0138	
18		30 min	0143-0213	
15		30 min	0218-0248	
12		30 min	0253-0323	
9	2 h		0328-0528	
6	2 h		0533-0733	
3	2 h		0738-0938	
Surface			0943	

Total table time 9 hours, 43 minutes

Table 53
Air Recompression Therapy

GAUGE DEPTH (metres)	STOPPAGES (hours (h) and minutes (min))		ELAPSED TIME (hours and minutes)	RATE OF ASCENT
50		30 min	0000-0030	5 minutes
42		12 min	0035-0047	between
36		12 min	0052-0104	stoppages
30		12 min	0109-0121	throughout
24		12 min	0126-0138	
18		30 min	0143-0213	
15		30 min	0218-0248	
12		30 min	0253-0323	
9	12 h		0328-1528	
6	2 h		1533-1733	
3	2 h		1738-1938	
Surface			1943	

Total table time 19 hours, 43 minutes

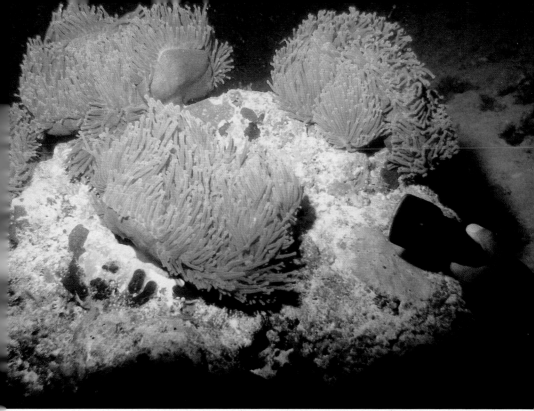

Sea anemones photographed during a night dive in the Maldives.

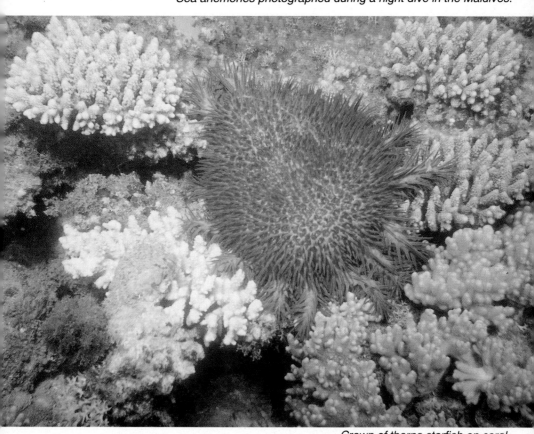

Crown of thorns starfish on coral.

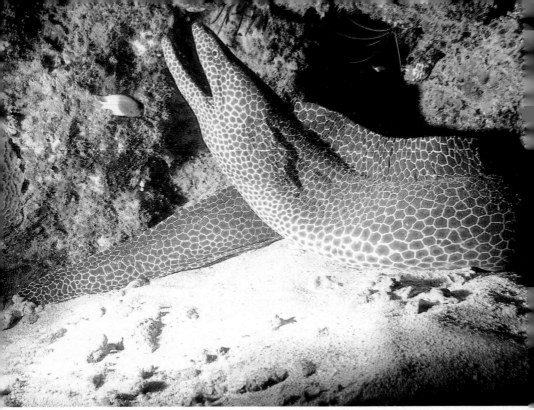

Moray eel emerging from its lair.

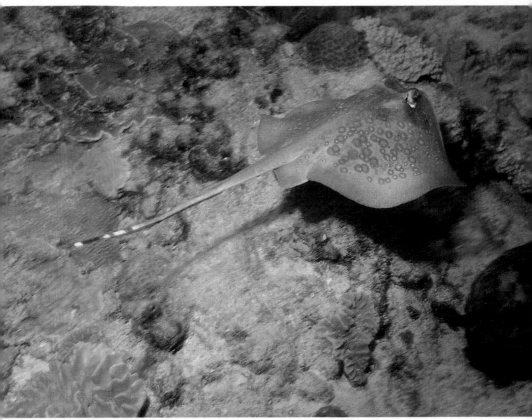

Stingray gliding over the reef, Sodwana

Table 54
Air Recompression Therapy

GAUGE DEPTH (metres)	STOPPAGES (hours (h) and minutes (min))	ELAPSED TIME (hours and minutes)	RATE OF ASCENT
50	2h	0000-0200	5 minutes
42	30 min	0205-0235	between
36	30 min	0240-0310	stoppages
30	30 min	0315-0345	throughout
24	30 min	0350-0420	
18	6 h	0425-1025	
15	6 h	1030-1630	
12	6 h	1635-2235	
9	11 h	2240-3340	
	1 h (O_2)	3340-3440	
6	1 h	3445-3545	
	1 h (O_2)	3545-3645	
3	1 h	3650-3750	
	1 h (O_2)	3750-3850	
Surface		3855	

Total table time 38 hours, 55 minutes

Table 55
Air Recompression Therapy

GAUGE DEPTH (metres)	STOPPAGES (hours (h) and minutes (min))	ELAPSED TIME (hours and minutes)	RATE OF ASCENT
50	2 h	0000-0200	5 minutes
42	30 min	0205-0235	between
36	30 min	0240-0310	stoppages
30	30 min	0315-0345	throughout
24	30 min	0350-0420	
18	6 h	0425-1025	
15	6 h	1030-1630	
12	6 h	1635-2235	
9	12 h	2240-3440	
6	4 h	3445-3845	
3	4 h	3850-4250	
Surface		4255	

Total table time 42 hours, 55 minutes

5518. Tables 61, 62: Oxygen recompression therapy

1. Tables 61 and 62 are employed when oxygen is available and is required for the greater part of the therapy.

2. These tables are applied as described in Article 5516, but with the following modifications:

28

(a) *Descent.* The descent is to take one to two minutes.
(b) *Ascent.* The ascent is to be conducted as follows:
  (i)   It is to be at a continuous bleed rate of three metres in 10 minutes.
  (ii) If the rate is slowed it is not to be compensated for by subsequent acceleration.
  (iii) The ascent should be halted if the rate is exceeded, or if the ascent cannot be controlled accurately during flushing of the chamber.
(c) *Oxygen.* Oxygen is to be breathed during descent. The attendant may remain on air unless it is a repetitive dive, when he must breathe oxygen for the final nine-metres ascent.

   To help prevent O_2 poisoning, the patient is to be kept at rest, lying down, during all oxygen breathing periods at 9 metres or deeper.

3. Oxygen poisoning is not likely to occur with these tables, but the supervisor must be prepared and take the following action if it does:
(a) If ascending, halt the ascent and maintain depth.
(b) Instruct the attendant to remove the oxygen mask and protect the tongue of the convulsing patient, and prevent him from injuring himself.
(c) Wait until 15 minutes after all symptoms of O_2 poisoning have subsided, then resume the O_2 treatment table at the point of interruption. In the unlikely event of a second episode of O_2 poisoning, act as in (b) above, then change to decompression on Table 55 or 73 from the same depth. However, if the patient is free of decompression sickness symptoms, and the depth is less than 9 m, continue the bleed to the surface on air.

Table 61

Oxygen Recompression Therapy

GAUGE DEPTH (metres)	STOPPAGES/ ASCENT (minutes)	ELAPSED TIME (hours and minutes)	RATE OF ASCENT (metres/minute)
18	20 (O_2)	0000-0020	—
18	5	0020-0025	—
18	20 (O_2)	0025-0045	—
18-9	30 (O_2)	0045-0115	3 m in 10 mins
9	5	0115-0120	—
9	20 (O_2)	0120-0140	—
9	5	0140-0145	—
9-0	30 (O_2)	0145-0215	3 m in 10 mins
Surface		0215	

Total table time 2 hours, 15 minutes

Table 62
Oxygen Recompression Therapy

GAUGE DEPTH *(metres)*	STOPPAGES/ ASCENT *(minutes)*	ELAPSED TIME *(hours and minutes)*	RATE OF ASCENT *(metres/minute)*
18	20 (O_2)	0000-0020	–
18	5	0020-0025	–
18	20 (O_2)	0025-0045	–
18	5	0045-0050	–
18	20 (O_2)	0050-0110	–
18	5	0110-0115	–
18-9	30 (O_2)	0115-0145	3 m in 10 mins
9	15	0145-0200	–
9	60 (O_2)	0200-0300	–
9	15	0300-0315	–
9	60 (O_2)	0315-0415	–
9-0	30 (O_2)	0415-0445	3 m in 10 mins
Surface		0445	

Total table time 4 hours, 45 minutes

5519. Table 63: Deep air-oxygen recompression therapy

1. In cases of definite arterial gas embolism, when the patient is completely relieved of symptoms within 25 min at 50 m, this table may be used.
2. The table is applied as in Art. 5516.
   (a) Rate of descent – as fast as tolerable.
   (b) Rate of ascent
      (i) From 50 to 18 m in 4 min.
      (ii) From 18 m to 9 m and 9 m to the surface: at 3 m in 10 min.
   (c) The oxygen part of the schedule is conducted as in Table 62, except that the attendant must always breathe O_2 during the final 9 m of ascent.

Table 63
Air-Oxygen Recompression Therapy

GAUGE DEPTH (metres)	STOPPAGES/ ASCENT (minutes)	ELAPSED TIME (hours and minutes)	RATE OF ASCENT (metres/minute)
50	30	0000-0030	–
50-18	4	0030-0034	8 m per min
18	20 (O_2)	0034-0054	–
18	5	0054-0059	–
18	20 (O_2)	0059-0119	–
18	5	0119-0124	–
18	20 (O_2)	0124-0144	–
18	5	0144-0149	–
18-9	30 (O_2)	0149-0219	3 m in 10 mins
9	15	0219-0234	–
9	60 (O_2)	0234-0334	–
9	15	0334-0349	–
9	60 (O_2)	0349-0449	–
9-0	30 (O_2)	0449-0519	3 m in 10 mins
Surface		0519	

Total table time 5 hours, 19 minutes

5520. Tables 71, 72, 73: Modified air-recompression therapy

1. Tables 71 and 72 can be used instead of the air recompression therapies, Tables 51 to 55, on the advice of a specialist medical officer.
2. Table 72 is applicable when multiple recompression of submarine survivors is called for (Article 5522).
3. Table 73 may be used in place of Tables 54 and 55. Although somewhat more difficult to accomplish, the smaller step size in the final 18 m is preferred, especially in cases of gas embolism or incomplete relief of decompression sickness. The table approximates the bleed rate of the final 18 m of Tables 71 and 72.
4. These tables are applied as described in Article 5516, but with the following modifications for Tables 71 and 72:
   (a) *Maximum pressure.* Maximum pressure may be less than that quoted and depends on the working pressure of the chamber available, which could be the fore-ends of a submarine.
   (b) *Ascent.* The ascent is to be conducted as follows:
      (i) It is to be a continuous bleed at the rates indicated.
      (ii) If the rate is slowed it is not to be compensated for by subsequent acceleration.
      (iii) The ascent should be halted if the rate is exceeded or if the ascent cannot be controlled accurately during flushing of the chamber.
   (c) *Oxygen.* Oxygen may be administered periodically to selected cases as advised by the medical officer.

Table 71

Modified Air Recompression Therapy

GAUGE DEPTH (metres)	STOPPAGES/ASCENT (hours (h) and minutes (min))	ELAPSED TIME (hours and minutes)	RATE OF ASCENT (metres/hour)
70	30 min	0000-0030	—
70-63	7 min	0030-0037	60
63-51	2 h	0037-0237	6
51-39	4 h	0237-0637	3
39-29	5 h	0637-1137	2
29-20	6 h	1137-1737	1.5
20-10	10 h	1737-2737	1
10-0	20 h	2737-4737	0.5
Surface		4737	

Total table time 47 hours, 37 minutes

Table 72

Modified Air Recompression Therapy

GAUGE DEPTH (metres)	STOPPAGES/ASCENT (hours (h) and minutes (min))	ELAPSED TIME (hours and minutes)	RATE OF ASCENT (metres/hour)
50	2 h (see note)	0000-0200	—
50-39	3 h 40 min	0200-0540	3
39-29	5 h	0540-1040	2
29-20	6 h	1040-1640	1.5
20-10	10 h	1640-2640	1
10-0	20 h	2640-4640	0.5
Surface		4640	

Total table time 46 hours, 40 minutes

Note: the period of 2 hours can be reduced and decompression started earlier if the patient's symptoms have cleared.

Table 73

Modified Air Recompression Therapy

GAUGE DEPTH (metres)	STOPPAGES (hours (h) and minutes (min))		ELAPSED TIME (hours and minutes)	RATE OF ASCENT
50	2 h		0000-0200	–
42		30 min	0205-0235	5 min between
36		30 min	0240-0310	stoppages
30		30 min	0315-0345	throughout
24		30 min	0350-0420	
18	6 h		0425-1025	
17		55 min	1030-1125	
16		55 min	1130-1225	
15		55 min	1230-1325	
14		55 min	1330-1425	
13		55 min	1430-1525	
12		55 min	1530-1625	
11		55 min	1630-1725	
10	1 h	55 min	1730-1925	
9	1 h	55 min	1930-2125	
8	1 h	55 min	2130-2325	
7	1 h	55 min	2330-2525	
6	1 h	55 min	2530-2725	
5	1 h	55 min	2730-2925	
4	1 h	55 min	2930-3125	
3	1 h	55 min	3130-3325	
2	1 h	55 min	3330-3525	
1	1 h	55 min	3530-3725	
Surface			3750	

Total table time 37 hours, 50 minutes

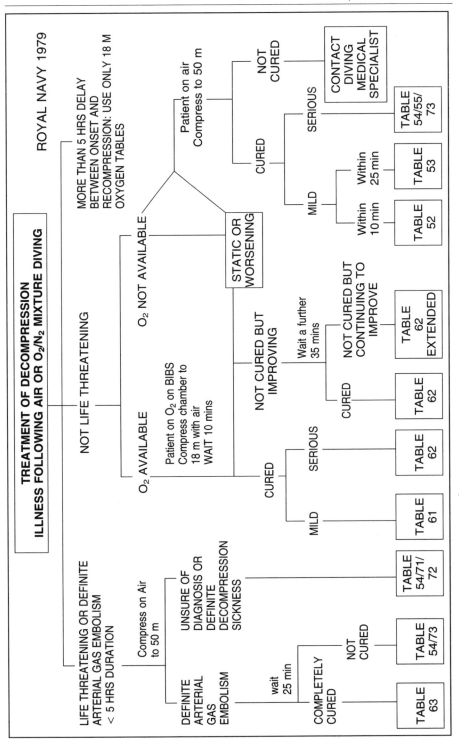

TREATMENT OF DECOMPRESSION
ILLNESS FOLLOWING AIR OR O₂/N₂ MIXTURE DIVING

ROYAL NAVY 1979

U.S. Navy Recompression Therapy Tables

Table 1A: Air treatment of pain-only decompression sickness — 100-foot treatment

1. Treatment of pain-only decompression sickness when oxygen unavailable and pain is relieved at a depth less than 66 feet.
2. Descent rate — 25 ft/min.
3. Ascent rate — 1 minute between stops.
4. Time at 100 feet — includes time from the surface.
5. If the piping configuration of the chamber does not allow it to return to atmospheric pressure from the 10 foot stop in the one minute specified, disregard the additional time required.

Depth (feet)	Time (minutes)	Breathing Media	Total Elapsed Time (hrs:min)
100	30	Air	0:30
80	12	Air	0:43
60	30	Air	1:14
50	30	Air	1:45
40	30	Air	2:16
30	60	Air	3:17
20	60	Air	4:18
10	120	Air	6:19
0	1	Air	6:20

Table 2A: Air treatment of pain-only decompression sickness — 165-foot treatment

1. Treatment of pain-only decompression sickness when oxygen unavailable and pain is relieved at a depth greater than 66 feet.
2. Descent rate — 25 ft/min.
3. Ascent rate — 1 minute between stops.
4. Time at 165 feet — includes time from the surface.

Depth (feet)	Time (minutes)	Breathing Media	Total Elapsed Time (hrs:min)
165	30	Air	0:30
140	12	Air	0:43
120	12	Air	0:56
100	12	Air	1:09
80	12	Air	1:22
60	30	Air	1:53
50	30	Air	2:24
40	30	Air	2:55
30	120	Air	4:56
20	120	Air	6:57
10	240	Air	10:58
1	1	Air	10:59

Table 3: Air treatment of serious decompression sickness or gas embolism

1. Treatment of serious symptoms or gas embolism when oxygen unavailable and symptoms are relieved within 30 minutes at 165 feet.
2. Descent rate — as rapidly as possible.
3. Ascent rate — 1 minute between stops.
4. Time at 165 feet — includes time from the surface.

Depth (feet)	Time	Breathing Media	Total Elapsed Time (hrs:min)
165	30 min	Air	0:30
140	12 min	Air	0:43
120	12 min	Air	0:56
100	12 min	Air	1:09
80	12 min	Air	1:22
60	30 min	Air	1:53
50	30 min	Air	2:24
40	30 min	Air	2:55
30	12 hr	Air	14:56
20	2 hr	Air	16:57
10	2 hr	Air	18:58
0	1 min	Air	18:59

Table 4: Air treatment of serious decompression sickness or gas embolism

1. Treatment of worsening symptoms during the first 20-minute oxygen breathing period at 60 feet on Table 6, or when symptoms are not relieved within 30 minutes at 165 feet using air treatment Table 3.
2. Descent rate — as rapidly as possible.
3. Ascent rate — 1 minute between stops.
4. Time at 165 feet — includes time from the surface.

Depth (feet)	Time	Breathing Media	Total Elapsed Time (hrs:min)
165	$^1/_2$ to 2 hr	Air	2:00
140	$^1/_2$ hr	Air	2:31
120	$^1/_2$ hr	Air	3:02
100	$^1/_2$ hr	Air	3:33
80	$^1/_2$ hr	Air	4:04
60	6 hr	Air	10:05
50	6 hr	Air	16:06
40	6 hr	Air	22:07
30	11 hr	Air	33:08
30	1 hr	Oxygen (or air)	34:08
20	1 hr	Air	35:09
20	1 hr	Oxygen (or air)	36:09
10	1 hr	Air	37:10
10	1 hr	Oxygen (or air)	38:10
0	1 min	Oxygen	38:11

Author's note: The air version alone is a classic attendant bender. Use the oxygen version i.e. oxygen from 30 ft (9 metres) if possible.

Table 5: Oxygen treatment of pain-only decompression sickness

1. Treatment of pain-only decompression sickness when symptoms are relieved within 10 minutes at 60 feet.
2. Descent rate — 25 ft/min.
3. Ascent rate — 1 ft/min. Do not compensate for slower ascent rates. Compensate for faster rates by halting the ascent.
4. Time at 60 feet begins on arrival at 60 feet.
5. If oxygen breathing must be interrupted, allow 15 minutes after the reaction has entirely subsided and resume schedule at point of interruption.
6. If oxygen breathing must be interrupted at 60 feet, switch to Table 6 upon arrival at the 30 foot stop.
7. Tender breathes air throughout. If treatment is a repetitive dive for the tender or tables are lengthened, tender should breathe oxygen during the last 30 minutes of ascent to the surface.

Depth (feet)	Time (minutes)	Breathing Media	Total Elapsed Time (hrs:min)
60	20	Oxygen	0:20
60	5	Air	0:25
60	20	Oxygen	0:45
60 to 30	30	Oxygen	1:15
30	5	Air	1:20
30	20	Oxygen	1:40
30	5	Air	1:45
30 to 0	30	Oxygen	2:15

Table 6: Oxygen treatment of serious decompression sickness

1. Treatment of serious or pain-only decompression sickness when symptoms are not relieved within 10 minutes at 60 feet.
2. Descent rate — 25 ft/min.
3. Ascent rate — 1 ft/min. Do not compensate for slower ascent rates. Compensate for faster rates by halting the ascent.
4. Time at 60 feet — begins on arrival at 60 feet.
5. If oxygen breathing must be interrupted, allow 15 minutes after the reaction has entirely subsided and resume schedule at point of interruption.
6. Tender breathes air throughout. If treatment is a repetitive dive for the tender or tables are lengthened, tender should breathe oxygen during the last 30 minutes of ascent to the surface.
7. Table 6 can be lengthened by an additional 25 minutes at 60 feet (20 minutes on oxygen and 5 minutes on air) or an additional 75 minutes at 30 feet (15 minutes on air and 60 minutes on oxygen), or both.

Depth (feet)	Time (minutes)	Breathing Media	Total Elapsed Time (hrs:min)
60	20	Oxygen	0:20
60	5	Air	0:25
60	20	Oxygen	0:45
60	5	Air	0:50
60	20	Oxygen	1:10
60	5	Air	1:15
60 to 30	30	Oxygen	1:45
30	15	Air	2:00
30	60	Oxygen	3:00
30	15	Air	3:15
30	60	Oxygen	4:15
30 to 0	30	Oxygen	4:45

Table 6A: Air and oxygen treatment of gas embolism

1. Treatment of gas embolism. Use also when unable to determine whether symptoms are caused by gas embolism or severe decompression sickness.
2. Descent rate — as fast as possible.
3. Ascent rate — 1 ft/min. Do not compensate for slower ascent rates. Compensate for faster ascent rates by halting the ascent.
4. Time at 165 feet — includes time from the surface.
5. If oxygen breathing must be interrupted, allow 15 minutes after the reaction has entirely subsided and resume schedule at point of interruption.
6. Tender breathes air throughout. If treatment is a repetitive dive for the tender or tables are lengthened, tender should breathe oxygen during the last 30 minutes of ascent to the surface.
7. Table 6A can be lengthened by an additional 25 minutes at 60 feet (20 minutes on oxygen and 5 minutes on air) or an additional 75 minutes at 30 feet (15 minutes on air and 60 minutes on oxygen), or both.

Depth (feet)	Time (minutes)	Breathing Media	Total Elapsed Time (hrs:min)
165	30	Air	0:30
165 to 60	4	Air	0:34
60	20	Oxygen	0:54
60	5	Air	0:59
60	20	Oxygen	1:19
60	5	Air	1:29
60	20	Oxygen	1:44
60	5	Air	1:49
60 to 30	30	Oxygen	2:19
30	15	Air	2:34
30	60	Oxygen	3:34
30	15	Air	3:49
30	60	Oxygen	4:49
30 to 0	30	Oxygen	5:19

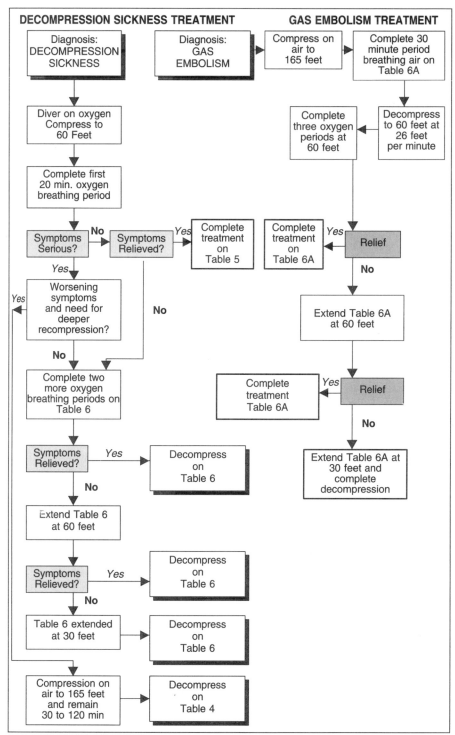

DECOMPRESSION SICKNESS TREATMENT

GAS EMBOLISM TREATMENT

Diagnosis: DECOMPRESSION SICKNESS

Diagnosis: GAS EMBOLISM

Compress on air to 165 feet

Complete 30 minute period breathing air on Table 6A

Diver on oxygen Compress to 60 Feet

Complete three oxygen periods at 60 feet

Decompress to 60 feet at 26 feet per minute

Complete first 20 min. oxygen breathing period

Symptoms Serious? — **No** → Symptoms Relieved? — *Yes* → Complete treatment on Table 5

Complete treatment on Table 6A ← *Yes* — Relief — **No**

Yes ↓

Worsening symptoms and need for deeper recompression? — **No**

Extend Table 6A at 60 feet

Complete two more oxygen breathing periods on Table 6

Complete treatment Table 6A ← *Yes* — Relief — **No**

Symptoms Relieved? — *Yes* → Decompress on Table 6 — **No**

Extend Table 6A at 30 feet and complete decompression

Extend Table 6 at 60 feet

Symptoms Relieved? — *Yes* → Decompress on Table 6 — **No**

Table 6 extended at 30 feet → Decompress on Table 6

Compression on air to 165 feet and remain 30 to 120 min → Decompress on Table 4

NOTE FOR EXTENDING TABLES:
A. Tables 6 and 6A may be extended by an additional 25 minutes at 60 feet (20 minutes on oxygen and 5 minutes on air) or an additional 75 minutes at 30 feet (15 minutes on air and 60 minutes on oxygen), or both.
B. No extension of Table 4 is permitted except by a qualified Diving Medical Officer.

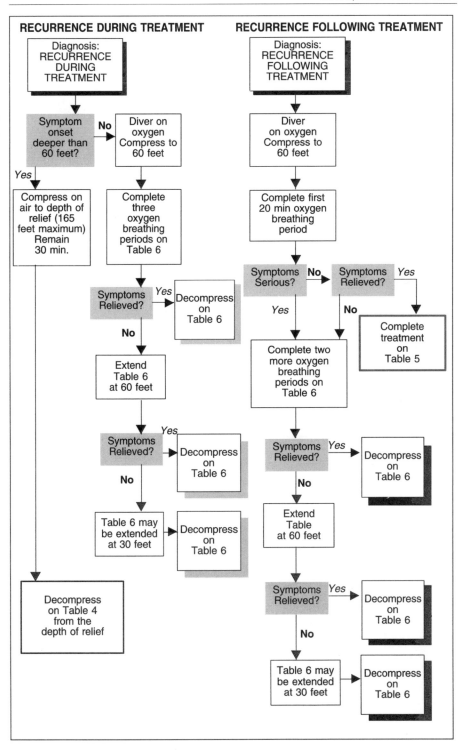

RECURRENCE DURING TREATMENT

Diagnosis:
RECURRENCE
DURING
TREATMENT

Symptom onset deeper than 60 feet? — **No** → Diver on oxygen Compress to 60 feet

Yes → Compress on air to depth of relief (165 feet maximum) Remain 30 min.

Diver on oxygen Compress to 60 feet → Complete three oxygen breathing periods on Table 6

Symptoms Relieved? — *Yes* → Decompress on Table 6

No → Extend Table 6 at 60 feet

Symptoms Relieved? — *Yes* → Decompress on Table 6

No → Table 6 may be extended at 30 feet → Decompress on Table 6

Decompress on Table 4 from the depth of relief

RECURRENCE FOLLOWING TREATMENT

Diagnosis:
RECURRENCE
FOLLOWING
TREATMENT

Diver on oxygen Compress to 60 feet → Complete first 20 min oxygen breathing period

Symptoms Serious? — **No** → Symptoms Relieved? — *Yes* → Complete treatment on Table 5

Yes ↓   **No** ↓

Complete two more oxygen breathing periods on Table 6

Symptoms Relieved? — *Yes* → Decompress on Table 6

No → Extend Table at 60 feet

Symptoms Relieved? — *Yes* → Decompress on Table 6

No → Table 6 may be extended at 30 feet → Decompress on Table 6

Acknowledgements

The author and publisher thank the following:

Professor A A Buehlmann for permission to reproduce the tables on pp 165-166;
the National Association of Underwater Instructors (NAUI) for permission to reproduce the Dive Tables on pp 277-278;
the Royal Navy and the US Navy for permission to reproduce the Recompression Therapy Tables and the Standard Air Decompression Tables on pp 279-307;
Dr W G J Kloeck, National Chairman of the Resuscitation Council of Southern Africa for permission to reproduce the life-support CPR pictorial flow diagrams on pp 176-177. The diagrams originally appeared in an article by Dr Kloeck entitled 'New recommendations for basic life support in adults, children and infants' published in *Trauma and Emergency Medicine*, January/February 1993, pp 738-748;
Ciba-Geigy Limited, Basle (Switzerland) for permission to reproduce anatomical drawings from the *Netter Atlas of Human Anatomy;*
Dr Leon Greenbaum, Executive Director of the Undersea and Hyperbaric Medical Society, for reading the proofs and writing the Foreword.

Source List

BEST, C.H., TAYLOR, N.B. 1961. *The physiological basis of medical practice.* 7th ed. Baltimore: Williams and Wilkins.

BOIES, L.R., HILGER, J.A., PRIEST, R.A. 1964. *Fundamentals of otolaryngology.* 4th ed. Philadelphia: W.B. Saunders Company.

BOVE, A.A. 1983. An approach to medical evaluation of the sport diver. *SPUMS J.* 2: 3-17.

BOVE, A.A. 1992. If the O_2 doesn't get you the CO_2 will. *Skin Diver* Nov.: 8-9.

BOVE, A.A. 1992. Diving science in '92. *Skin Diver* Dec.: 18-19.

BUEHLMANN, A.A. 1987. Decompression after repeated dives. *Undersea Biomedical Research* 14(1): 59-66.

BUTLER, F.K. Jr., THALMANN, E.D. 1986. Central nervous system oxygen toxicity in closed circuit scuba divers II. *Undersea Biomedical Research* 13 (2): 193-223.

CLARK, J.M., LAMBERTSEN, C.J. 1971. Pulmonary oxygen toxicity: a review. *Pharmacology Review* 23 (2): 37-133.

COUSTEAU, J.Y., COUSTEAU, P. 1970. *The shark: splendid savage of the sea.* New York: Doubleday & Co., Inc.

CROSS, E.R. 1992. Why I won't use nitrox for recreational diving. *Skin Diver* Nov.: 10-11.

DANIELS, S., HALSEY, M.J., SMITH, E.B. 1980. Techniques for diving deeper than 1,500 feet. *The twenty-third undersea medical society workshop.* 19-21 Mar. 1980. Bethesda: Undersea Medical Society, Inc.

DAVIS, B. 1983. Lecture on shark attacks at Aqua-Medic Disaster Symposium. Wild Coast SA: Personal observations.

DAVIS, J.C. 1986. *Medical examination of sport scuba divers.* 2nd ed. San Antonio, Texas: Medical Seminars Inc.

DAVIS, R.H. 1955. *Deep diving and submarine operations.* London: St. Catherine's Press.

DIVING MEDICAL ADVISORY COMMITTEE WORKSHOP. 1981. *Thermal stress in relation to diving.* 19-20 Mar. 1981. Institute of Naval Medicine, Gosport, Hants: Undersea Medical Society, Inc.

DUEKER, C.W. 1970. *Medical aspects of sport diving.* London: A. S. Barnes & Co.

EDMONDS, C., LOWRY, C., PENNEFATHER, J. 1981. *Diving and subaquatic medicine.* 2nd ed. N.S.W. Australia: Diving medical centre.

EGSTROM, G.H., BACHRACH, A. 1971. Diver Panic. *Skin Diver Magazine* Nov. 1971.

ENCYCLOPAEDIA BRITANNICA. 1970. *Diving, deep-sea.* 7: 507-510D. Chicago: William Benton.

EUROPEAN UNDERSEA BIOMEDICAL SOCIETY. 1991. *Proceedings XVIIth annual meeting on diving and hyberbaric medicine.* 29 Sept. – 3 Oct. 1991. Heraklion/Crete: EUBS.

FRANCIS, T.J.R., DUTKA, A.J. 1989. Methyl prednisolone in the treatment of acute spinal cord decompression sickness. *Undersea Biomedical Research* 16(2): 165-172.

GLEASON, B. 1992. Just say no to nitrox? *Skin Diver* Nov.: 6-7.

GRAVER, D.K. 1993. Flying and diving. *Skin Diver* Aug.: 23-24.

GRIMSTAD, J. ed. 1979. *5th Annual Scientific Meeting* 5-6 July 1979 – Bergen/Norway: European Undersea Biomedical Society.

HALSTEAD, B.W. 1980. *Dangerous marine animals.* 2nd ed. Maryland: Cornell Maritime Press.

HAMILTON, R.W. 1975. Development of decompression procedures for depths in excess of 400 feet. *The ninth undersea medical society workshop.* 21-23 Feb. 1975. Bethesda: Undersea Medical Society, Inc.

HAMILTON, R.W. *et al.* 1988. *REPEX: Development of Repetitive Excursions, surfacing techniques, and oxygen procedures for habitat diving.* National Undersea Research Program. Technical reports 88-1A & 88-1B. Maryland: National Oceanic and Atmosphere Administration, US Dept. Commerce.

HARRISON, T.R. *et al.* 1962. *Principles of internal medicine.* 4th ed. New York: McGraw Hill.

HICKEY, D.D. 1984. Outline of medical standards for divers. *Undersea Biomedical Research* 11(4): 407-430.

JENKINS, C., ANDERSON, S.D., WONG, R., VEALE, A. 1993. Compressed air diving and respiratory disease. *The Medical Journal of Australia* 158: 276-279.

KAYLE, A. 1982. Skindivers, whales and things. *Fathoms* 3 (6): 5-6.

KAYLE, A. 1992. Decompression disorders. *Divestyle* 14: 8.

KAYLE, A. 1992. Divers and life assurance. *Divestyle* 16: 14.

KAYLE, A. 1992. Victims of near-drowning. *Divestyle* 17: 8.

KAYLE, A. 1992. Demons of the deep. *Divestyle* 19: 8.

KAYLE, A. 1992. Diving with a duplicate. *Divestyle* 19: 14.

KAYLE, A. 1993. Back pain problems. *Divestyle* 20: 8.

KAYLE, A. 1993. Thermal stress — the dangers of being too cold. *Divestyle* 22: 5.

KAYLE, A. 1993. Cholesterol and diving. *Divestyle* 23: 8.

KENT, M.B. ed. 1980. Effects of diving on pregnancy. *The nineteenth undersea medical society workshop*. 2-3 Nov. 1978. Bethesda: Undersea Medical Society, Inc.

KENT, M.B. ed. 1979. Emergency ascent training. *The fifteenth undersea medical society workshop*. 10-11 Dec. 1977. Bethesda: Undersea Medical Society, Inc.

KLOECK, W.G.J. 1993. New recommendations for basic life support in adults, children and infants. *CME*. April 11(4):763-780.

KLOECK, W.G.J. 1993. Choking. *South African Family Practice Manual*. Jun.-Aug. 6:06.

KUEHN, L.A. ed. 1980. Thermal constraints in diving. *The twenty-fourth undersea medical society workshop*. 3-4 Sept. 1980. Bethesda: Undersea Medical Society, Inc.

LANDSBERG, P.G. 1988. Hyperventilation: an unpredictable danger to the sports diver. Chapter 18: 292-305. *South Africa's second underwater handbook* ed. A.J. Venter. Rivonia, Johannesburg: Ashanti Press.

LANPHIER, E.H. ed. 1980. The unconscious diver: Respiratory control and other contributing factors. *The twenty-fifth undersea medical society workshop*. 18-20 Sept. 1980. Bethesda: Undersea Medical Society, Inc.

LEE, H.C., NIU, K.C., CHEN, S.H. *et al.* 1991. Therapeutic effects of different tables on Type II decompression sickness. *J. Hyperbaric Medicine* 6(1): 11-17.

LLOYD'S REGISTER OF SHIPPING. 1980. *Rules and regulations for the construction and classification of submersibles and diving systems*. London: Lloyd's Register Printing House.

LUNDGREN, C.E.G. ed. 1978. Monitoring vital signs in the diver. *The sixteenth undersea medical society workshop*. 17-18 Mar. 1978. Bethesda: Undersea Medical Society, Inc.

MELAMED, Y., SHUPAK, A., BITTERMAN, H. 1992. Medical problems associated with underwater diving. *The New England Journal of Medicine* Jan. 2 1992: 30-33.

MILLER, J.W. ed. *et al*. 1976. *Vertical excursions breathing air from nitrogen-oxygen or air saturation exposures*. National Oceanic and Atmosphere Administration, Washington, D.C.: US Government Printing Office.

MINISTRY OF DEFENCE. 1972. *Diving manual* B.R. 2806. London: Ministry of Defence (Navy).

MOON, R.E., CAMPORESI, E.M., KISSLO, J.A. 1989. Patent foramen ovale and decompression sickness in divers. *Lancet* 1(8637): 513-514.

MURPHY, G. 1992. Nitrox ban in the Caribbean. *Skin Diver* Nov: 12.

MURPHY, G. 1992. Nitrox: Miracle gas or double jeopardy? *Skin Diver* Dec.: 30-31, 167.

PAYLING WRIGHT, G. 1960. *An introduction to pathology*. 3rd ed. London: Longmans.

SHILLING, C.W., STORY, P. 1982. *Man in the cold environment*. A bibliography. Bethesda: Undersea Medical Society, Inc.

SMITH, D.J., FRANCIS, T.J.R. 1991. A descriptive approach to reclassifying the decompression disorders. *Proceedings XVIIth annual meeting on diving and hyperbaric medicine*. 29 Sept. − 3 Oct. 1991. Heraklion/Crete: EUBS.

SMITH, E. 1993. Malaria treatment and prophylaxis. *Modern Medicine of South Africa*. June: 53-66.

STRAUSS, R.H. ed. 1976. *Diving medicine*. New York: Grune & Stratton.

TEICHLER, M. ed. 1993. Burns. *South African Family Practice Manual*. Jun.-Aug. 6:48-49.

TUERK, G.M. ed. 1975. *Emergency medical technician/diver workshop*. Bethesda: Undersea Medical Society, Inc.

UNDERSEA MEDICAL SOCIETY. 1978. Decompression theory. *The seventeenth undersea medical society workshop*. 6-7 Sept. 1978. Bethesda: Undersea Medical Society, Inc.

US NAVY DIVING MANUAL. 1979. Washington, D.C.: US Govt. Printing Office.

WALSH, J.M. ed. 1980. Interaction of drugs in the hyperbaric environment. *The twenty-first undersea medical society workshop*. 13-14 Sept. 1979. Bethesda: Undersea Medical Society, Inc.

Index